T0263291

Current Topics in Molecular Diagnostics and Precision Medicine

Editor

GREGORY J. TSONGALIS

CLINICS IN LABORATORY MEDICINE

www.labmed.theclinics.com

Consulting Editor
MILENKO JOVAN TANASIJEVIC

December 2022 • Volume 42 • Number 4

ELSEVIER

1600 John F. Kennedy Boulevard • Suite 1800 • Philadelphia, Pennsylvania, 19103-2899

http://www.theclinics.com

CLINICS IN LABORATORY MEDICINE Volume 42, Number 4
December 2022 ISSN 0272-2712, ISBN-13: 978-0-443-18310-2

Editor: Taylor Hayes
Developmental Editor: Ann Gielou M. Posedio

© **2022 Elsevier Inc. All rights reserved.**

This periodical and the individual contributions contained in it are protected under copyright by Elsevier, and the following terms and conditions apply to their use:

Photocopying
Single photocopies of single articles may be made for personal use as allowed by national copyright laws. Permission of the Publisher and payment of a fee is required for all other photocopying, including multiple or systematic copying, copying for advertising or promotional purposes, resale, and all forms of document delivery. Special rates are available for educational institutions that wish to make photocopies for non-profit educational classroom use. For information on how to seek permission visit www.elsevier.com/permissions or call: (+44) 1865 843830 (UK)/(+1) 215 239 3804 (USA).

Derivative Works
Subscribers may reproduce tables of contents or prepare lists of articles including abstracts for internal circulation within their institutions. Permission of the Publisher is required for resale or distribution outside the institution. Permission of the Publisher is required for all other derivative works, including compilations and translations (please consult www.elsevier.com/permissions).

Electronic Storage or Usage
Permission of the Publisher is required to store or use electronically anymaterial contained in this periodical, including any article or part of an article (please consult www.elsevier.com/permissions). Except as outlined above, no part of this publication may be reproduced, stored in a retrieval system or transmitted in any form or by any means, electronic, mechanical, photocopying, recording or otherwise, without prior written permission of the Publisher.

Notice
No responsibility is assumed by the Publisher for any injury and/or damage to persons or property as a matter of products liability, negligence or otherwise, or from any use or operation of any methods, products, instructions or ideas contained in the material herein. Because of rapid advances in the medical sciences, in particular, independent verification of diagnoses and drug dosages should be made.

Although all advertising material is expected to conform to ethical (medical) standards, inclusion in this publication does not constitute a guarantee or endorsement of the quality or value of such product or of the claims made of it by its manufacturer.

Reprints. For copies of 100 or more, of articles in this publication, please contact the Commercial Reprints Department, Elsevier Inc., 360 Park Avenue South, New York, New York 10010-1710. Tel. 212-633-3874, Fax: 212-633-3820, E-mail: reprints@elsevier.com.

Clinics in Laboratory Medicine (ISSN 0272-2712) is published quarterly by Elsevier Inc., 360 Park Avenue South, New York, NY 10010-1710. Months of issue are March, June, September, and December. Business and Editorial offices: 1600 John F. Kennedy Blvd., Suite 1800, Philadelphia, PA 19103-2899. Periodicals postage paid at NewYork, NY and additional mailing offices. Subscription prices are $283.00 per year (US individuals), $753.00 per year (US institutions), $100.00 per year (US students), $363.00 per year (Canadian individuals), $776.00 per year (Canadian institutions), $100.00 per year (Canadian students), $404.00 per year (international individuals), $776.00 per year (international institutions), $185.00 (international students). Foreign air speed delivery is included in all Clinics subscription prices. All prices are subject to change without notice. POSTMASTER: Send address changes to *Clinics in Laboratory Medicine*, Elsevier Health Sciences Division, Subscription Customer Service, 3251 Riverport Lane, Maryland Heights, MO 63043. **Customer Service: 1-800-654-2452 (US). From outside of the US and Canada, call 1-314-447-8871. Fax: 1-314-447-8029. E-mail: journalscustomerservice-usa@elsevier.com (for print support) or journalsonlinesupport-usa@elsevier.com (for online support).**

Clinics in Laboratory Medicine is covered in *EMBASE/Exerpta Medica, MEDLINE/PubMed (Index Medicus), Cinahl, Current Contents/Clinical Medicine, BIOSIS and ISI/BIOMED.*

Contributors

EDITOR

GREGORY J. TSONGALIS, PhD, HCLD
Medical Director, Clinical Genomics and Advanced Technology, Vice Chair for Research and Professor, Department of Pathology and Laboratory Medicine, Dartmouth Hitchcock Memorial Hospital, Lebanon, New Hampshire; Audrey and Theodore Geisel School of Medicine, Hanover, New Hampshire

AUTHORS

APRIL N. ABBOTT, PhD, D(ABMM)
Department of Laboratory Medicine, Deaconess Hospital, Evansville, Indiana, USA

MIR B. ALIKHAN, MD
Department of Pathology and Laboratory Medicine, NorthShore University HealthSystem, Evanston, Illinois, USA

JENNIFER A. CAMPBELL, PharmD
Associate Dean of Academic Programs, Manchester University, College of Pharmacy, Natural, and Health Sciences, Fort Wayne, Indiana, USA

GERALD A. CAPRARO, PhD, D(ABMM)
Director, Clinical Microbiology Laboratory, Carolinas Pathology Group, Atrium Health, Charlotte, North Carolina, USA

LARISA H. CAVALLARI, PharmD
Associate Professor, Department of Pharmacotherapy and Translational Research, Associate Director, Director, Center for Pharmacogenomics and Precision Medicine, University of Florida, Gainesville, Florida, USA

MARK A. CERVINSKI, PhD
Associate Professor, Department of Pathology and Laboratory Medicine, Dartmouth-Hitchcock Medical Center, Lebanon, New Hampshire, USA

JENSYN K. CONE SULLIVAN, MD
Department of Pathology, Associate Director of Transfusion Medicine and The Neely Cell Therapy Center, Tufts Medical Center, Assistant Professor of Pathology, Tufts University School of Medicine, Boston, Massachusetts, USA

CALEB CORNABY, PhD
McLendon Clinical Laboratories, UNC Hospitals, Chapel Hill, North Carolina, USA

NICHOLAS GLEADALL, PhD
Postdoctoral Research Associate, Department of Haematology, University of Cambridge, University of Cambridge Biomedical Campus, Cambridge, United Kingdom

HENK-JAN GUCHELAAR, PharmD, PhD
Professor of Clinical Pharmacy and Department Head, Department of Clinical Pharmacy and Toxicology, Leiden University Medical Center, Leiden Network for Personalised Therapeutics, Leiden, The Netherlands

CARRIE C. HOEFER, PhD, MBA
Director of Pharmacogenomics, Assistant Professor of Pharmaceutical Sciences, James L Winkle School of Pharmacy and Pharmaceutical Sciences, University of Cincinnati, Cincinnati, Ohio, USA

LEAH K. HOLLON, ND, MPH, CEO
Richmond Natural Medicine, National University of Natural Medicine Residency, Distant Site Supervisor and Board of Directors Member, Richmond, Virginia, USA

JACQUELINE A. HUBBARD, PhD
Assistant Professor, Department of Pathology and Laboratory Medicine, Dartmouth-Hitchcock Medical Center, Lebanon, New Hampshire, USA

NORA JOSEPH, MD
Department of Pathology and Laboratory Medicine, NorthShore University HealthSystem, Evanston, Illinois, USA

KAREN L. KAUL, MD PhD
Department of Pathology and Laboratory Medicine, NorthShore University HealthSystem, Evanston, Illinois, USA

WAHAB A. KHAN, PhD, FACMG
Department of Pathology and Laboratory Medicine, Dartmouth-Hitchcock Medical Center, Lebanon, New Hampshire, USA; Assistant Professor, Dartmouth Geisel School of Medicine, Dartmouth College, Hanover, New Hampshire, USA

WILLIAM J. LANE, MD, PhD
Assistant Medical Director Tissue Typing Lab, Department of Pathology, Brigham and Women's Hospital, Hale Building for Transformative Medicine, Associate Professor, Harvard Medical School, Boston, Massachusetts, USA

KATHY A. MANGOLD, PhD
Department of Pathology and Laboratory Medicine, NorthShore University HealthSystem, Evanston, Illinois, USA

ROBERT D. NERENZ, PhD
Assistant Professor, Department of Pathology and Laboratory Medicine, Dartmouth-Hitchcock Medical Center, Lebanon, New Hampshire, USA

ZHIYU PENG, PhD
BGI Genomics, BGI-Shenzhen, Shenzhen, China; College of Life Sciences, University of Chinese Academy of Sciences, Beijing, China

VICTORIA M. PRATT, PhD
Director, Pharmacogenomics and Molecular Genetics Laboratories, Optum Genomics, Eden Praire, Minnesota, USA

KALPANA S. REDDY, MD
Department of Pathology and Laboratory Medicine, NorthShore University HealthSystem, Evanston, Illinois, USA

RYAN F. RELICH, PhD, D(ABMM), MLS(ASCP)SM
Division of Clinical Microbiology, Indiana University Health Pathology Laboratory, Indiana University Health and Indiana University School of Medicine, Indianapolis, Indiana, USA

LINDA M. SABATINI, PhD
Department of Pathology and Laboratory Medicine, NorthShore University HealthSystem, Evanston, Illinois, USA

PATRICIA J. SIMNER, PhD, D(ABMM)
Associate Professor of Pathology, Director of Bacteriology and Parasitology, Division of Medical Microbiology, Department of Pathology, Johns Hopkins School of Medicine, Baltimore, Maryland, USA

LIRON BARNEA SLONIM, MD
Department of Pathology and Laboratory Medicine, NorthShore University HealthSystem, Evanston, Illinois, USA

JESSE J. SWEN, PharmD, PhD
Associate Professor of Pharmacogenomics and Section Head Laboratory, Department of Clinical Pharmacy and Toxicology, Leiden University Medical Center, Leiden Network for Personalised Therapeutics, Leiden, The Netherlands

GAIL H. VANCE, MD, FCAP, FACMG
Department of Medical and Molecular Genetics, Indiana University School of Medicine, Professor, Pathology and Laboratory Medicine, Indiana University School of Medicine, Indianapolis, Indiana, USA

CATHELIJNE H. VAN DER WOUDEN, PharmD
PhD Candidate U-PGx Consortium, Department of Clinical Pharmacy and Toxicology, Leiden University Medical Center, Leiden Network for Personalised Therapeutics, Leiden, The Netherlands

ERIC T. WEIMER, PhD
McLendon Clinical Laboratories, UNC Hospitals, Department of Pathology and Laboratory Medicine, University of North Carolina at Chapel Hill School of Medicine, Chapel Hill, North Carolina, USA

JIALE XIANG, MS
BGI Genomics, BGI-Shenzhen, Shenzhen, China; College of Life Sciences, University of Chinese Academy of Sciences, Beijing, China

REBECCA YEE, PhD, D(ABMM)
Division of Medical Microbiology, Department of Pathology, Johns Hopkins School of Medicine, Baltimore, Maryland, USA

Contents

CLINICS IN LABORATORY MEDICINE

SERIES OF RELATED INTEREST

Surgical Pathology Clinics
Available at: https://www.surgpath.theclinics.com/

THE CLINICS ARE NOW AVAILABLE ONLINE!
Access your subscription at:
www.theclinics.com

Preface

Current Topics in Molecular Diagnostics and Precision Medicine

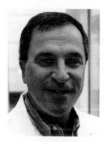

Gregory J. Tsongalis, PhD, HCLD
Editor

At the time of the writing of this editorial, the United States and for that matter the world were finally seeing the COVID-19 pandemic begin to dwindle to the lowest levels of SARS-CoV-2–driven mortality and decreases in new numbers of infections. Over the course of the past two years, laboratory testing became a household topic of discussion, yet most do not recognize that the vast majority of clinical decisions are made based on a lab test result. Nonetheless, the pandemic brought laboratory testing into the limelight, and the heroic efforts of laboratory staff everywhere were acknowledged by those who once saw the lab as a black box.

It has been almost 70 years since the first published description of the structure of DNA by Watson and Crick. No other section of laboratory medicine has experienced the explosive growth in molecular technologies and clinical applications as we have seen in molecular diagnostics. Beginning with relatively simple Southern blot transfer analyses and end-point polymerase chain reactions (PCR) through highly complex microarrays, digital PCR, and massively parallel sequencing, molecular technologies have impacted all facets of medical practice. Dramatic decreases in cost, vast improvements in turnaround times, and the ability to decentralize molecular technologies for use at point of care have resulted in unprecedented growth in implementation, reimbursement, and clinical utility.

As universal technologies, molecular techniques have become accepted as standard of care and routinely applied to the detection of nucleic acids for the identification of disease-causing variants, for the presence of pathogens, and to direct therapeutic selection as a means to inform precision medicine across the spectrum of human disease. From viral load testing where molecular disease monitoring made its debut to

Clin Lab Med 42 (2022) xi–xii
https://doi.org/10.1016/j.cll.2022.09.019
0272-2712/22/© 2022 Published by Elsevier Inc.   **labmed.theclinics.com**

current applications of liquid biopsy to assess cell-free DNA, the trend has been to provide complex information from the least-invasive sample possible. In addition, there is a huge need to democratize these technologies by developing rapid, user-friendly, low-cost mechanisms of testing for deployment outside of a central lab to point of care and at-home testing, which was so clearly evident during the pandemic.

The field of molecular diagnostics has matured. No longer do providers question the use of a molecular technique, they ask for it. Payors continue to improve reimbursement rates for those tests and technologies that offer the most cost-effective and clinically useful results, realizing that downstream savings in the management of a patient are real and significant. Federal regulators continue to review and approve testing for clinical use, and as we saw with the pandemic, recognized the need to allow labs to develop tests and follow guidance under the Emergency Use Authorization ruling. The public has become more engaged and educated in their health care needs/wants through the Internet and continue to participate in direct-to-consumer testing of various types. Together these attributes have made molecular diagnostic testing the standard of practice for many clinical diagnostic and management strategies.

In this special issue of Clinics in Laboratory Medicine titled "Current Topics in Molecular Diagnostics and Precision Medicine," we explore the application of molecular technologies to a variety of human disease conditions. Articles by experts in their individual subspecialties highlight the utility of molecular technologies in understanding and detecting the cause of disease. I would like to thank the many contributors for sharing their thoughts in their excellent articles. There is no doubt that molecular diagnostics will continue to contribute to a better health care delivery system.

Gregory J. Tsongalis, PhD, HCLD
Clinical Genomics and Advanced Technology
Department of Pathology and Laboratory Medicine
Dartmouth Hitchcock Medical Center
1 Medical Center Drive
Lebanon, NH 03756, USA

Audrey and Theodore Geisel School of Medicine
Hanover, NH 03755, USA

E-mail address:
Gregory.J.Tsongalis@hitchcock.org

Syndromic and Point-of-Care Molecular Testing

Ryan F. Relich, PhD, D(ABMM), MLS(ASCP)SM[a],*, April N. Abbott, PhD, D(ABMM)[b]

KEYWORDS

- Syndromic panels • Point-of-care molecular diagnostics • Multiplex PCR
- Group A *Streptococcus* • Influenza-like illness • Meningitis • Gastroenteritis
- Blood stream infections

KEY POINTS

- Syndromic and point-of-care molecular diagnostic testing methods have revolutionized infectious disease testing by permitting the simultaneous detection of multiple pathogens and drug resistance mechanisms directly from clinical specimens and positive blood cultures.
- Syndromic testing panels currently include those designed for the detection of pathogens responsible for bloodstream, central nervous system, gastrointestinal tract, and respiratory tract infections as well as some biothreat agents.
- Point-of-care molecular diagnostic systems afford providers the ability to generate laboratory-quality results without the need for confirmatory testing of negative specimens.
- Implementation of syndromic and point-of-care molecular infectious disease testing methods has curbed the unnecessary use of antibiotics, strengthening antimicrobial stewardship practices.
- Development of methods for the detection of infectious diseases beyond those that are detectable by current technologies is an area of investigation.

INTRODUCTION

For decades, the clinical laboratory diagnosis of many infectious diseases relied solely on time-consuming and often labor-intensive manual cultivation-based, microscopic, and immunoserologic methods that required experienced technical personnel to perform and interpret. The introduction of semiautomated and fully automated microbial phenotyping systems in the later part of the 20th century vastly improved the

This article originally appeared in *Advances in Molecular Pathology*, Volume 1, Issue 1, November 2018.

[a] Division of Clinical Microbiology, Indiana University Health Pathology Laboratory, Indiana University Health and Indiana University School of Medicine, Suite 6027E, 350 West 11th Street, Indianapolis, IN 46202, USA; [b] Department of Laboratory Medicine, Deaconess Hospital, 600 Mary Street, Evansville, IN 47747, USA
* Corresponding author.
E-mail address: rrelich@iupui.edu

Clin Lab Med 42 (2022) 507–531
https://doi.org/10.1016/j.cll.2022.09.008
0272-2712/22/© 2022 Elsevier Inc. All rights reserved.

processes of bacterial and yeast isolate workup by decreasing identification and antimicrobial susceptibility testing turnaround times (TATs); however, the detection of many viruses and parasites still required traditional techniques. Subsequent improvements to automated platforms, including the refinement of the automated expert systems used by these devices to generate and interpret data, led to further decreases in TATs and a concomitant increase in culture throughput.

In the 1990s, the era of molecular diagnostics was ushered in with the introduction of nucleic acid analysis methods, including the hybridization protection assay (eg, AccuProbe, Salem, MA) for the identification of isolates and polymerase chain reaction (PCR) for the detection of pathogens directly from patient specimens [1–7]. Later, the implementation of real-time nucleic acid amplification chemistries permitted both faster pathogen detection and the enablement of nucleic acid quantitation [8]. These methods quickly migrated from research laboratories into clinical laboratories, first as laboratory-developed tests or so-called home brew tests. This revolution enabled laboratorians to more precisely identify the causes of infectious diseases by detecting pathogen-specific nucleotide sequences in cultured isolates and clinical specimens. Many of these methods proved to be far superior in terms of accuracy and result TAT compared with cultivation-dependent approaches, especially for the identification of viruses. Over time, these methods also underwent refinements that included the adaptation of several assays to automated platforms, allowing users to minimize the manual handling of specimens and reaction components.

One recent advancement in pathogen detection is the syndromic approach in which groups of pathogens are tested for simultaneously in a single reaction vessel. These assays incorporate components of older methods, including real-time PCR; however, rather than ordering separate tests for various pathogens, the syndromic tests allow simultaneous detection of a variety of agents that are associated with a specific disease syndrome [9].

The newest systems are those that allow users to perform laboratory-quality molecular testing at the point of patient care, a major advancement that has moved molecular pathology to the forefront of modern diagnostics. Many Clinical Laboratory Improvement Amendments (CLIA)-waived point-of-care (POC) systems are now available and permit rapid result reporting, enabling prescription of targeted treatment at the time of clinic visit. The current assays on these platforms largely target infections diagnosed in the ambulatory setting such as influenza and streptococcal pharyngitis.

SIGNIFICANCE

Syndromic and POC molecular testing methods have revolutionized the diagnosis of infectious diseases by increasing the accuracy of microbial detection, substantially decreasing the time needed to generate clinically useful laboratory test results, and enabling the performance of laboratory-quality testing at or near the point of care by nonlaboratorians [9]. In return, patients are able to receive appropriate treatment sooner, avoiding prolonged exposure to unnecessary antimicrobial drugs, thereby avoiding the selection of drug-resistant pathogens and strengthening antimicrobial stewardship practices [9–11]. In addition, many of these methods permit the rapid detection of pathogens that pose significant infection control and public health hazards, including high-consequence and travel-related pathogens (eg, *Bacillus anthracis*, Ebola virus, and *Plasmodium* spp.) that can be associated with either naturally acquired infections or infections resulting from the deliberate release of these agents. As a consequence of the rapid TATs of these tests, containment and epidemiologic interventions can be instituted very soon after specimen acquisition.

In addition to the syndromic and POC molecular testing solutions available for aiding in the identification of pathogens, many test panels are also capable of detecting antimicrobial resistance mechanisms [9,12,13], the rapid detection of which affords clinicians and infection control practitioners the ability to quickly implement appropriate therapies and infection control precautions. The diagnostic power of these technologies coupled with their user friendliness have made them highly attractive alternatives to traditional methods that rely on the procurement of isolates. As a consequence, methods such as viral culture and direct immunofluorescence have largely disappeared from modern clinical microbiology laboratories. With these methods removed, many laboratories have streamlined the workup of clinical specimens by using one syndromic testing platform for the analysis of a variety of specimen types for a large array of pathogens.

PRESENT RELEVANCE AND FUTURE AVENUES TO CONSIDER/INVESTIGATE

Currently, numerous diagnostic product manufacturers market infectious disease syndromic panels and POC molecular tests that are available in a variety of formats, including customizable panels, single-analyte tests, and CLIA-waived and moderate complexity systems. These tests were designed to provide all of the advantages that traditional molecular diagnostic tests offer plus the benefits of rapid result delivery, portability, and ease of use. The ability of many of these test platforms to be successfully used by nonlaboratorians have made them amenable to deployment in patient care facilities such as clinics and hospital emergency departments, which are traditionally not staffed by medical laboratory scientists.

Several syndromic and POC testing systems that provide qualitative results are described herein. Please note that not all available systems are mentioned, but those with a visible market presence in the United States are discussed.

Currently Available Syndromic Panel Platforms

BD MAX system

The BD MAX System (BD Diagnostics, Quebec, Canada; **Fig. 1**) is an automated real-time PCR platform using TaqMan hydrolysis probes for detection. In addition to syndromic panels (see **Table 1** and **Table 3**), the system is designed to run singleplex and user-defined assays. To perform testing, specimens in sample buffer, reagents, extraction wells, pipette tips, and a real-time PCR microfluidic cartridge is placed on board the BD MAX instrument, which automates all sample handling and real-time PCR steps (see **Fig. 1**). Up to 24 assays can be run simultaneously and results are available within 3 hours. Panel performance characteristics are reviewed in refs. [14–17].

ePlex, ePlex NP, and eSensor XT-8 systems

The ePlex, ePlex NP, and XT-8 systems (GenMark Diagnostics, Inc., Carlsbad, CA; **Fig. 2**) use patented eSensor technology to detect a variety of pathogens directly from patient specimens (ePlex and ePlex NP systems) and amplified nucleic acid mixtures (eSensor XT-8 system).

For the ePlex system, the specimen in a buffer solution is added to the ePlex panel in which all liquid handling steps are performed by digital microfluidics technology (electrowetting) [14]. Electrochemical detection of ferrocene-labeled PCR amplicons occurs via capture probes that have been immobilized on gold-plated electrodes [15]. Results are generally available within 90 minutes, and anywhere from 3 to 24 assays can be ran simultaneously, depending on the instrument configuration (the ePlex NP performs a maximum of 3 tests at once). In contrast, the eSensor XT-8 system, the predecessor of

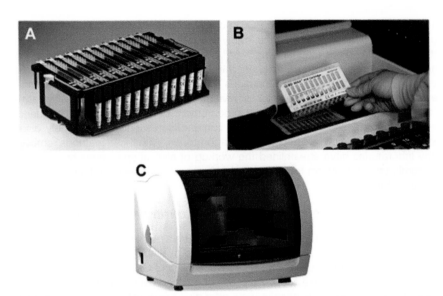

Fig. 1. The BD MAX System, which is comprised of (*A*) a rack for holding specimens (blue-capped tubes in front) and reagent strip, (*B*) the PCR cartridge, and (*C*) the BD MAX instrument. (*Courtesy of* BD, Sparks, MD; with permission.)

the ePlex system, is designed to simultaneously interrogate up to 24 samples that have undergone offline nucleic acid amplification; results are available within 30 minutes [15]. Analytes detectable by the current panels are listed in **Table 2** and performance characteristics and impacts of these systems are discussed in refs. [18–21].

FilmArray system

The FilmArray system (BioFire Diagnostics and BioFire Defense, LLC, Salt Lake City, UT; **Fig. 3**) family of syndromic panels includes several assays that are cleared by the US Food and Drug Administration (FDA) and several research use only assays (**Box 1**, see **Table 2**; **Tables 3** and **4**). Of note, BioFire Defense offers research-use-only reagents panels that are designed for detection of high-consequence and emerging pathogens whose detection could signal possible bioterrorism events, and for pathogens associated with travel to areas of the world where certain infectious diseases that are rare in the United States are endemic (**Table 5**).

The FilmArray System incorporates lyophilized reagents and assay reaction vessels on a small plastic film pouch topped by a solid plastic reagent housing (**Fig. 3**A). After reagent rehydration, the sample in buffer is added to a pouch that is then loaded into a FilmArray instrument for automated nucleic acid extraction, real-time PCR, detection, and high-resolution melt steps. The hands-on time of this system is minimal (approximately 2 minutes) and results are generally available in approximately 60 minutes [18]. Like the ePlex system, the FilmArray 2.0 and Torch instruments are scalable. With the exception of the FilmArray BCID Panel, which is meant for testing blood culture broths, all other panels are amenable to the direct testing of clinical specimens. The FilmArray BioThreat Panel, BioThreat-E Test, and Global Fever Panel are designed to test a variety of sample types, which are listed in the notes in **Box 1**. Numerous studies describing the performance characteristics and benefits of the FilmArray System have been published; examples can be found in refs. [13,22–31].

Table 1
Overview of Analytes Detected by the BD MAX Women's Health Panels, CT/GC/TV, and Vaginal Panel

Analyte	FDA Cleared?	Atopobium vaginae	Bacterial Vaginosis-Associated Bacteria-2	Candida spp.[a]	Chlamydia trachomatis	Gardnerella vaginalis	Lactobacillus spp.[b]	Megasphaera-1	Neisseria gonorrhoeae	Trichomonas vaginalis
BD MAX CT/GC/TV	+	−	−	−	+	−	−	−	+	+
BD MAX Vaginal Panel[c]	+	+	+	+	−	+	+	+	−	+

Abbreviations: CT/GC/VT, Chlamydia trachomatis/gonococcus (Neisseria gonorrhoeae)/Trichomonas vaginalis; FDA, US Food and Drug Administration.

Symbols: +, yes or present on panel; −, no or absent from panel.

[a] The BD MAX vaginal panel detects Candida albicans, C dubliniensis, C glabrata, C krusei, C parapsilosis, and C tropicalis but reports them as "Candida group" for all except C glabrata and C krusei, which it reports individually.

[b] The BD MAX Vaginal Panel detects Lactobacillus crispatus and L jensenii, which are grouped as Lactobacillus species.

[c] Detection of 1 or more bacterial analytes are reported as positive or negative for bacterial vaginosis.

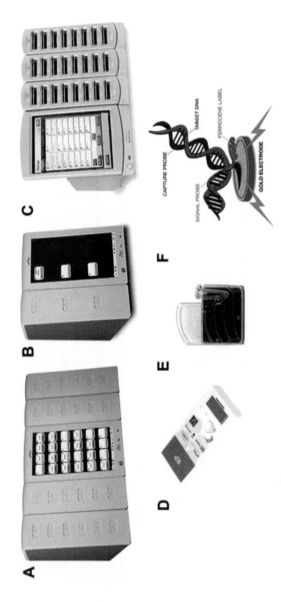

Fig. 2. The ePlex (*A*), ePlex NP (*B*), and eSensor XT-8 (*C*) systems available from GenMark Diagnostics. Also shown are examples of ePlex (*D*) and XT-8 (*E*) panels. The nucleic acid hybridization complex described in the text is shown in (*F*). (*Courtesy of GenMark Diagnostics, Carlsbad, CA; with permission.*)

Table 2
Syndromic Panels that Are Currently Available in the United States for the Detection of Upper Respiratory Tract Pathogens

Analyte	FDA Cleared?	Adenovirus	Adenovirus Subtyping	Bordetella bronchiseptica	Bordetella holmesii	Bordetella pertussis/B. parapertussis	Chlamydophila pneumoniae	Coronavirus HKU1	Coronavirus NL63	Coronavirus 229E	Coronavirus OC43	Enterovirus/Rhinovirus	Human Bocavirus	Human Metapneumovirus	Human Metapneumovirus Subtyping	Human Parainfluenza Virus 1	Human Parainfluenza Virus 2	Human Parainfluenza Virus 3	Human Parainfluenza Virus 4	Influenza A	Influenza A Subtyping	Influenza B	Legionella pneumophila	Mycoplasma pneumoniae	Respiratory Syncytial Virus	Respiratory Syncytial Virus Subtyping
ePlex RP	+	+	−	−	−	−/	+	+	+	+	+	+	−	+	−	+	+	+	+	+	+	+	−	+	+	+
eSensor RVP	+	+	+	−	−	−	−	−	−	−	−	+[c]	−	+	−	+	+	+	−	+	+	+	−	−	+	+
FilmArray RP Panel	+	+	−	−	−	−/	+	+	+	+	+	+	−	+	−	+	+	+	+	+	+	+	−	+	+	−
FilmArray RP2 Panel	+	+	−	−	−	+/	+	+	+	+	+	+/	−	+	−	+	+	+	+	+	+	+	−	+	+	−
FilmArray RP EZ[a]	+	+	−	−	−	+/	+	+	+	+	+	+/	−	+	−	+	+	+	+	+	+	+	−	+	+	−
NxTAG RPP[b]	+	+	−	−	−	−/	+	+	+	+	+	+	+	+	−	+	+	+	+	+	+	+	−	−	+	+
VERIGENE RP Flex[b]	+	+	−	+	+	+/	−	−	−	−	−	+[c]	−	+	−	+	+	+	+	+	+	+	−	−	+	+

Abbreviations: FDA, US Food and Drug Administration; RPP, respiratory pathogen panel.
Symbols: +, yes or present on panel; −, no or absent from panel.
[a] The FilmArray RP EZ assay tests for human coronaviruses HKU1, NL63, 229E, and OC43 and human parainfluenza viruses 1, 2, 3, and 4, but it reports those analytes as coronavirus and parainfluenza virus, respectively.
[b] The NxTAG and VERIGENE RP *flex* assays allow users to selectively report targets.
[c] Rhinovirus alone is reported by the eSensor RVP, VERIGENE RP *flex*, US versions of the NxTAG RVP assays.

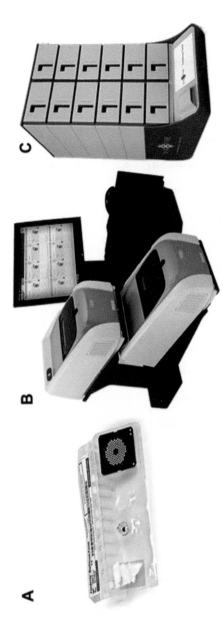

Fig. 3. The FilmArray system. The FilmArray pouch (*A*) and (*B*) the FilmArray 2.0 and (*C*) Torch instruments. (*Courtesy of* BioFire Diagnostics, Salt Lake City, UT; with permission.)

Box 1
Central Nervous System Pathogens Detected by the FilmArray ME Panel

Bacteria

Escherichia coli K1

Haemophilus influenzae

Listeria monocytogenes

Neisseria meningitidis

Streptococcus agalactiae

Streptococcus pneumoniae

Fungi[a]

Cryptococcus neoformans/C gattii

Viruses

Cytomegalovirus

Enterovirus

Herpes simplex virus 1

Herpes simplex virus 2

Human herpes virus 6

Human parechovirus

Varicella-zoster virus

[a] The FilmArray ME Panel detects *C neoformans* and *C gattii* but reports them together as *C neoformans/C gattii.*

Unyvero system

The Unyvero Lower Respiratory Tract Panel (Curetis USA Inc., San Diego, CA; **Fig. 4**), known as the Pneumonia Panel in Europe, is the first multiplex lower respiratory tract infection testing system to receive FDA clearance as of April 2018. This system uses PCR to detect an array of bacterial pathogens and antimicrobial resistance genes (**Table 6**) directly from tracheal aspirates in 4 to 5 hours. The Unyvero system is composed of 3 hardware components: a sample lysis device (Unyvero L4 Lysator), a panel analyzer (Unyvero A50 Analyzer), and a touchscreen computer interface and barcode scanner (Unyvero C8 Cockpit). Performance characteristics are described in refs. [32,33].

VERIGENE system

The VERIGENE system (Luminex Corporation. Austin, TX; **Fig. 5**) consists of VERIGENE Processor *SP* modules and the VERIGENE Reader, designed around a family of FDA-cleared syndromic panels. Multiple Processor *SP* units can be combined with a single Reader to accommodate the simultaneous testing of multiple samples. The extraction tray containing the sample, test cartridge (see **Tables 2** and **3** for cartridges and analytes), tip holder assembly, and utility tray are loaded into the Processor *SP* for automated nucleic acid extraction, purification, target amplification (if required by the specific assay), and hybridization of the target molecules to a glass detection array in the test cartridge. NanoGrid Technology is used to capture, detect, and identify target molecules. After the processing step, the test cartridge array is

Table 3
Syndromic Panels that Are Currently Available in the United States for the Detection of Gastrointestinal Tract Pathogens

Analyte	FDA Cleared?	Adenovirus F 40/41	Astrovirus	Campylobacter spp.	Clostridium difficile (Toxin A/B)	Cryptosporidium spp.	Cyclospora cayetanensis	Entamoeba histolytica	Escherichia coli O157	E coli (EAEC)	E coli (EPEC)	E coli (EIEC)	E coli (ETEC)	E coli (STEC) or stx1 and stx2	Giardia intestinalis (G lamblia)	Norovirus	Plesiomonas shigelloides	Rotavirus	Salmonella spp.	Sapovirus	Shigella spp.	Vibrio cholerae	Vibrio parahaemolyticus	Vibrio vulnificus	Yersinia enterocolitica
BD MAX Enteric Bacterial Panel	+	–	–	+	–	–	–	–	+	–	–	+	–	+	–	–	–	–	+	–	+	–	–	–	–
BD MAX Extended Enteric Bacterial Panel	+	–	–	+	–	–	–	–	+	–	–	–	+	+	–	–	+	–	+	–	+	+	+	+	+
BD MAX Enteric Parasite Panel	+	–	–	–	–	+	+	+	–	–	–	–	–	–	+	–	–	–	–	–	–	–	–	–	–
FilmArray GI Panel[a]	+	+	+	+	+	+	–	+	+	+	+	+	+	+	+	+	+	+	+	+	+	+	+	+	+
VERIGENE EP Test[b]	+	–	–	+	–	–	–	–	–	–	–	–	–	+	–	+	–	+	+	–	+	+	+	–	+
xTAG GPP[c]	+	+	–	+	+	+	–	+	+	–	–	–	+	+	+	+	–	+	+	–	+	+	–	–	–

Abbreviations: EIEC, *Shigella/*enteroinvasive *E coli;* EAEC, Enteroaggregative *E coli;* EPEC, Enteropathogenic *E coli;* ETEC, Enterotoxigenic *E coli;* STEC, Shiga Toxin-producing *E coli;* FDA, US Food and Drug Administration; GI, gastrointestinal; GPP, gastrointestinal pathogen panel.

Symbols: +, yes or present on panel; –, no or absent from panel.

a The FilmArray GI panel detects *Campylobacter jejuni, C coli,* and *C upsaliensis* and reports them as "*Campylobacter* (*jejuni, coli* and *upsaliensis*)." *Shigella* spp. are reported along with *E coli* (EIEC) as "*Shigella/*enteroinvasive *E coli* (EIEC)." *V cholerae, V parahaemolyticus,* and *V vulnificus* are detected and are reported as "*Vibrio* (*parahaemolyticus, vulnificus* and *cholerae*)"; however, *V cholerae* is also reported independently if it alone is detected. Norovirus genogroups I and II are detected, and astrovirus genotypes I, II, IV, and V are detected.

b The *VERIGENE* EP test detects *C jejuni, C coli,* and *C lari* and reports them as *Campylobacter* group. *Shigella boydii, S dysenteriae, S flexneri,* and *S sonnei* are detected and reported as *Shigella* spp. *V cholerae* and *V parahaemolyticus* are detected and reported as *Vibrio* group. Norovirus genogroups I and II are detected.

c The xTAG GPP detects *C jejuni, C coli,* and *C lari* and reports them as *Campylobacter; Cryptosporidium parvum* and *C hominis,* and reports them as *Cryptosporidium;* and *S boydii, S dysenteriae, S flexneri,* and *S sonnei,* and reports them as *Shigella.*

placed into the VERIGENE Reader to obtain results, which may be selectively reported. Total hands-on, automated processing, and test interpretation time is less than 3 hours. Performance characteristics are described in refs. [34,35].

xTAG technology

In addition to the VERIGENE system, Luminex offers FDA-cleared bead hybridization-based (xTAG) assays that require offline nucleic acid extraction followed by multiplex PCR and bead hybridization in 96-well plates. Analysis of beads is carried out by the MAGPIX instrument (**Fig. 6**). The MAGPIX instrument interrogates beads in each well of the reaction plate to detect fluorescent reporters that are linked to bead-hybridized target molecules. The total time required to perform a run is approximately 5 hours, so batch testing of samples is required. The NxTAG next-generation Respiratory Pathogen Panel allows users to selectively report analytes (see **Table 2**) whereas the xTAG Gastrointestinal Pathogen Panel (see **Table 3**) does not. See refs. [36–38] for performance characteristics.

Brief Description of Currently Available Syndromic Panels

Blood culture

Accurate diagnosis and early, appropriate treatment of sepsis is a life-saving event. Syndromic panels are designed to use the exponential growth of organisms in broth-based blood culture systems to detect the most common causes of bacteremia and key resistance mechanisms that would alter therapeutic management (eg, methicillin resistance). The performance of these systems has been thoroughly reviewed elsewhere [39]. Of note, FilmArray and VERIGENE correctly detect more than 95% of identifiable organisms in monomicrobial cultures when compared with conventional methods. The Achilles heel of blood culture syndromic panels is miscalls, which are associated with polymicrobial cultures and, more specifically, those errors associated with antimicrobial resistance.

Central nervous system

Infectious meningitis and encephalitis are often medical emergencies requiring prompt and accurate diagnosis and intervention for favorable outcomes. Culture is suboptimal for detecting many etiologies; however, most laboratories lack the infrastructure to perform laboratory-developed molecular tests and, therefore, rely on reference laboratories for viral detection in the cerebrospinal fluid or when the patient is on antimicrobials. Widespread early adoption has been plagued by concerns around performance in a setting where misdiagnosis could be catastrophic. As with the respiratory panel, the correlation of results without a sensitive and specific gold standard is challenging. A multicenter evaluation established a high percent agreement (>99%) with comparator testing; however, the percent agreement for positive results was only 84.4% [40]. Furthermore, reports of false-negative (eg, potential suboptimal detection of herpesviruses and *Cryptococcus*) and false-positive results (eg, *Streptococcus pneumoniae* and herpes simplex virus-1) have resulted in delayed or missed meningitis diagnoses [41].

Gastrointestinal

Acute gastroenteritis presents a clinical and public health dilemma because the symptoms of infectious and noninfectious causes of diarrhea overlap. Traditional diagnostics (eg, culture, microscopy, antigen detection) are time consuming and may require multiple specimens for optimal sensitivity. Studies have reproducibly shown that 2 to 3 times more pathogens are detected when a molecular assay is used, compared with traditional methods [39]. This is due in part to an enhanced range of the targets, an

Table 4
Syndromic Panels that Are Currently Available in the United States for the Detection of Bloodstream Infection Pathogens

Analyte	FilmArray BCID Panel	VERIGENE GN BC Test	VERIGENE GP BC Test
FDA Cleared?	+	+	+
Acinetobacter baumannii or Acinetobacter spp.	+	+	×
Candida spp.	+	×	×
Citrobacter spp.	−	+	×
Enterobacteriaceae	+	−	×
Enterobacter spp.	+	−	×
Enterococcus spp.	+	×	+
Escherichia coli	+	+	×
Haemophilus influenzae	+	−	×
Klebsiella oxytoca	+	−	×
Klebsiella pneumoniae	+	+	×
Listeria spp.	+	×	×
Micrococcus spp.	−	×	+
Neisseria meningitidis	+	−	×
Proteus spp.	+	+	×
Pseudomonas aeruginosa	+	+	×
Serratia spp.	+	+	×
Staphylococcus spp.	+	×	+
Staphylococcus aureus	+	×	+
Streptococcus spp.	+	×	+
Streptococcus agalactiae	+	×	+
Streptococcus pneumoniae	+	×	+
Streptococcus pyogenes	+	×	+
Carbapenemase Genes	+	+	×
Extended-Spectrum β-Lactamase Genes	−	+	×
mecA	+	×	+
vanA/vanB	+	×	+

Abbreviation: FDA, US Food and Drug Administration.
Symbols: +, yes or present on panel; −, no or absent from panel.

Table 5
Multiplex Nucleic Acid Amplification Panels Available for the Detection of High-Consequence and Travel-Associated Pathogens

Analyte	FDA Cleared?	Bacillus anthracis	Brucella melitensis	Burkholderia mallei /B pseudomallei	Chikungunya Virus	Clostridium botulinum	Coxiella burnetii	Crimean-Congo Hemorrhagic Fever Virus	Dengue Virus	Ebola Virus (Zaire ebolavirus)	EEE Virus	Francisella tularensis	Lassa Virus	Leptospira spp.	Leishmania spp.	Marburg Virus	Orthopox Virus	Plasmodium spp.	Ricinus communis	Rickettsia prowazekii	Salmonella enterica Serovar. Paratyphi A	S enterica Serovar. Typhi	Variola Virus	VEE Virus	WEE Virus	Yellow Fever Virus	Yersinia pestis	West Nile Virus	Zika Virus
FilmArray BioThreat Panel[a]	–	+	+	+	–	+	+	–	–	+	+	+	–	–	–	+	+	–	+	+	–	–	+	+	+	–	+	–	–
FilmArray BioThreat – E Test[b]	–[c]	–	–	–	–	–	–	–	–	+	–	–	–	–	–	–	–	–	–	–	–	–	–	–	–	–	–	–	–
FilmArray Global Fever Panel[d]	–	+	–	–	+	–	–	+	+	+	–	+	+	+	+	+	–	+[e]	–	–	+	+	–	–	–	+	–	+	+

Abbreviations: EEE virus, eastern equine encephalitis virus; FDA, US Food and Drug Administration; VEE virus, Venezuelan equine encephalitis virus; WEE, western equine encephalitis virus.

Symbols: +, yes or present on panel/test; -, no or absent from panel/test.

[a] The FilmArray BioThreat Panel is designed to detect analytes from swab, liquid, culture, and powder samples.

[b] The FilmArray BioThreat-E Test is designed to detect Ebola virus (*Zaire ebolavirus*) in blood and urine samples.

[c] The FilmArray BioThreat-E Test was granted FDA EUA status in 2014 and it is only authorized for use by CLIA moderate and high complexity laboratories throughout the duration of the EUA. This test is intended to detect Ebola virus (*Zaire ebolavirus*) from blood and urine specimens.

[d] The FilmArray Global Fever Panel is designed to detect analytes in whole blood.

[e] The FilmArray Global Fever Panel detects and reports *Plasmodium* spp. and it also distinguishes *Plasmodium falciparum* from *Plasmodium ovale*/*Plasmodium vivax* and reports them as such.

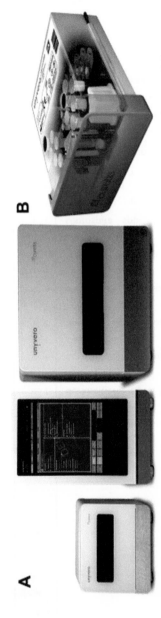

Fig. 4. The Curetis Unyvero system, composed of the Unyvero L4 Lysator (*A, left*), the Unyvero C8 Cockpit (*A, middle*), and the Unyvero A50 Analyzer (*A, right*), and the Unyvero LRT panel (*B*). (*Courtesy of* Curetis, San Diego, CA; with permission.)

Table 6 Curetis Unyvero Lower Respiratory Tract Panel for the Diagnosis of Community-Acquired and Health Care-Associated Pneumonia	
Microbial Targets	**Antimicrobial Resistance Genes**
Acinetobacter spp.	bla_{TEM}
Chlamydophila pneumoniae	bla_{SHV}
Citrobacter freundii	bla_{VIM}
Enterobacter cloacae complex	bla_{NDM}
Escherichia coli	bla_{KPC}
Haemophilus influenzae	bla_{CTX-M}
Klebsiella oxytoca	bla_{OXA-23}
Klebsiella pneumoniae	bla_{OXA-24}
Klebsiella variicola	bla_{OXA-48}
Legionella pneumophila	bla_{OXA-58}
Moraxella catarrhalis	*gyrA*83 mutation (of *Escherichia coli*)
Morganella morganii	*gyrA*87 mutation (of *E coli*)
Mycoplasma pneumoniae	*gyrA*83 mutation (of *Pseudomonas aeruginosa*)
Proteus spp.	*gyrA*87 mutation (of *P aeruginosa*)
Pseudomonas aeruginosa	*mecA*
Serratia marcescens	
Staphylococcus aureus	
Stenotrophomonas maltophilia	
Streptococcus pneumoniae	

increase in sensitivity of the assays over traditional methods, and the recognition of co-infections that were previously unrecognized. Sensitivity and specificity of these assays, overall, is high, with few exceptions. Notably, detection of rotavirus, *Campylobacter* spp., and *Salmonella* spp. may be problematic with VERIGENE; one publication noted false positivity with norovirus using BioFire. Overall, these platforms allow timely, accurate diagnosis of diarrhea and can assist with pathogen-directed therapy [42].

Respiratory

Owing to a relative paucity of accurate and rapid diagnostics, pathogen determination in acute respiratory illness had traditionally fallen to clinical presentation, despite its poor prognostic value. Rapid, accurate diagnosis is critical for antibiotic stewardship, informing the clinician if antivirals are warranted, and infection control initiatives (eg, isolation, cohorting). Unsurprisingly, respiratory illness has been a key target for syndromic testing (see **Table 2**). Performance characteristics have been reviewed in depth elsewhere [39], with key attributes highlighted herein. All commercially available respiratory panels significantly outperform traditional methods of detection and have expanded our recognition of coinfections (approximately 5% of samples tested). At present, no gold standard method for comparison of these assays has hampered exact determination of performance; however, the generally accepted overall agreement between molecular methods is between 85% and 99% for each target, with some exceptions. Accurate detection of adenovirus is problematic in many first-generation assays; however, a multicenter analysis of the FilmArray RP2 [43] indicates increased sensitivity with this assay.

Sexually transmitted infections/women's health

Sexually transmitted infections, bacterial vaginosis, and vaginal yeast infections are associated with significant morbidity and can have long-term consequences, including infertility. The diagnosis of these highly prevalent infectious diseases once

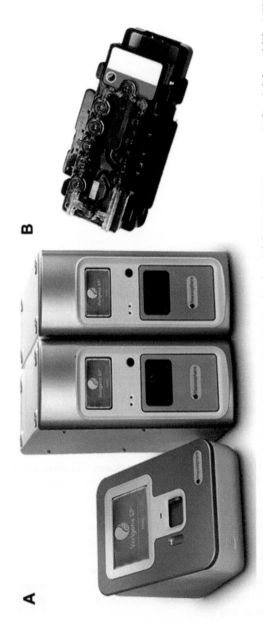

Fig. 5. The Luminex VERIGENE system, composed of (**A**, *left*) the VERIGENE Reader, (**A**, *right*) VERIGENE Processor *SP* (**A**, *right*), and (**B**) a VERIGENE Test Cartridge. (*Courtesy of* Luminex, Austin, TX; with permission.)

required the use of multiple testing methods such as microscopy, culture, and nucleic acid amplification testing; however, the advent of syndromic testing systems for these pathogens (eg, BD MAX CT/GC/TV and BD MAX Vaginal Panel; see **Table 1**) has streamlined their detection. Overall, both of the assays listed in **Table 1** outperform traditional methods, including *Chlamydia trachomatis* culture and microscopic screening for bacterial vaginosis, candidiasis, and trichomoniasis. In one study that evaluated the performance of the BD MAX CT/GC/TV assay, the sensitivities for detection of all three analytes were 91.5% or greater and the specificities were 98.6% or greater [14]. According to clinical trial data of the BD MAX Vaginal Panel, the sensitivities for analytes ranged from 75.9% (analyte [collection method]: *Candida glabrata* [clinician-collected specimens]) to 100% (*C glabrata* [simulated specimens] and *Candida krusei* [simulated specimens]) and specificities ranged from 84.5% (bacterial vaginosis [self-collected specimens]) to 100% (*C glabrata* [simulated specimens] and *C krusei* [self-collected and simulated specimens]) [44]. Overall, sexually transmitted infection/women's health syndromic panels outperform traditional methods in terms of sensitivity, specificity, and TATs.

Currently Available Point-of-Care Molecular Methods

The push to get faster diagnostic answers to guide admission or discharge strategies and therapeutics is likely to propel multiplex testing into the realm of POC testing. At present, issues with contamination, quality control performance and monitoring, interpretation of results, and overall good laboratory practices as technologies migrate into a less controlled setting is an obvious concern. Current CLIA-waived platforms are discussed briefly, because these systems may be readily adaptable to multiplex syndromic testing in the POC setting.

Alere i

The Alere i (Alere Scarborough, Inc., Scarborough, ME; **Fig. 7**) system uses nicking enzyme amplification reaction technology, an isothermal amplification method, to detect nucleic acids of target pathogens, including influenza A and B viruses, respiratory syncytial virus, and group A *Streptococcus*, either directly from swabs or from swab eluates in transport media. The consumable is a 3-component system that consists of a reagent base, elution buffer container, and transfer cartridge that is assembled on the Alere i instrument. Positive results are available within 8 to 15 minutes (depending on the assay type). Performance characteristics and additional details are described in refs. [45–50].

cobas Liat system

The cobas Liat System (Roche Diagnostics, Indianapolis, IN; **Fig. 8**) integrates all reagents necessary for nucleic acid purification and amplification (by real-time PCR) into a segmented soft plastic tube housed within a rigid plastic frame. After specimen collection (eg, nasopharyngeal swab) and elution into a suitable specimen transport medium (eg, viral transport medium), a small aliquot of the specimen is pipetted into the tube, the tube is capped, and the entire tube-frame assembly is loaded into the cobas Liat instrument, which automates all reaction and amplicon detection steps. Results for influenza detection are available within 20 minutes, and those for group A *Streptococcus* are available within 15 minutes of assay initiation. Currently, three FDA-cleared, CLIA-waived assays are available for the detection of influenza A/B viruses alone, influenza A/B viruses and respiratory syncytial virus, and group A *Streptococcus*. Performance characteristics are discussed in refs. [45,51–53].

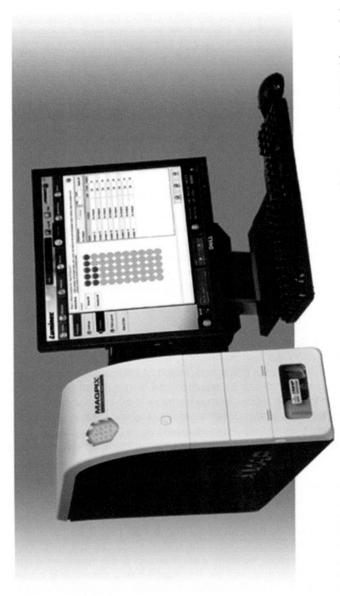

Fig. 6. The Luminex MAGPIX instrument and computer for NxTAG and xTAG assays. (*Courtesy of* Luminex, Austin, TX; with permission.)

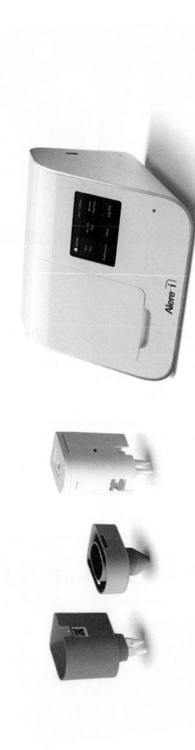

Fig. 7. The Alere i system, including the 3-part test cartridge (*left*) and the Alere i instrument (*right*). (*Courtesy of* Alere, Waltham, MA; with permission.)

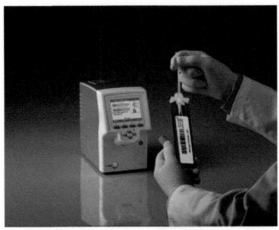

Fig. 8. The cobas Liat system from Roche Diagnostics includes the test cartridge (*foreground*) and the Liat instrument (*background*). (*Courtesy of* Roche Diagnostics, Indianapolis, IN; with permission.)

Solana

The Solana system (Quidel Corporation, San Diego, CA; **Fig. 9**) uses isothermal, helicase-dependent amplification and fluorescent-probe detection of target nucleic acids. Currently, FDA-approved assays are available for the detection of *Clostridium difficile*, groups A and B streptococci, herpes simplex viruses, varicella-zoster virus, influenza viruses, respiratory syncytial virus, human metapneumovirus, and *Trichomonas vaginalis*.

To perform testing, a patient specimen (eg, nasal swab in viral transport medium) in Process Buffer is heated before transfer to a reaction tube. The reaction tube contains all reagents needed for amplification and detection in a lyophilized form. The reaction tube is next inserted into the Solana instrument where amplification and detection are performed. Results are available in 30 minutes or less. Up to 12 Solana diagnostic

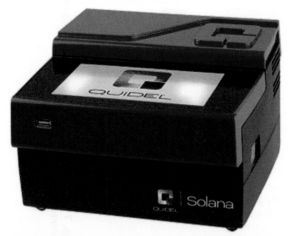

Fig. 9. The Quidel Solana instrument. (*Courtesy of* Quidel, San Diego, CA; with permission.)

assays can be analyzed simultaneously. Relevant performance characteristics are described in ref. [54] and in assay package inserts available on the Quidel website (https://www.quidel.com).

The Future of Syndromic Testing and Point-of-Care Molecular Diagnostics

Each of these systems, plus those that have not been described herein, are constantly undergoing refinement to ensure their continued relevance in the molecular diagnostics marketplace. Test systems are continuously challenged with new strains of pathogens and antimicrobial resistance mechanisms to evaluate their inclusivity and/or exclusivity, and panels are frequently updated to include additional analytes. Also, new assays that enable detection and quantitation of pathogens associated with disease processes besides those mentioned previously are in development. The goal of most manufacturers is to offer infectious disease diagnostic testing solutions that allow identification of the greatest breadth of pathogens associated with a specific disease process or syndrome. To that end, future applications of these technologies include the enhancement of currently available systems, the development of additional panels that are amenable to the diagnosis other infectious processes, and the development of tests that enable users to comprehensively profile the antimicrobial susceptibility of pathogens.

SUMMARY

The use of multiplex panels for pathogen detection provides several advantages over traditional laboratory diagnostic approach. Providers tout multiplex assays as a means to simplify the ordering process, decrease the number of required specimens, detect pathogens that may not be part of the initial diagnostic differential owing to rarity of the agent or inaccessibility of an alternative in-house test method, and provide results in a clinically actionable timeframe. The incorporation of molecular multiplex panels is of financial and logistical benefit to the laboratory. Specifically, one can decrease the number of methods needed to detect the same diversity of infectious agents and decrease technologist hands-on time, which results in a simplified workflow for the purposes of training, competency, use, and often cost. For the patient, these assays provide superior accuracy over traditional approaches and a greater breadth of targeted pathogens, which may decrease the number of medical visits, interventions, and durations of diagnosis. Certain multiplex assays provide benefits beyond direct patient care, such as early recognition of drug-resistant pathogens for swift implementation of infection control measures or improved detection of gastrointestinal pathogens that may impact outbreak investigations. Finally, rapid pathogen detection and the potential for improved, early intervention has been shown to positively impact associated costs by aiding in selective test use and reduced length of stay [39].

Taken together, the benefits of molecular syndromic panels and POC tests vastly outweigh any disadvantages, which is centered around cost to the health care system, namely, to the hospital or patient. The claim that this so-called shotgun approach adds unnecessary cost to the patient is an oversimplification. Although molecular multiplex assays are often more costly in terms of reagents and patient billing compared with a single culture- or serology-based assay, when multiple diagnostic tests are ordered, the multiplex assay is often less expensive than the full battery of traditional tests. Anecdotally, physicians desire to provide the patient with a definitive diagnosis and treatment plan, which may inadvertently lead to the overuse of medical resources such as injudicious antibiotic use and additional diagnostic tests (eg, imaging) to help establish a diagnosis when the causative pathogen is not easily identified. Therefore, the ability to rapidly and accurately provide a cause for the patient's illness may improve both physician and patient satisfaction.

At present, FDA-cleared syndromic and POC molecular assays center around a few syndromes; however, this menu is likely to expand in the coming years as laboratories rapidly adopt this approach to testing. When combined with consultation (eg, antimicrobial stewardship intervention), the implementation of these assays has been shown to decrease the time to appropriate therapy, improve patient survival, and decrease overall health care-associated costs [9]. Care must be taken in the selection and appropriate use of multiplex panels. Specifically, one must balance the potential for increased laboratory reagent and equipment costs against the potential for reduced labor costs and increased revenue. To provide the highest quality of care while limiting unnecessary expense, laboratories must develop algorithms that assist providers in test ordering and use.

REFERENCES

1. Daly JA, Clifton NL, Seskin KC, et al. Use of rapid, nonradioactive DNA probes in culture confirmation tests to detect *Streptococcus agalactiae, Haemophilus influenza*, and *Enterococcus* spp. from pediatric patients with significant infections. J Clin Microbiol 1991;29:80–2.

2. Davis TE, Fuller DD. Direct identification of bacterial isolates in blood cultures by using a DNA probe. J Clin Microbiol 1991;29:2193–6.

3. Lumb R, Lanser JA, Lim IS. Rapid identification of mycobacteria by the Gen-Probe Accuprobe system. Pathology 1993;25:313–5.

4. Padhye AA, Smith G, Standard PG, et al. Comparative evaluation of chemilluminescent DNA probe assays and exoantigen tests for rapid identification of *Blastomyces dermatitidis* and *Coccidioides immitis*. J Clin Microbiol 1994;32:867–70.

5. Sninsky JJ. The polymerase chain reaction (PCR): a valuable method for retroviral detection. Lymphology 1990;23:92–7.

6. Persing DH, Mathiesen D, Marshall WF, et al. Detection of *Babesia microti* by polymerase chain reaction. J Clin Microbiol 1992;30:2097–103.

7. Karron RA, Froehlich JL, Bobo L, et al. Rapid detection of parainfluenza virus type 3 RNA in respiratory specimens: use of reverse-transcription-PCR-enzyme immunoassay. J Clin Microbiol 1994;32:484–8.

8. Orlando C, Pinzani P, Pazzagli M. Developments in quantitative PCR. Clin Chem Lab Med 1998;36:255–69.

9. Abbott AN, Fang FC. Clinical impact of multiplex syndromic panels in the diagnosis of bloodstream, gastrointestinal, respiratory, and central nervous system infections. Clin Microbiol Newsl 2017;39:133–42.

10. Messacar K, Hurst AL, Child J, et al. Clinical impact and provider acceptability of real-time antimicrobial stewardship decision support for rapid diagnostics in children with positive blood culture results. J Pediatric Infect Dis Soc 2016;6:267–74.

11. Rappo U, Schuetz AN, Jenkins SG, et al. Impact of early detection of respiratory viruses by multiplex PCR assay on clinical outcomes in adult patients. J Clin Microbiol 2016;54:2096–103.

12. Ward C, Stocker K, Begum J, et al. Performance evaluation of the Verigene® (Nanosphere) and FilmArray® (BioFire®) molecular assays for identification of causative organisms in bacterial bloodstream infections. Eur J Clin Microbiol Infect Dis 2015;34:487–96.

13. Salimnia H, Fairfax MR, Lephart PR, et al. Evaluation of the FilmArray blood culture identification panel: results of a multicenter controlled trial. J Clin Microbiol 2016;54:687–98.
14. Van Der Pol B. Profile of the triplex assay for detection of chlamydia, gonorrhea, and trichomonas using the BD MAX system. Expert Rev Mol Diagn 2017;17: 539–47.
15. Madison-Antenucci S, Relich RF, Doyle L, et al. Multicenter evaluation of the BD MAX enteric parasite real-time PCR assay for detection of *Giardia duodenalis, Cryptosporidium hominis, Cryptosporidium parvum,* and *Entamoeba histolytica.* J Clin Microbiol 2016;54:2681–8.
16. Knabl L, Grutsch I, Orth-Höller D. Comparison of the BD MAX enteric pathogen panel with conventional diagnostic procedures in diarrheal stool samples. Eur J Clin Microbiol Infect Dis 2016;35:131–6.
17. Simner PJ, Oethinger M, Stellrecht KA, et al. Multisite evaluation of the BD MAX extended enteric bacterial panel for detection of *Yersinia enterocolitica,* enterotoxigenic *Escherichia coli, Vibrio,* and *Plesiomonas shigelloides* from stool specimens. J Clin Microbiol 2017;55:3258–66.
18. Nijhuis RHT, Guerendiain D, Claas ECJ. Comparison of the ePlex respiratory pathogen panel with laboratory-developed real-time PCR assays for detection of respiratory pathogens. J Clin Microbiol 2017;55:1938–45.
19. Pierce VM, Hodinka RL. Comparison of the GenMark diagnostics eSensor respiratory viral panel to real-time PCR for detection of respiratory viruses in children. J Clin Microbiol 2012;50:3458–65.
20. Babady NE, England MR, Jurcic Smith KL, et al. Multicenter evaluation of the ePlex respiratory pathogen panel for the detection of viral and bacterial respiratory tract pathogens in nasopharyngeal swabs. J Clin Microbiol 2018;56 [pii: e01658-17].
21. Van Rijn AL, Nijhuis RHT, Bekker V, et al. Clinical implications of rapid ePlex respiratory pathogen panel testing compared to laboratory-developed real-time PCR. Eur J Clin Microbiol Infect Dis 2018;37:571–7.
22. McCoy MH, Relich RF, Davis TE, et al. Performance of the FilmArray blood culture identification panel utilized by non-expert staff compared to conventional microbial identification and antimicrobial resistance gene detection from positive blood cultures. J Med Microbiol 2016;65:619–25.
23. Rogers BB, Shankar P, Jerris RC, et al. Impact of a rapid respiratory panel test on patient outcomes. Arch Pathol Lab Med 2015;139:636–41.
24. Kanack KJ. Rapid respiratory panel testing influences patient management and clinical outcomes. MLO Med Lab Obs 2014;46:16.
25. MacVane SH, Nolte FS. Benefits of adding a rapid PCR-based blood culture identification panel to an established antimicrobial stewardship program. J Clin Microbiol 2016;54:2455–63.
26. Southern TR, Van Schooneveld TC, Bannister DL, et al. Implementation and performance of the BioFire FilmArray blood culture identification panel with antimicrobial treatment recommendations for bloodstream infections at a midwestern academic tertiary hospital. Diagn Microbiol Infect Dis 2015;81:96–101.
27. Buss SN, Leber A, Chapin K, et al. Multicenter evaluation of the BioFire FilmArray gastrointestinal panel for etiologic diagnosis of infectious gastroenteritis. J Clin Microbiol 2015;53:915–25.
28. Prakash VP, LeBlanc L, Alexander-Scott NE, et al. Use of a culture-independent gastrointestinal multiplex PCR panel during a shigellosis outbreak: considerations for clinical laboratories and public health. J Clin Microbiol 2015;53:1048–9.

29. Hanson KE, Slechta ES, Killpack JA, et al. Preclinical assessment of a fully auto-mated multiplex PCR panel for detection of central nervous system pathogens. J Clin Microbiol 2016;54:785–7.

30. Duff S, Hasbun R, Ginocchio CC, et al. Economic analysis of rapid multiplex po-lymerase chain reaction testing for meningitis/encephalitis in pediatric patients. Future Microbiol 2018;13:617–29.

31. Gay-Andrieu F, Magassouba N, Picto V, et al. Clinical evaluation of the BioFire Fil-mArray BioThreat-E test for the diagnosis of Ebola virus disease in Guinea. J Clin Virol 2017;92:20–4.

32. Papan C, Meyer-Buehn M, Laniado G, et al. Assessment of the multiplex PCR-based assay Unyvero pneumonia application for detection of bacterial patho-gens and antibiotic resistance genes in children and neonates. Infection 2018; 46:189–96.

33. Personne Y, Ozongwu C, Platt G, et al. 'Sample-in, answer-out'? Evaluation and comprehensive analysis of the Unyvero P50 pneumonia assay. Diagn Microbiol Infect Dis 2016;86:5–10.

34. Ledeboer NA, Lopansri BK, Dhiman N, et al. Identification of Gram-negative bac-teria and genetic resistance determinants from positive blood culture broths by use of the Verigene Gram-negative blood culture multiplex microarray-based mo-lecular assay. J Clin Microbiol 2015;53:2460–72.

35. Buchan BW, Ginocchio CC, Manii R, et al. Multiplex identification of Gram-positive bacteria and resistance determinants directly from positive blood culture broths: evaluation of an automated microarray-based nucleic acid test. PLoS Med 2013;10:e1001478.

36. Esposito S, Principi N. The role of the NxTAG respiratory pathogen panel assay and other multiplex platforms in clinical practice. Expert Rev Mol Diagn 2017; 17:9–17.

37. Tang YW, Gonsalves S, Sun JY, et al. Clinical evaluation of the Luminex NxTAG respiratory pathogen panel. J Clin Microbiol 2016;54:1912–4.

38. Huang RS, Johnson CL, Pritchard L, et al. Performance of the Verigene enteric pathogens test, BioFire FilmArray gastrointestinal panel and Luminex xTAG gastrointestinal pathogen panel for detection of common enteric pathogens. Di-agn Microbiol Infect Dis 2016;86:336–9.

39. Ramanan P, Bryson AL, Binnicker MJ, et al. Syndromic panel-based testing in clinical microbiology. Clin Microbiol Rev 2017;31 [pii:e00024-17].

40. Leber AL, Everhart K, Balada-Llasat JM, et al. Multicenter evaluation of BioFire FilmArray Meningitis/Encephalitis Panel for detection of bacteria, viruses, and yeast in cerebrospinal fluid specimens. J Clin Microbiol 2016;54(9):2251–61.

41. Dien Bard J, Alby K. Point-counterpoint: meningitis/encephalitis syndromic testing in the clinical laboratory. J Clin Microbiol 2018;56(4) [pii:e00018-18].

42. Cybulski RJ Jr, Bateman AC, Bourassa L, et al. Clinical impact of a multiplex gastrointestinal PCR panel in patients with acute gastroenteritis. Clin Infect Dis 2018. https://doi.org/10.1093/cid/ciy357.

43. Leber AL, Everhart K, Daly JA, et al. Multicenter evaluation of BioFire FilmArray Respiratory Panel 2 for detection of viruses and bacteria in nasopharyngeal swab samples. J Clin Microbiol 2018;25(6):56 [pii:e01945-17].

44. Kawa D, Paradis S, Yu JH, et al. Evaluating the standard of care for women's health: the BD MAX Vaginal Panel and management of vaginal infections (white paper). 2017. Available at: http://moleculardiagnostics.bd.com/wp-content/uploads/2017/08/MAX-Vaginal-Panel-Whitepaper.pdf. Accessed June 25, 2018.

45. Young S, Illescas P, Nicasio J, et al. Diagnostic accuracy of the real-time PCR co-bas Liat influenza A/B assay and the Alere i influenza A&B NEAR isothermal nucleic acid amplification assay for the detection of influenza using adult nasopharyngeal specimens. J Clin Virol 2017;94:86–90.

46. Davis S, Allen AJ, O'Leary R, et al. Diagnostic accuracy and cost analysis of the Alere i influenza A&B near-patient test using throat swabs. J Hosp Infect 2017;97:301–9.

47. Hassan F, Hays LM, Bonner A, et al. Multicenter clinical evaluation of the Alere i respiratory syncytial virus isothermal nucleic acid amplification assay. J Clin Microbiol 2018;56 [pii:e01777-17].

48. Schnee SV, Pfeil J, Ihling CM, et al. Performance of the Alere i RSV assay for point-of-care detection of respiratory syncytial virus in children. BMC Infect Dis 2017;17:767.

49. Cohen DM, Russo ME, Jaggi P, et al. Multicenter clinical evaluation of the novel Alere i Strep A isothermal nucleic acid amplification test. J Clin Microbiol 2015;53:2258–61.

50. Berry GJ, Miller CR, Prats MM, et al. Comparison of the Alere i Strep A test and the BD Veritor system in the detection of group A *Streptococcus* and the hypothetical impact of results on antibiotic utilization. J Clin Microbiol 2018;56 [pii:e01310-17].

51. Melchers WJG, Kuijpers J, Sickler JJ, et al. Lab-in-a-tube: real-time molecular point-of-care diagnostics for influenza A and B using the cobas Liat system. J Med Virol 2017;89:1382–6.

52. Gibson J, Schechter-Perkins EM, Mitchell P, et al. Multi-center evaluation of the cobas Liat Influenza A/B & RSV assay for rapid point of care diagnosis. J Clin Virol 2017;95:5–9.

53. Ling L, Kaplan SE, Lopez JC, et al. Parallel validation of three molecular devices for simultaneous detection and identification of influenza A and B and respiratory syncytial viruses. J Clin Microbiol 2018;56 [pii:e01691-17].

54. Gaydos CA, Schwebke J, Dombrowski J, et al. Clinical performance of the Solana point-of-care trichomonas assay from clinician-collected vaginal swabs and urine specimens from symptomatic and asymptomatic women. Expert Rev Mol Diagn 2017;17:303–6.

Building Evidence for Clinical Use of Pharmacogenomics and Reimbursement for Testing

Larisa H. Cavallari, PharmD[a],*, Victoria M. Pratt, PhD[b]

KEYWORDS

• Pharmacogenomics • Genotype • Evidence • Outcomes • Reimbursement

KEY POINTS

- The evidence gap in outcomes with pharmacogenomic testing and testing reimbursement are major challenges to pharmacogenomic implementation.
- Although randomized controlled trials (RCTs) are considered the gold standard for establishing clinical utility and informing treatment guidelines, few have been done in pharmacogenomics.
- Conducting an RCT for each gene-drug pair is impractical from a time and cost perspective, and more efficient approaches are needed for evidence generation.
- Outcomes data with pharmacogenomic testing are emerging from pragmatic and observational studies, and further data are expected from ongoing pragmatic clinical trials.
- It is expected that reimbursement will follow evidence for benefit with pharmacogenomic testing.

INTRODUCTION

In his 2015 State of the Union Address, former President Obama announced the Precision Medicine Initiative signaling continued United States government support toward individualized disease detection, prevention, and management strategies [1]. Pharmacogenomics is one component of precision medicine and promises to optimize drug therapy through the incorporation of an individual's genetic information in

This article originally appeared in Advances in Molecular Pathology, Volume 1, Issue 1, November 2018.

Disclosure: The authors have nothing to disclose.

Funding: This work is supported by NIH/NHGRI grant U01 HG007269 and NIH/NCATS grant UL1 TR001427 to L.H. Cavallari.

[a] Department of Pharmacotherapy and Translational Research, Center for Pharmacogenomics and Precision Medicine, University of Florida, PO Box 100486, Gainesville, FL 32610-0486, USA; [b] Optum Genomics, 11000 Optum Circle, Eden Praire, MN 55344, USA

* Corresponding author.

E-mail address: lcavallari@cop.ufl.edu

drug prescribing decisions. Genotype specifically influences pharmacokinetics and pharmacodynamics and allows for prediction of risk for adverse drug effects and likelihood of drug effectiveness.

Following decades of research into genetic determinants of drug response, pharmacogenomics is entering clinical practice at institutions across the US and Europe [2–11]. Guidelines by the Clinical Pharmacogenetics Implementation Consortium (CPIC) and Dutch Pharmacogenetics Working Group (DPWG) have facilitated the adoption of genotype-guided therapy by informing implementation priorities and strategies [12,13]. These guidelines specifically provide recommendations for how to translate genotype results to prescribing decisions for gene-drug pairs with evidence supporting their incorporation in clinical practice.

Clinical validity is well established for gene-drug pairs addressed by the CPIC and DPGW. However, evidence supporting the clinical utility of testing is much more limited. Although randomized controlled trials (RCTs) are considered the gold standard for establishing clinical utility and informing treatment guidelines, few have been done in pharmacogenomics. Some in fact argue that RCTs should not be the level of evidentiary support required for pharmacogenomic implementation [14–16]. Rather, genotype may be viewed as one of the several patient-specific factors that influence drug response, as shown in **Fig. 1**. Laboratory tests such as serum creatinine, hemoglobin, and serum potassium are routinely ordered before initiating drug therapy to guide drug and dose selection in the absence of RCT evidence to support this approach. Genotype is essentially another laboratory test that can be considered in the context of other patient-specific factors to enable individualized drug therapy. Nonetheless, demonstrating value with genotype-guided therapy is needed to influence policy makers and key stakeholders in genomic medicine, including providers and third party payers. In this article, the authors discuss existing data and ongoing efforts to generate evidence in support of genotype-guided therapy approaches and reimbursement for pharmacogenomic testing.

BUILDING EVIDENCE TO SUPPORT PHARMACOGENOMIC IMPLEMENTATION
Randomized Controlled Trial Evidence

Table 1 summarizes gene-drug pairs investigated in RCTs, which include *HLA-B*57:01*-abacavir, *TPMT*-thiopurines, and *CYP2C9/VKORC1*-warfarin. In the case of

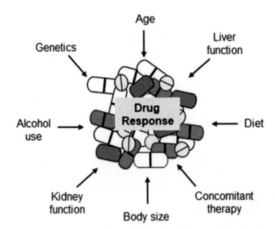

Fig. 1. Patient-specific factors commonly influencing drug response.

Table 1
Examples of Randomized Controlled Trials of Genotype-Guided Therapies

Gene-Drug Pair	Trial Acronym	Patient Population	Summary of Results
*HLA-B*57:01*-Abacavir	PREDICT-1 [17]	1956 patients with HIV randomized to prospective genetic screening with avoidance of abacavir in patients screening positive or to abacavir use without screening	Immunologically confirmed hypersensitivity occurred in 0% of patients in the prospective-screening group vs 2.7% of controls, *P*<.001
TPMT-Thiopurines	TOPIC [20]	783 patients with inflammatory bowel disease randomized to pretreatment screening with thiopurine dose reduction in carriers of a variant allele according to DPWG guidelines or to usual thiopurine dosing without screening	Adverse hematologic reactions did not differ between genotype vs control patients in the population overall, but were less common in *TPMT* variant allele carriers in the genotype vs control group (2.6% vs 22.9%, RR, 0.11, 95% CI 0.01–0.85)
CYP2C9/VKORC1-warfarin	COAG [22]	1015 patients randomized to genotype-guided dosing or clinically guided dosing	Mean percent of time in therapeutic range in the first 4 wk was similar between the genotype- and clinically guided groups (45.2% and 45.4%) for the population overall. Among Blacks, the mean time in range was lower with genotype- vs clinically guided dosing (35.2% vs 43.5%, *P* = .01)
	EU-PACT [23]	455 patients randomized to genotype-guided dosing or fixed dosing (5–10 mg day 1, then 5 mg/d days 2–3, then adjustment based on INR)	Mean percent of time in therapeutic range in the initial 12 wk was lower in the control group vs the genotype group (60.3% vs 67.4%, *P*<.001)
	GIFT [24]	1650 older patients (≥65 y) undergoing elective hip or knee arthroplasty randomized to genotype-guided dosing or clinically guided dosing	The rate of the composite outcome of death, venous thromboembolism, major bleeding, or INR ≥4 during the initial 4–6 wk was 10.8% in the genotype-guided arm and 14.7% in the clinically guided arm, representing a 27% relative rate reduction in the primary endpoint

(continued on next page)

Table 1
(continued)

Gene-Drug Pair	Trial Acronym	Patient Population	Summary of Results
CYP3A5-Tacrolimus	Not available	280 renal transplant recipients randomized to CYP3A5-guided tacrolimus dosing or standard dosing [60]	A higher proportion of patients in the genotype-guided group achieved therapeutic tacrolimus levels at day 10 post-transplant compared with those in the standard dosing group (43.2% vs 29.1%, $P = .03$).
CYP2C19-clopidogrel	TAILOR-PCI (ClinicalTrials.gov ID NCT01742117)	5270 patients undergoing PCI for an acute coronary syndrome or stable coronary disease randomized to CYP2C19 genotype–guided antiplatelet therapy, with clopidogrel avoided in carriers of a nonfunctional allele, or to routine clopidogrel	Estimated to be completed in 2020. The primary outcome is the occurrence of a major adverse cardiovascular event, defined as nonfatal myocardial infarction, nonfatal stroke, cardiovascular mortality, severe recurrent ischemia, and stent thrombosis at 1 year
	POPular Genetics (ClinicalTrials.gov ID NCT01761786) [44]	2700 patients with ST-segment elevation myocardial infarction undergoing PCI randomized to CYP2C19 genotype–guided antiplatelet therapy, with clopidogrel avoided in carriers of a nonfunctional allele, or to routine ticagrelor or prasugrel	Estimated to be completed in 2019. The primary endpoint is the composite of death, myocardial infarction, stent thrombosis, stroke, and major bleeding at 1 year

Abbreviations: CI, confidence interval; DPWG, Dutch Pharmacogenetics Working Group; HIV, human immunodeficiency virus; INR, international normalized ratio; PCI, percutaneous coronary intervention; RR, relative risk.

abacavir, the PREDICT-1 trial of nearly 2000 patients showed that prospective screening for the *HLA-B*57:01* allele, with avoidance of abacavir in patients testing positive for the allele, resulted in a significant reduction in the risk for immunologically confirmed hypersensitivity reactions, with a 100% negative predictive value [17]. Based on these data, the Food and Drug Administration (FDA), European Medicines Agency, CPIC, DPWG, and Human Immunodeficiency Virus treatment guidelines recommend *HLA-B*57:01* screening before initiation of abacavir-containing regimens [18]. Similarly, *TPMT*-guided thiopurine dosing was shown to reduce the risk for adverse hematologic reactions in variant allele carriers, with CPIC and DPWG guidelines available and *TPMT* genotyping routinely incorporated into thiopurine dosing decisions at many institutions [3,7,8,19–21].

Genotype-guided warfarin dosing is probably the most extensively studied pharmacogenomic intervention, with 3 large RCTs investigating the efficacy of genotype-guided warfarin dosing [22–24]. Only the most recent trial, Genetics InFormatics Trial (GIFT), had sufficient power to examine clinical outcomes with warfarin pharmacogenomics, whereas previous trials focused on the endpoint of time in therapeutic range. Among patients who underwent elective hip or knee arthroplasty, GIFT demonstrated a 27% relative risk reduction in the composite outcome of death, venous thromboembolism, major bleeding, or an international normalized ratio (INR) greater than or equal to 4 with a genotype-guided dosing approach versus dosing based on clinical factors [24]. These findings are consistent with data from the EU-PACT trial, which demonstrated greater time in the therapeutic INR range with genotype-guided dosing compared with a traditional dosing approach [23]. In contrast, the Classification of Optimal Anticoagulation Through Genetics (COAG) trial, which included a more racially diverse population than either the EU-PACT trial or GIFT, found no difference in time in therapeutic INR range between genotype-guided dosing versus clinically guided dosing [22]. In the subset of African Americans, genotype-guided dosing led to lower time in therapeutic range compared with clinical dosing, which is probably because the study did not genotype for many of the variants influencing warfarin dose requirements in African Americans [25]. Other factors that may have contributed to disparate findings across studies are summarized elsewhere [26,27].

CPIC guidelines for genotype-guided warfarin dosing were originally published in 2011 before the release of data from large RCTs [28]. Even so, the guidelines strongly recommended using genotype data to dose warfarin when such data are available based on the strong and consistent evidence that genotype influences dose requirements. The guidelines were updated in 2017 to emphasize the importance of genotyping persons of African ancestry for variants important in this population [29]. However, based on the disparate results of the EU-PACT and COAG trials and controversy generated, there are few examples of genotype-guided warfarin dosing in practice, and most of these involve pharmacogenomic panel-based testing where warfarin-related genotypes are included among numerous other genotypes with implications for other drug responses [2,6,8,30].

Alternative Methods of Evidence Generation

With the rapidly growing number of discoveries in pharmacogenomics, conducting an RCT for each gene-drug pair is impractical from a time and cost perspective, and a more efficient approach is needed to generate evidence to support translation into patient care. Pharmacogenomic clinical trials are especially challenging because for any given gene-drug pair only a small portion of the population carries a variant allele associated with drug toxicity or ineffectiveness. Otherwise the drug would never have reached the market. In this regard, pharmacogenomics is a study of outliers, and very large study populations may be needed to detect significant effects. An RCT may also be unethical when the consequences of drug exposure in a genetically predisposed patient can be life-threatening. Such is the case with the HLA-B*15:02 allele, which is found most often in persons of southeastern Asian ancestry and significantly increases the risk for carbamazepine-induced Stevens–Johnson syndrome and toxic epidermal necrolysis. In lieu of an RCT, a prospective cohort study of 4877 carbamazepine candidates was conducted and showed that, compared with historical incidence rates, genetic screening with avoidance of carbamazepine in HLA*15:02 positive patients significantly reduced the occurrence of severe cutaneous reactions [31]. The FDA-approved carbamazepine labeling includes a boxed warning about the risk for severe cutaneous reactions in individuals with the HLA-B*15:02 allele and states that genotyping should be done before carbamazepine use in at-risk populations (ie, southeast Asian populations). Similar data exist with HLA-B*58:01 screening to predict risk for severe cutaneous adverse reactions to allopurinol [32]. Guidelines by both CPIC and the Canadian Pharmacogenomics Network for Drug Safety address risk associated with the HLA-B genotype for carbamazepine, and CPIC provides additional guidelines for allopurinol [33–35].

One alternative approach to an RCT is to gather evidence as part of continuing clinical care in a learning health system model through practice-based pragmatic studies [36,37]. Unlike RCTs, pragmatic studies are conducted in the context of clinical practice and reflect the effectiveness of an intervention in a real-world setting [38]. As such, an advantage of pragmatic study results is that they are more generalizable than those from RCTs, which often have strict eligibility criteria and are conducted in controlled settings to minimize selection bias and confounding and maximize internal validity [39]. Pragmatic studies are also less rigorous by nature and thus more efficient to conduct. On the other hand, the major limitation with pragmatic studies is that there is less control for sources of bias creating greater uncertainty and necessitating statistical techniques such as propensity score matching to account for differences between treatment groups [39].

Pragmatic and Observational Studies of CYP2C19-Guided Antiplatelet Prescribing

CYP2C19-clopidogrel is an example of a gene-drug pair with evidence of benefit from pragmatic studies. Clopidogrel is a prodrug, and the CYP2C19 enzyme has a critical role in clopidogrel bioactivation. Approximately 30% of White and African American individuals and up to 60% of Asian individuals carry a nonfunctional CYP2C19 allele leading to impaired clopidogrel bioactivation and lesser clopidogrel-mediated effects, the consequences of which are greatest for patients undergoing percutaneous coronary intervention (PCI) [40–42]. Specifically, numerous studies have demonstrated an increased risk for adverse cardiovascular events after PCI in clopidogrel-treated patients with a nonfunctional allele compared with similarly treated patients with normal or increased function alleles [41,43]. Two RCTs investigating the clinical utility of CYP2C19-guided clopidogrel prescribing after PCI are ongoing but not expected to be completed until 2019 to 2020 (ClinicalTrials.gov Identifier: NCT01742117 and NCT01761786) [44].

Several institutions have clinically implemented CYP2C19 testing to guide post-PCI antiplatelet therapy ahead of clinical trial results [45]. In fact, CYP2C19-clopidogrel is one of the most common gene-drug pairs implemented in practice [8]. As part of the National Institutes of Health–funded Implementing GeNomics In pracTicE (IGNITE) Network Pharmacogenomics Working Group, 7 US institutions pooled data for 1815 patients who were genotyped for CYP2C19 variants at the time of emergent or elective PCI, with genotype results placed in the electronic health record [8,46,47]. Consistent with a pragmatic study design, alternative antiplatelet therapy (eg, prasugrel or ticagrelor) was recommended in patients with 1 or 2 nonfunctional alleles (ie, interme-diate or poor metabolizers), but the ultimate prescribing decision was left to the discre-tion of the physician. Thirty-one percent of patients had a nonfunctional allele, and alternative therapy was prescribed in 61% of these patients, whereas the remainders were treated with clopidogrel. In contrast, only 15.5% of patients without a nonfunc-tional allele were prescribed prasugrel or ticagrelor. After propensity scoring to ac-count for differences between groups, the risk for major adverse cardiovascular events (defined as the composite outcome of death, myocardial infarction, and ischemic stroke) over a median follow-up of approximately 5 months was significantly higher in carriers of a nonfunctional allele who were prescribed clopidogrel versus alternative therapy (adjusted hazard ratio 2.26, 95% confidence interval 1.18–4.32). There was no difference in risk for cardiovascular events between carriers of a nonfunctional allele prescribed alternative therapy and those without a nonfunctional allele. The group is currently conducting a cost-effectiveness study based on these data.

These data are consistent with findings from a Dutch study of patients genotyped at the time of elective PCI [9]. In contrast to the US study, alternative antiplatelet therapy was only recommended in poor metabolizers (with 2 nonfunctional alleles). Over an 18-month follow-up period, there were significantly more adverse cardiovascular events in poor metabolizers treated with clopidogrel versus alternative antiplatelet therapy. An additional study, conducted in Spain, compared outcomes between pa-tients who received genotype-guided antiplatelet therapy after PCI and historical con-trols who were mostly treated with clopidogrel [10]. Both *CYP2C19* and *ABCB1* genotypes were determined, and alternative therapy was prescribed to patients with either a *CYP2C19* nonfunctional allele or the *ABCB1* rs1045642 TT genotype. Compared with controls who underwent PCI before genotype implementation, there were significantly fewer cardiovascular events in the genotype group.

Pragmatic Trials of Pharmacogenomic-Guided Treatment of Depression and Anxiety

Both the *CYP2D6* and *CYP2C19* genes influence the pharmacokinetics and response to multiple antidepressants, and there are other genes in the serotonergic pathway with potential effects on antidepressant drug response [48,49]. The clinical effectiveness of genotype-guided management of depression and anxiety has been the subject of several pragmatic clinical trials and observational studies [50–52]. In a recent multicenter study, 685 patients with depression and/or anxiety, who were either new to treatment or had inadequately controlled symptoms, were randomized to a genotype-guided approach to therapy or usual care [50]. Patients were blinded to treatment assignment. Patients in the genotype group were tested using a commercially available panel of 10 genes, including *CYP2D6* and *CYP2C19*. Genotype results were provided to the physician to consider when making drug prescribing decisions. Patients in the geno-type arm reported greater response rates for both depression and anxiety at 8 and 12 weeks compared with those in the control group. A smaller pragmatic trial [52] and observational study [51] also showed favorable effects with a genotype-guided strategy of antidepressant prescribing.

Pragmatic Trials of Panel-Based Pharmacogenomic Testing

The examples discussed earlier focus on individual drugs or drug classes. As of early 2018, CPIC and DPWG guidelines are available for at least 19 gene-drug pairs. Thus, a panel-based approach to testing whereby multiple variants with implications for mul-tiple drugs are tested at once has been proposed as a more practical approach to pharmacogenomic testing than testing genes one at a time. More than 90% of the population is estimated to have at least one variant associated with reduced drug response or increased risk for toxicity, supporting a panel-based approach done preemptively so that genotype data are readily available to inform prescribing decisions across a person's lifetime [53].

Initial efforts have established the feasibility of incorporating multiple genotypes from panel-based testing into clinical care [2,3,5]. This includes the Mayo Clinic Right Drug, Right Dose, Right Time-Using Genomic Data to Individualize Treatment (RIGHT) pilot project, whereby actionable variants in 4 genes from a next-generation sequencing panel plus CYP2D6 genotype were integrated into the electronic health records for more than 1000 patients along with point-of-care clinical decision support [54]. An expansion of the project is underway, with preemptive testing of 13 pharmacogenes in 10,000 patients who receive care at Mayo Clinic with the goal of examining the clinical and economic impact of this approach in addition to providing genetic data for discovery purposes.

Pragmatic trials are examining the clinical utility of panel-based testing [6,11]. The INdiana GENomics Implementation: an Opportunity for the UnderServed (INGENIOUS) trial, funded by NHGRI, is examining the economic impact of genotyping for 43 variants in 14 pharmacogenes on the incidence of adverse events and health care cost [6]. The Ubiquitous Pharmacogenomics Consortium, funded by the European Commission's Horizon-2929 program, is examining similar outcomes with panel-based pharmacogenomic testing in the PREemptive Pharmacogenomics testing for prevention of Adverse drug REactions (PREPARE) trial [11]. The trial is being conducted in 7 European countries using a block-randomized design. Participating countries are randomized to an 18-month block of pharmacogenomics-guided prescribing or standard of care, after which they switch to the opposite strategy for a second 18-month block. The trial is targeting enrollment of 4050 total patients during each block. The pharmacogenomics panel includes 50 variants in 13 genes, and drug therapy recommendations are provided according to DPWG guidelines.

REIMBURSEMENT FOR PHARMACOGENETIC TESTING

Reimbursement for pharmacogenomics testing involves many constantly moving parts. First, there must be evidence (ie, clinical validity) to obtain a Current Procedural Terminology (CPT) code. Once a CPT code is obtained, such as a catalog number, a value must be assigned to it. Then payers, whether governmental or private, decide whether or not to reimburse the pharmacogenomics test (or panel). This section provides an overview of evidence needed for reimbursement for pharmacogenomics.

Billing and reimbursement for medical services including pharmacogenetics testing are codified by a code set that is maintained and administered by the American Medical Association (AMA). CPT codes are considered level 1 Healthcare Common Procedure Coding System (HCPCS, pronounced as "hickspicks"), which is overseen by the Centers for Medicare and Medicaid Services (CMS). To obtain a CPT code, the medical service must demonstrate clinical validity (**Fig. 2**). CPT codes are assigned categories. Category I include procedures that are consistent with contemporary medical practice and are widely performed. Category III include temporary codes for emerging technology, services, and procedures. For molecular pathology procedures in which pharmacogenomics falls, the AMA created additional criteria to help guide category I status as follows [55].

- For Mendelian and somatic disorders, there is a demonstrated relationship between biomarker and phenotype (ie, clinical validity).

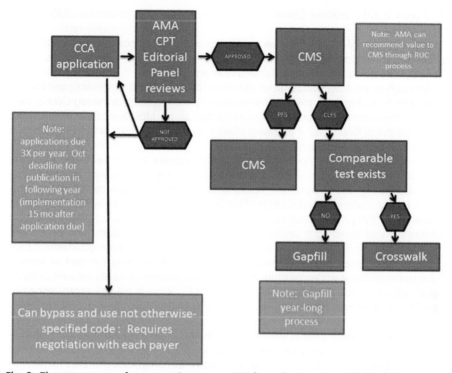

Fig. 2. The process map for requesting a new CPT from the American Medical Association (AMA) with how the US governmental payer determines a reimbursement value. CCA, coding change application; CLFS, clinical lab fee schedule; CMS, Centers for Medicare and Medicaid Services; PFS, physician fee schedule; RUC, specialty society relative value scale update committee or relative value update committee (pronounced "ruck").

- Biomarkers (eg, SNPs) that have an association but not a proven causative effect to a known clinical phenotype should have demonstrated clinical usefulness (eg, high positive predictive value, high negative predictive value, directing therapy/management).

The US government, through programs such as CMS, pays for approximately half of the country's health care [56]. CMS uses Medicare Administrative Contractors (MACs), who are private health care insurers, to administer the Medicare program. The MACs are responsible for various geographic jurisdictions to process Medicare Part A and Part B (A/B) medical claims such as pharmacogenomic testing for Medicare fee-for-service beneficiaries. Medicare Part A is hospital insurance, which includes, but is not limited to, inpatient care in hospitals, nursing homes, skilled nursing facilities, and critical access hospitals. Medicare Part B covers 2 types of services: (1) medically necessary services that are needed to diagnose or treat a medical condition and that meet accepted standards of medical practice and (2) preventive services. Pharmacogenomics testing can occur in both inpatient and outpatient settings and would be covered in Part A/B. Title XVIII of the Social Security Act, Section 1862(a) (1) (A) prohibits Medicare payment "…for items or services which are not reasonable and necessary (often equated to clinical validity) for the diagnosis and treatment of illness or injury…." with certain exceptions. The MACs use a process called Local Coverage Determinations (LCDs) to determine whether they will cover a particular service on a

MAC-wide basis. National Coverage Decisions (NCDs) are issued by CMS for the entire country.

Most, if not all, MACs have issued LCDs limiting pharmacogenomics testing reimbursement to few medications and associated gene testing [57]. For a medical test, the MACs are using the concept of reasonable and necessary to equate to clinical utility. Although there is no standardized definition for clinical utility, in its simplest form, it is equated to a change in medical management. Testing for pharmacogenomic variants can determine if a medication is predicted to be effective at current dosage, should be discontinued, or if a dosing change is needed, which should equate to a change in medical management of a patient.

Government reimbursement has an impact on private insurance. Often when the MACs or CMS make LCDs or NCDs to limit coverage on services such as pharmacogenomics testing due to not being reasonable or necessary, private insurance companies follow these same decisions. This is usually determined by the employer's contract with the private insurance companies. In some instances, employers have determined that covering a service may make them a differentiator and save them money in the long term. In addition, because reimbursements from government programs such as Medicare and Medicaid are lower than the average cost of serving those patients, laboratories or other providers may charge privately insured patients higher rates in order to recoup their costs. This increase in private sector prices to adjust for government payment levels is called "cost-shifting" and is a controversial concept.

CPIC evaluates both clinical and research studies of pharmacogenes and administered medications and publishes the drug-gene pair clinical validity [12]. The stance of CPIC is to guide medication dosing or selection if the pharmacogenomic results are already present in the medical record. They do not make statements on whether or not pharmacogenomics testing should be performed before or concurrently with medication administration. This is left to the US FDA in the package insert for a medication and to the prescriber to follow. The FDA can also make determinations of a boxed warning, commonly referred to as a "black box" warning, for prescribers about serious adverse reactions. It is still up to the medical practice of the prescriber based on their knowledge of the patient to follow (or not) boxed warnings. Even with a boxed warning for pharmacogenomic testing, there is no requirement for testing to be performed. As such, payers would prefer that CPIC support preemptive testing in their guidelines [58].

PRESENT RELEVANCE AND FUTURE AVENUES TO CONSIDER OR TO INVESTIGATE

Data from a limited number of RCTs and prospective cohort and pragmatic studies provide support for clinical implementation of various gene-drug pairs. Research projects such as the National Institutes of Health–sponsored IGNITE Network and the Ubiquitous Pharmacogenomics Consortium PREPARE trial are using pragmatic trial designs to build further evidence of clinical utility of pharmacogenomics as well as other genomics. Although the IGNITE network as a whole aims to identify and address barriers to implementing genomics, the Pharmacogenetics Working Group is examining outcomes with pharmacogenomic testing across network sites. In addition, the IGNITE INGenious project when completed will look at the economic value of panel-based pharmacogenomics testing [59]. Similarly, outcomes and cost-effectiveness data are expected from the PREPARE trial. Together, these data may demonstrate improved patient outcomes and cost savings to the health care system with pharmacogenomic testing and further drive the field forward.

SUMMARY

Pharmacogenomic research and implementation continues to be an active area in molecular medicine. In some cases such as with abacavir and *HLA-B*57:01*, pharmacogenomics can help reduce the frequency of adverse drug reactions by allowing preemptive identification of at-risk individuals in whom the drug can be avoided. In other cases, such as with clopidogrel and *CYP2C19* testing, pharmacogenomics allows for predicting patients unlikely to respond in whom alternative therapy may be initiated. Together, such examples can have a tremendously positive impact on morbidity and mortality of patients. The trial-and-error approach to prescribing where one-drug-fits-all that is current practice, all too often results in a medication being ineffective, thus causing wasted treatment time, high health care and drug costs, and, most importantly, therapeutic failures or alternatively in a medication causing toxicity, also causing significant medical expenditure and threatening patient life and well-being. As additional evidence is gained for the clinical benefit of genotype-guided therapy, it is expected that reimbursement for pharmacogenomic testing will follow of which both are critical to support broader adoption and sustainability of pharmacogenomics in practice.

REFERENCES

1. Collins FS, Varmus H. A new initiative on precision medicine. N Engl J Med 2015; 372:793–5.
2. O'Donnell PH, Wadhwa N, Danahey K, et al. Pharmacogenomics-based point-of-care clinical decision support significantly alters drug prescribing. Clin Pharmacol Ther 2017;102:859–69.
3. Hoffman JM, Haidar CE, Wilkinson MR, et al. PG4KDS: a model for the clinical implementation of pre-emptive pharmacogenetics. Am J Med Genet C Semin Med Genet 2014;166C:45–55.
4. Peterson JF, Field JR, Unertl KM, et al. Physician response to implementation of genotype-tailored antiplatelet therapy. Clin Pharmacol Ther 2016;100:67–74.
5. Pulley JM, Denny JC, Peterson JF, et al. Operational implementation of prospective genotyping for personalized medicine: the design of the vanderbilt PREDICT project. Clin Pharmacol Ther 2012;92:87–95.
6. Eadon MT, Desta Z, Levy KD, et al. Implementation of a pharmacogenomics consult service to support the INGENIOUS trial. Clin Pharmacol Ther 2016;100:63–6.
7. Hicks JK, Stowe D, Willner MA, et al. Implementation of clinical pharmacogenomics within a large health system: from electronic health record decision support to consultation services. Pharmacotherapy 2016;36:940–8.
8. Cavallari LH, Beitelshees AL, Blake KV, et al. The IGNITE pharmacogenetics working group: an opportunity for building evidence with pharmacogenetic implementation in a real-world setting. Clin Transl Sci 2017;10:143–6.
9. Deiman BA, Tonino PA, Kouhestani K, et al. Reduced number of cardiovascular events and increased cost-effectiveness by genotype-guided antiplatelet therapy in patients undergoing percutaneous coronary interventions in the Netherlands. Neth Heart J 2016;24:589–99.
10. Sanchez-Ramos J, Davila-Fajardo CL, Toledo Frias P, et al. Results of genotype-guided antiplatelet therapy in patients who undergone percutaneous coronary intervention with stent. Int J Cardiol 2016;225:289–95.
11. van der Wouden CH, Cambon-Thomsen A, Cecchin E, et al. Implementing pharmacogenomics in Europe: design and implementation strategy of the ubiquitous pharmacogenomics consortium. Clin Pharmacol Ther 2017;101:341–58.

12. Relling MV, Klein TE. CPIC: clinical pharmacogenetics implementation consortium of the pharmacogenomics research network. Clin Pharmacol Ther 2011;89:464–7.

13. Swen JJ, Nijenhuis M, de Boer A, et al. Pharmacogenetics: from bench to byte–an update of guidelines. Clin Pharmacol Ther 2011;89:662–73.

14. Relling MV, Altman RB, Goetz MP, et al. Clinical implementation of pharmacogenomics: overcoming genetic exceptionalism. Lancet Oncol 2010;11:507–9.

15. Khoury MJ. Dealing with the evidence dilemma in genomics and personalized medicine. Clin Pharmacol Ther 2010;87:635–8.

16. van der Wouden CH, Swen JJ, Samwald M, et al. A brighter future for the implementation of pharmacogenomic testing. Eur J Hum Genet 2016;24:1658–60.

17. Mallal S, Phillips E, Carosi G, et al. HLA-B*5701 screening for hypersensitivity to abacavir. N Engl J Med 2008;358:568–79.

18. Guidelines for the use of antiretroviral agents in adults and adolescents living with HIV. Department of Health and Human Services. Panel on antiretroviral guidelines for adults and adolescents. Available at: http://www.aidsinfo.nih.gov/ContentFiles/AdultandAdolescentGL.pdf. Accessed February 28, 2018.

19. Relling MV, Gardner EE, Sandborn WJ, et al. Clinical Pharmacogenetics Implementation Consortium guidelines for thiopurine methyltransferase genotype and thiopurine dosing. Clin Pharmacol Ther 2011;89:387–91.

20. Coenen MJ, de Jong DJ, van Marrewijk CJ, et al. Identification of patients with variants in TPMT and dose reduction reduces hematologic events during thiopurine treatment of inflammatory bowel disease. Gastroenterology 2015;149: 907–17.e7.

21. Weitzel KW, Smith DM, Elsey AR, et al. Implementation of standardized clinical processes for TPMT testing in a diverse multidisciplinary population: challenges and lessons learned. Clin Transl Sci 2018;11(2):175–81.

22. Kimmel SE, French B, Kasner SE, et al. A pharmacogenetic versus a clinical algorithm for warfarin dosing. N Engl J Med 2013;369:2283–93.

23. Pirmohamed M, Burnside G, Eriksson N, et al. A randomized trial of genotype-guided dosing of warfarin. N Engl J Med 2013;369:2294–303.

24. Gage BF, Bass AR, Lin H, et al. Effect of genotype-guided warfarin dosing on clinical events and anticoagulation control among patients undergoing hip or knee arthroplasty: the GIFT randomized clinical trial. JAMA 2017;318:1115–24.

25. Drozda K, Wong S, Patel SR, et al. Poor warfarin dose prediction with pharmacogenetic algorithms that exclude genotypes important for African Americans. Pharmacogenet Genomics 2015;25:73–81.

26. Cavallari LH. Time to revisit warfarin pharmacogenetics. Future Cardiol 2017;13: 511–3.

27. Johnson JA, Cavallari LH. Warfarin pharmacogenetics. Trends Cardiovasc Med 2015;25:33–41.

28. Johnson JA, Gong L, Whirl-Carrillo M, et al. Clinical pharmacogenetics implementation consortium guidelines for CYP2C9 and VKORC1 genotypes and warfarin dosing. Clin Pharmacol Ther 2011;90:625–9.

29. Johnson JA, Caudle KE, Gong L, et al. Clinical Pharmacogenetics Implementation Consortium (CPIC) guideline for pharmacogenetics-guided warfarin dosing: 2017 update. Clin Pharmacol Ther 2017;102:397–404.

30. Nutescu EA, Drozda K, Bress AP, et al. Feasibility of implementing a comprehensive warfarin pharmacogenetics service. Pharmacotherapy 2013;33:1156–64.

31. Chen P, Lin JJ, Lu CS, et al. Carbamazepine-induced toxic effects and HLA-B*1502 screening in Taiwan. N Engl J Med 2011;364:1126–33.

32. Ko TM, Tsai CY, Chen SY, et al. Use of HLA-B*58:01 genotyping to prevent allo-purinol induced severe cutaneous adverse reactions in Taiwan: national prospective cohort study. BMJ 2015;351:h4848.

33. Phillips EJ, Sukasem C, Whirl-Carrillo M, et al. Clinical pharmacogenetics implementation consortium guideline for HLA genotype and use of carbamazepine and oxcarbazepine: 2017 update. Clin Pharmacol Ther 2018;103(4):574–81.

34. Saito Y, Stamp LK, Caudle KE, et al, Clinical Pharmacogenetics Implementation Consortium. Clinical Pharmacogenetics Implementation Consortium (CPIC) guidelines for human leukocyte antigen B (HLA-B) genotype and allopurinol dosing: 2015 update. Clin Pharmacol Ther 2016;99:36–7.

35. Amstutz U, Shear NH, Rieder MJ, et al, CPNDS clinical recommendation group. Recommendations for HLA-B*15:02 and HLA-A*31:01 genetic testing to reduce the risk of carbamazepine-induced hypersensitivity reactions. Epilepsia 2014; 55:496–506.

36. Ginsburg G. Medical genomics: gather and use genetic data in health care. Nature 2014;508:451–3.

37. Rosenthal GE. The role of pragmatic clinical trials in the evolution of learning health systems. Trans Am Clin Climatol Assoc 2014;125:204–16 [discussion: 17–8].

38. Patsopoulos NA. A pragmatic view on pragmatic trials. Dialogues Clin Neurosci 2011;13:217–24.

39. Terry SF. An evidence framework for genetic testing. Genet Test Mol Biomarkers 2017;21:407–8.

40. Mega JL, Close SL, Wiviott SD, et al. Cytochrome p-450 polymorphisms and response to clopidogrel. N Engl J Med 2009;360:354–62.

41. Scott SA, Sangkuhl K, Stein CM, et al. Clinical Pharmacogenetics Implementation Consortium guidelines for CYP2C19 genotype and clopidogrel therapy: 2013 update. Clin Pharmacol Ther 2013;94:317–23.

42. Sorich MJ, Rowland A, McKinnon RA, et al. CYP2C19 genotype has a greater effect on adverse cardiovascular outcomes following percutaneous coronary intervention and in Asian populations treated with clopidogrel: a meta-analysis. Circ Cardiovasc Genet 2014;7:895–902.

43. Mega JL, Simon T, Collet JP, et al. Reduced-function CYP2C19 genotype and risk of adverse clinical outcomes among patients treated with clopidogrel predominantly for PCI: a meta-analysis. JAMA 2010;304:1821–30.

44. Bergmeijer TO, Janssen PW, Schipper JC, et al. CYP2C19 genotype-guided antiplatelet therapy in ST-segment elevation myocardial infarction patients-Rationale and design of the Patient Outcome after primary PCI (POPular) Genetics study. Am Heart J 2014;168:16–22 e1.

45. Empey PE, Stevenson JM, Tuteja S, et al, IGNITE Network. Multisite investigation of strategies for the implementation of CYP2C19 genotype-guided antiplatelet therapy. Clin Pharmacol Ther 2018;104:664–74.

46. Weitzel KW, Alexander M, Bernhardt BA, et al. The IGNITE network: a model for genomic medicine implementation and research. BMC Med Genomics 2016;9:1.

47. Cavallari LH, Lee CR, Beitelshees AL, et al, IGNITE Network. Multisite investigation of outcomes with implementation of CYP2C19 genotype-guided antiplatelet therapy after percutaneous coronary intervention. JACC Cardiovasc Interv 2018;11:181–91.

48. Hicks JK, Bishop JR, Sangkuhl K, et al, Clinical Pharmacogenetics Implementation Consortium. Clinical Pharmacogenetics Implementation Consortium (CPIC)

guideline for CYP2D6 and CYP2C19 genotypes and dosing of selective serotonin reuptake inhibitors. Clin Pharmacol Ther 2015;98:127–34.

49. Hicks JK, Sangkuhl K, Swen JJ, et al. Clinical pharmacogenetics implementation consortium guideline (CPIC) for CYP2D6 and CYP2C19 genotypes and dosing of tricyclic antidepressants: 2016 update. Clin Pharmacol Ther 2016;102:37–44.

50. Bradley P, Shiekh M, Mehra V, et al. Improved efficacy with targeted pharmacogenetic-guided treatment of patients with depression and anxiety: a randomized clinical trial demonstrating clinical utility. J Psychiatr Res 2018;96:100–7.

51. Brennan FX, Gardner KR, Lombard J, et al. A naturalistic study of the effectiveness of pharmacogenetic testing to guide treatment in psychiatric patients with mood and anxiety disorders. Prim Care Companion CNS Disord 2015;17.

52. Perez V, Salavert A, Espadaler J, et al. Efficacy of prospective pharmacogenetic testing in the treatment of major depressive disorder: results of a randomized, double-blind clinical trial. BMC Psychiatry 2017;17:250.

53. Van Driest SL, Shi Y, Bowton EA, et al. Clinically actionable genotypes among 10,000 patients with preemptive pharmacogenomic testing. Clin Pharmacol Ther 2014;95:423–31.

54. Ji Y, Skierka JM, Blommel JH, et al. Preemptive pharmacogenomic testing for precision medicine: a comprehensive analysis of five actionable pharmacogenomic genes using next-generation DNA sequencing and a customized CYP2D6 genotyping cascade. J Mol Diagn 2016;18:438–45.

55. CPT Code Application. American Medical Association. Available at: https://www.ama-assn.org/practice-management/applying-cpt-codes. Accessed February 25, 2018.

56. NHE Fact Sheet. Center for medicare & medicaid services. Available at: https://www.cms.gov/research-statistics-data-and-systems/statistics-trends-and-reports/nationalhealthexpenddata/nhe-fact-sheet.html. Accessed February 25, 2018.

57. Medicare Coverage Database. Center for medicare & medicaid services. Available at: https://www.cms.gov/medicare-coverage-database. Accessed February 25, 2018.

58. Keeling NJ, Rosenthal MM, West-Strum D, et al. Preemptive pharmacogenetic testing: exploring the knowledge and perspectives of US payers. Genet Med 2019;21:1224–32.

59. Rosenman MB, Decker B, Levy KD, et al. Lessons learned when introducing pharmacogenomic panel testing into clinical practice. Value Health 2017;20:54–9.

60. Thervet E, Loriot MA, Barbier S, et al. Optimization of initial tacrolimus dose using pharmacogenetic testing. Clin Pharmacol Ther 2010;87:721–6.

Replacement of Culture with Molecular Testing for Diagnosis Infectious Diseases

Gerald A. Capraro, PhD

KEYWORDS

- Molecular diagnostics • PCR • Culture • Turnaround time • Improvement • Quality

KEY POINTS

- Molecular diagnostics are more sensitive and specific than traditional culture-based testing and there are many successful examples where nucleic acid amplification testing has replaced culture.
- Current, commercially available molecular testing has the capability to be performed in traditional microbiology laboratories, but laboratories would have to decide what makes sense for their facility.
- A thoughtful approach to the implementation of molecular testing is necessary when deciding to transition from culture to molecular testing.

INTRODUCTION

Despite significant advances in molecular testing platforms, in vitro cultivation of microbial pathogens on artificial media remains a hallmark of infectious disease diagnostics. Culture-based approaches allow for the recovery, identification, and antimicrobial susceptibility testing of a specific pathogen. However, there are many limitations to the use of culture. The growth of an organism can take days to weeks; definitive testing for identification can be performed only on pure culture or isolated colony, which may introduce additional delays; some organisms cannot be cultivated in vitro (eg, some viruses, parasites) or have specialized growth requirements that cannot be met by most routine clinical microbiology laboratories (eg, *Mycoplasma* species). Ultimately, culture is labor intensive and is associated with long turnaround

This article originally appeared in *Advances in Molecular Pathology*, Volume 1, Issue 1, November 2018.

Disclosure Statement: The author serves on Advisory Boards for DiaSorin Molecular, BioRad, BD, and Roche Diagnostics. He has received research funding from Quidel, DiaSorin Molecular, and DiaGenode and speaking honoraria from Quidel.

Clinical Microbiology Laboratory, Carolinas Pathology Group, Atrium Health, 5040 Airport Center Parkway, Building H, Suite A, Charlotte, NC 28208, USA

E-mail address: gerald.capraro@carolinashealthcare.org

0272-2712/22/© 2022 Elsevier Inc. All rights reserved.

times. Molecular testing has exquisite sensitivity and specificity and is associated with faster turnaround times. Limitations of molecular assays include high cost, the need for specific primer sequences based on an a priori knowledge of the pathogen target sequence, and laboratory personnel with specific expertise in molecular techniques. Nonetheless, there are many areas where laboratories have transitioned away from culture-based pathogen detection to molecular methods. This article discusses the considerations for adoption of molecular assays as a replacement (in whole or in part) for culture, and to highlight examples where this approach has been successfully implemented.

DISCUSSION

The movement away from culture-based testing to molecular testing for infectious diseases largely began in academic medical centers and specialized reference laboratories, which implemented laboratory-developed molecular testing. Recently, there has been a shift in adoption of commercially available, sample-to-answer testing platforms for more routine pathogens. The nature of these tests allows use by smaller community hospitals and other laboratories located outside of large systems and academic centers. The decision to migrate culture-based diagnostic testing to molecular testing must include an assessment of several factors, including test volume, analytical performance, workflow and throughput, availability of trained personnel, and cost. Regulatory and accreditation factors must also be taken into consideration.

Early adoption of molecular testing as a replacement for culture occurred in the diagnostic virology laboratory. The ability to read cytopathic effect in cell culture and identify specific viruses based on the cytopathic effect observed in various cell lines is an expert skill that has waned in laboratories over time owing to staff attrition and a shortage of new medical laboratory scientists who are interested in microbiology. This situation has caused a shift in virology testing to shorter turnaround time and shell vial cultures, which require their own level of expertise to read immunofluorescent stains. The loss of skilled personnel and the inability to propagate some viruses in culture in vitro led to the replacement of culture-based virology testing with molecular testing. Viruses such as human immunodeficiency virus, hepatitis A, hepatitis B, and hepatitis C were among the first molecular tests used both for the diagnosis of infection and monitoring of viral load over time to determine the effectiveness of antiviral therapy. Testing for other clinically important viruses soon shifted to molecular testing. Respiratory virus testing, for example, has largely transitioned to multiplex molecular panels that allow for a diagnosis of influenza virus A, influenza virus B, and respiratory syncytial virus (as well as other respiratory viruses for which there are no specific antiviral therapies, such as human metapneumovirus) from a single specimen in a single test. The diagnosis of infectious diarrhea has also shifted from culture, specialized microscopy, and rapid antigen testing methods to multiplex molecular gastrointestinal panels. Etiologic causes of infectious gastroenteritis include bacteria, viruses, and parasites, and clinical presentation typically does not allow for a specific diagnosis because diarrhea is the predominant symptom. Therefore, a battery of tests must be ordered, yet often the causative agent remains unidentified. Gastrointestinal panels provide the laboratory with a single test for a single specimen and yield results for a breadth of infectious agents. Performance of these culture-independent diagnostic tests is reported to be excellent[1,2], with a sensitivity of greater than 95% and a specificity of greater than 97%. Despite the improved turnaround time and improvement in the use of infection control practices[3], culture-independent diagnostic tests have created a quandary with regard to the public health[4]. The replacement of culture with culture-independent diagnostic tests has resulted in laboratories no longer routinely recovering isolates of *Salmonella* and other pathogens of public health importance, which must be submitted to public health laboratories for outbreak tracking and other epidemiologic purposes. Some states continue to require submission of an isolate to the public health laboratory, whereas others have allowed submission of the primary specimen that tested positive by a culture-independent diagnostic test. As laboratories work through this diagnostic transitional period, it is critical that the lines of communication between diagnostic laboratories and public health laboratories remain open.

One of the earliest transitions to molecular diagnostics for bacteria was for the sexually transmitted pathogens *Neisseria gonorrhoeae* and *Chlamydia trachomatis*. Molecular probe assays and polymerase chain reaction provide exquisite sensitivity and specificity and provide faster time to result compared with culture. Most laboratories now use molecular methods for the screening of patients with suspected *C trachomatis-N gonorrhoeae* infection. Several molecular assays cleared by the US Food and Drug Administration (FDA) are commercially available and demonstrate excellent performance for urogenital specimens from both males and females (**Table 1**). Infections in men who have sex with men and other high-risk patients can be diagnosed by testing oropharyngeal, ocular, and/or rectal specimens[5,6]. These alternative specimen types have not received FDA clearance; therefore, testing would require validation by individual laboratories. The drawback to molecular testing for these pathogens is that there is no isolate available for antimicrobial susceptibility testing. However, current standard therapeutic regimens recommended by the Centers for Disease Control and Prevention include ceftriaxone, 250 mg administered intramuscularly, and azithromycin, 1 g orally, for uncomplicated infection[7]. The gonococcal isolate surveillance project tracks resistance patterns in the United States by partnering with sexually transmitted disease clinics and publishing resistance patterns for various regions. Clinicians in these locales may rely on gonococcal isolate surveillance project data to provide appropriate empiric therapy of suspected gonorrhea infections. In cases of suspected failure of empiric treatment, the Centers for Disease Control and Prevention recommend culture of appropriate specimens, with antimicrobial susceptibility testing of recovered gonococcal isolates[7]; however, with the transition to molecular testing, many laboratories no longer have the expertise or reagents to perform this testing on site and would have to send specimens to a reference laboratory.

The evolution of diagnostic tests for *Clostridioides difficile*[8] continues today. Anaerobic toxigenic culture methods were time consuming, and results were often reported too late during a patient's hospital course to make clinically actionable decisions. To shorten the turnaround time, culture was removed from the testing strategy, and toxin neutralization testing performed directly on filtered liquid stool became standard of care. However, this approach was labor intensive and was fraught with false-negative results. A liquid-based, enzyme-linked immunosorbent assay to determine the presence of *C difficile* toxin in a filtered stool specimen was fast and easy to perform and soon replaced toxin neutralization as the diagnostic modality of choice. This test was associated with an unacceptable rate of both false-positive and false-negative results, so to achieve an acceptable level of analytical sensitivity, 3 patient specimens were required. The lack of confidence in this test by clinicians led to a culture of repeat testing for *C difficile*, and the order for "Cdiff × 3" is something that laboratories still contend with. Currently, many laboratories have implemented a 2-step diagnostic algorithm for laboratory detection of *C difficile*[9] using an immunochromatographic cartridge to determine the presence of both the glutamate dehydrogenase enzyme and toxins A and B as a primary screen for *C difficile* infection, and molecular

Table 1
Commercially Available Nucleic Acid Amplification Tests for the Detection of *Neisseria gonorrhoeae* and *Chlamydia trachomatis*

Test Name	Manufacturer	Method	Specimen Types	Sensitivity (%)	Specificity (%)	References
BD ProbeTec	BD	SDA	U, ECS, US, V	>96	>99	27
Aptima Combo 2	Hologic	TMA	U, ECS, US, V	>94	>97	28
Abbott RealTime CT/NG	Abbott Molecular	PCR	U, ECS, US, V	>92	>99	29
Cobas 4800 CT/NG	Roche Molecular	PCR	U, ECS, V	>98	>99	30
Cepheid CT/NG Xpert	Cepheid	PCR	U, ECS, V	>95	>99	31

Abbreviations: ECS, endocervical swab; PCR, polymerase chain reaction; SDA, strand displacement amplification; TMA, transcription-mediated amplification; U, urine; US, urethral swab; V, vaginal swab.

testing as the confirmatory assay for indeterminate results (ie, GDH-positive, toxin A/B-negative). The American Society for Microbiology and the Infectious Diseases Society of America have issued guidance documents to assist laboratories in this testing strategy[10,11]. The use of molecular testing as a standalone assay for *C difficile* detection has shown to be of benefit and can shorten the turnaround time compared with the multistep diagnostic algorithm; however, as with all *C difficile* testing, it is incumbent on the laboratory to restrict these tests to diarrheal stools only and to reject nonliquid stool specimens.

The use of molecular testing for *Mycobacterium tuberculosis* (MTB) complex organisms, which cause pulmonary disease, would not replace conventional culture methods, per se. It would, however, provide a rapid result to the clinician and infection preventionist and allow for the appropriate isolation of only those patients who test positive for MTB by molecular testing. Culture of the specimen would continue to be required to obtain an isolate for antimicrobial susceptibility testing. Molecular testing for MTB has performed well compared with culture, with a reported sensitivity and specificity of 98.6% and 100%, respectively[12]. Use of the Xpert MTB/RIF Ultra assay (Cepheid, Sunnyvale, CA), a second-generation molecular test with a shorter turnaround time was shown to have a sensitivity of 87.5% and a specificity of 98.7% compared with culture when used at the point of care[13]. This assay has decreased sensitivity against smear-negative pulmonary specimens; however, in cases of culture-confirmed tuberculosis where the acid fast bacillus smear was reported as negative, the Xpert MTB/RIF assay had a sensitivity of 73.1%, an improvement of 36.5%, and may be used to accurately diagnose pulmonary tuberculosis in low prevalence areas[14]. One limitation of the commercially available molecular tests for MTB is that only respiratory specimens have received FDA clearance. Individual laboratories would be required to self-validate other clinically relevant specimen types (eg, cerebrospinal fluid, kidney biopsy material) to report results obtained from these specimens, because this use of the test would be considered off label.

There are several commercially available nucleic acid amplification tests (NAATs) for the detection of *Streptococcus agalactiae* (group B *Streptococcus* [GBS]). Except for one, each of these requires a specimen to be inoculated to an enrichment broth, such as Todd Hewitt, Todd Hewitt with Colistin, and Nalidixic Acid (LIM Broth), or Carrot Broth, for an overnight incubation before being tested by the molecular assay, to allow for maximum analytical sensitivity and specificity. The lone commercial assay for the direct detection of GBS in clinical specimens is the Xpert GBS assay (Cepheid) and has a reported sensitivity of between 78% and 86% in published studies[15,16], which is inferior to polymerase chain reaction assays performed on enriched specimens. Other commercially available molecular assays for detection of GBS are shown in**Table 2**. The benefit to molecular detection of GBS is improved turnaround time and laboratory workflow, particularly if a colorimetric enrichment broth or other enhanced culture method is used[17–19]. Laboratories would need to continue to provide culture and susceptibility testing results for isolates from patients with penicillin allergy, so the complete replacement of GBS culture with molecular techniques may not be possible.

In a similar fashion, molecular tests for *Streptococcus pyogenes* (group A *Streptococcus*) are commercially available and present a significant improvement in turnaround time. Studies have shown these assays to have superior analytical performance as compared with rapid antigen detection assays[20,21] and they can be placed in the laboratory or located at the point of care (**Table 3**). With improved sensitivity, the need for culture confirmation of negative results may no longer be necessary[22].

Table 2
Commercially Available Nucleic Acid Amplification Tests for the Detection of *Streptococcus agalactiae* (Group B *Streptococcus*)

Test Name	Manufacturer	Method	Sensitivity (%)	Specificity (%)	References
ARIES GBS Assay	Luminex	PCR	96	91	[32]
BD Max GBS Assay	BD	PCR	100	95.8	[33]
Xpert GBS Assay LB	Cepheid	PCR	99	92.4	[15]
Solana GBS Assay	Quidel	HDA	100	95.9	PI
Illumigene GBS Assay	Meridian Bioscience	LAMP	90.9	97.9	[33]

Abbreviations: HDA, helicase-dependent amplification; LAMP, loop-mediated isothermal amplification; PCR, polymerase chain reaction; PI, package insert (assay recently cleared by the US Food and Drug Administration).

From an infection prevention perspective, the use of molecular testing over culture for surveillance of specific pathogens presents the opportunity to act quickly to prevent the spread of communicable diseases and/or antimicrobial resistance mechanisms. Methicillin-resistant *Staphylococcus aureus*, vancomycin-resistant *Enterococcus* species, *C difficile*, carbapenem-resistant *Enterobacteriaceae*, and other multidrug-resistant organisms present significant threats to the health care environment. Hand hygiene plays a role in mitigating the spread of these organisms; however, organism-specific surveillance strategies can augment infection prevention strategies[23,24]. Some hospitals have chosen to screen patients upon admission and at certain regular frequencies to isolate or cohort colonized patients. Support from the microbiology laboratory is essential to the success of infection prevention strategies. Culture-based surveillance has been the presumed gold standard owing to its excellent specificity and relatively low cost to perform. Molecular assays for these organisms are now available and present improvements over culture in analytical performance, turnaround time, and laboratory workflow. Many results can be available in approximately 1 hour from receipt of the specimen, which allows for the rapid isolation of colonized patients and deisolation of patients found to be negative for colonization with multidrug-resistant organisms. In a similar fashion, patients scheduled for orthopedic or cardiac surgery may be screened for methicillin-resistant *S aureus* colonization. If found to be colonized, a treatment regimen including chlorhexidine and

Table 3
Commercially Available Nucleic Acid Amplification Tests for the Detection of *Streptococcus pyogenes* (Group A *Streptococcus*)

Test Name	Manufacturer	Method	Sensitivity (%)	Specificity (%)	References
Simplexa GAS Direct	DiaSorin Molecular	PCR	100	100	[34]
Cobas LIAT Strep A	Roche Molecular	PCR	97.7	93.3	[10]
Xpert Xpress Strep A	Cepheid	PCR	100	94.1	PI
Solana GAS Assay	Quidel	HDA	98.2	97.2	[35]
Illumigene GAS Assay	Meridian Bioscience	LAMP	100	99.2	[36]

Abbreviations: HDA, helicase-dependent amplification; LAMP, loop-mediated isothermal amplification; PCR, polymerase chain reaction; PI, package insert (assay recently cleared by the US Food and Drug Administration).

mupirocin leads to decolonization before the surgical procedure and has been shown to mitigate surgical site infections with methicillin-resistant *S aureus*[25,26].

Molecular diagnostic assays are replacing conventional, culture-based methods for the diagnosis of infectious diseases. NAATs are associated with higher sensitivity and specificity, shorter turnaround times, and the use of NAATs for diagnosis of infectious diseases is associated with improved patient outcomes. However, the implementation of NAATs as a replacement for culture must be done in a thoughtful way by laboratories that have considered the costs associated with these improved tests, the level of technical expertise that must be perpetually available in the laboratory, the amount of clinician education that is necessary for appropriate use of these tests, and the regulatory and accreditation requirements necessary for performance of molecular testing.

REFERENCES

1. Buss SN, Leber A, Chapin K, et al. Multicenter evaluation of the BioFire FilmArray Gastrointestinal Panel for etiologic diagnosis of infectious gastroenteritis. J Clin Microbiol 2015;53:915–25.
2. Binnicker MJ. Multiplex molecular panels for diagnosis of gastrointestinal infection: performance, result interpretation, and cost-effectiveness. J Clin Microbiol 2015;53:3723–8.
3. Rand KH, Tremblay EE, Hoidal M, et al. Multiplex gastrointestinal pathogen panels: implications for infection control. Diagn Microbiol Infect Dis 2015;82:154–7.
4. Prakash VP, LeBlanc L, Alexander-Scott NE, et al. Use of a culture-independent gastrointestinal multiplex PCR panel during a shigellosis outbreak: considerations for clinical laboratories and public health. J Clin Microbiol 2015;53:1048–9.
5. Cosentino LA, Danby CS, Rabe LK, et al. Use of nucleic acid amplification testing for diagnosis of extragenital sexually transmitted infections. J Clin Microbiol 2017;55:2801–7.
6. Dize L, West SK, Mkocha H, et al. Evaluation of pooled ocular and vaginal swabs by the Cepheid GeneXper CT/NG assay for the detection of Chlamydia trachomatis and Neisseria gonorrhoeae compared to the GenProbe Aptima Combo 2 assay. Diagn Microbiol Infect Dis 2015;81:102–4.
7. CDC. Sexually transmitted diseases treatment guidelines. MMWR Recomm Rep 2015;64(No. 3).
8. Lawson PA, Citron DM, Tyrrell KL, et al. Reclassification of Clostridium difficile as Clostridioides difficile (Hall and O'Toole 1935) Prevot 1938. Anaerobe 2016;40:95–9.
9. Culbreath K, Ager E, Nemeyer RJ, et al. Evolution of testing algorithms at a university hospital for detection of Clostridium difficile infections. J Clin Microbiol 2012;50:3073–6.
10. ASM. A practical guidance document for the laboratory detection of toxigenic Clostridium difficile. 2010.
11. McDonald LC, Gerding DN, Johnson S, et al. Clinical practice guidelines for Clostridium difficile infection in adults and children: 2017 update by the Infectious Diseases Society of America (IDSA) and Society for Healthcare Epidemiology of America (SHEA). Clin Infect Dis 2018;66:987–94.
12. Pandey P, Pant ND, Rijal KR, et al. Diagnostic accuracy of GeneXpert MTB/RIF assay in comparison to conventional drug susceptibility testing method for the diagnosis of multidrug-resistant tuberculosis. PLoS One 2017;12:e0169798.

13. Chakravorty S, Simmons AM, Rowneki M, et al. The new Xpert MTB/RIF Ultra: improving detection of Mycobacterium tuberculosis and resistance to rifampin in an assay suitable for point-of-care testing. Mbio 2017;29:812–7.

14. Lombardi G, DiGregori V, Girometti N, et al. Diagnosis of smear-negative tuberculosis is greatly improved by Xpert MTB/RIF. PLoS One 2017;12:e0176186.

15. Buchan BW, Faron ML, Fuller D, et al. Multicenter clinical evaluation of the Xpert GBS LB assay for detection of group B Streptococcus in prenatal screening specimens. J Clin Microbiol 2015;53:443–8.

16. Plainvert C, Al Alaoui F, Tazi A, et al. Intrapartum group B Streptococcus screening in the labor ward by Xpert GBS real-time PCR. Eur J Clin Microbiol Infect Dis 2018;37:265–70.

17. Church DL, Baxter H, Lloyd T, et al. Evaluation of StrepB carrot broth versus Lim broth for detection of group B Streptococcus colonization status of near-term pregnant women. J Clin Microbiol 2008;46:2780–2.

18. da Gloria Carvalho M, Facklam R, Jackson D, et al. Evaluation of three commercial broth media for pigment detection and identification of a group B Streptococcus (Streptococcus agalactiae). J Clin Microbiol 2009;47:4161–3.

19. Berg BR, Houseman JL, Garrasi MA, et al. Culture-based method with performance comparable to that of PCR-based methods for detection of Group B Streptococcus in screening samples from pregnant women. J Clin Microbiol 2013;51:1253–5.

20. Cohen DM, Russo ME, Jaggi P, et al. Multicenter clinical evaluation of the novel Alere i Strep A isothermal nucleic acid amplification test. J Clin Microbiol 2015; 53:2258–61.

21. Wang F, Tian Y, Chen L, et al. Accurate detection of Streptococcus pyogenes at the point of care using the Cobas Liat Strep A nucleic acid test. Clin Pediatr (Phila) 2017;56:1128–34.

22. Webb KH, Needham CA, Kurtz SR. Use of a high-sensitivity rapid strep test without culture confirmation of negative results: 2 years' experience. J Fam Pract 2000;49:34–8.

23. McLaws ML. The relationship between hand hygiene and health care-associated infection: it's complicated. Infect Drug Resist 2015;8:7–18.

24. Backman C, Zoutman DE, Marck PB. An integrative review of the current evidence on the relationship between hand hygiene interventions and the incidence of health care-associated infections. Am J Infect Control 2008;36:333–48.

25. Thompson P, Houston S. Decreasing methicillin-resistant Staphylococcus aureus surgical site infections with chlorhexidine and mupirocin. Am J Infect Control 2013;41:629–33.

26. George S, Leasure AR, Horstmanshof D. Effectiveness of decolonization with chlorhexidine and mupirocin in reducing surgical site infections: a systematic review. Dimens Crit Care Nurs 2016;35:204–22.

27. Van Der Pol B, Taylor SN, Lebar W, et al. Clinical evaluation of the BD ProbeTec Neisseria gonorrhoeae Qx amplified DNA assay on the BD Viper system with XTR technology. Sex Transm Dis 2012;39:147–53.

28. Gaydos CA, Quinn TC, Willis D, et al. Performance of the APTIMA Combo 2 assay for detection of Chlamydia trachomatis and Neisseria gonorrhoeae in female urine and endocervical swab specimens. J Clin Microbiol 2003;41:304–9.

29. Gaydos CA, Cartwright CP, Colaninno P, et al. Performance of the Abbott Real Time CT/NG for detection of Chlamydia trachomatis and Neisseria gonorrhoeae. J Clin Microbiol 2010;48:3236–43.

30. Bromhead C, Miller A, Jones M, et al. Comparison of the Cobas 4800 CT/NG test with culture for detecting Neisseria gonorrhoeae in genital and nongenital specimens in a low-prevalence population in New Zealand. J Clin Microbiol 2013;51: 1505–9.
31. Gaydos CA, Van Der Pol B, Jett-Goheen M, et al. Performance of the Cepheid CT/ NG Xpert Rapid PCR Test for detection of Chlamydia trachomatis and Neisseria gonorrhoeae. J Clin Microbiol 2013;51:1666–72.
32. Hernandez DR, Wolk DM, Walker KL, et al. Multicenter diagnostic accuracy evaluation of the Luminex ARIES Real-Time PCR Assay for Group B Streptococcus detection in Lim-enriched samples. J Clin Microbiol 2018. https://doi.org/10. 1128/JCM.01768-17.
33. Miller SA, Deak E, Humphries R. Comparison of the AmpliVue, BD Max System, and illumigene molecular assays for detection of group B Streptococcus in antenatal screening specimens. J Clin Microbiol 2015;53:1938–41.
34. Church DL, Lloyd T, Larios O, et al. Evaluation of Simplexa Group A Strep Direct kit compared to Hologic Group A Streptococcal Direct Assay for detection of Group A Streptococcus in throat swabs. J Clin Microbiol 2018;56 [pii:e01666-17].
35. Uphoff TS, Buchan BW, Ledeboer NA, et al. Multicenter evaluation of the Solana Group A Streptococcus assay: comparison with culture. J Clin Microbiol 2016;54: 2388–90.
36. Henson AM, Carter D, Todd K, et al. Detection of Streptococcus pyogenes by use of illumigene Group A Streptococcus assay. J Clin Microbiol 2013;51:4207–9.

Next-Generation Sequencing Approaches to Predicting Antimicrobial Susceptibility Testing Results

Rebecca Yee, PhD, D(ABMM), Patricia J. Simner, PhD, D(ABMM)*

KEYWORDS

- Whole genome sequencing (WGS) • Targeted NGS
- Metagenomic next-generation sequencing (mNGS) • Clinical microbiology
- Antimicrobial resistance • Predictions

KEY POINTS

- Next-generation sequencing (NGS) methods allow for a comprehensive detection of resistance genes within an organism or microbiome, known as the resistome.
- NGS-based detection of antimicrobial resistance can be further applied to predict phenotypic antimicrobial susceptibility testing (AST) using either a rule-based or a model-based approach.
- Most studies evaluating the accuracy of whole genome sequencing have applied second-generation, short-read sequencing methods, and have demonstrated good (>90%) predicted AST agreement for most antimicrobial agent-organism combinations.
- Newer, third-generation, long-read sequencing methods have increased applicability to patient care due to their real-time analysis capabilities.

INTRODUCTION

One of the largest global public health crises is the increase of antimicrobial-resistant infections. Internationally, more than 700,000 people (~23,000 Americans) die from antimicrobial-resistant infections annually. This number is projected to grow to 10

This article originally appeared in *Advances in Molecular Pathology*, Volume 2, Issue 1, November 2019.

Disclosure Statement: P.J. Simner reports grants and personal fees from Accelerate Diagnostics, grants from BD Diagnostics, Inc., grants from bioMerieux, Inc., grants from Check-Points Diagnostics, BV, grants from Hardy Diagnostics, personal fees from Roche Diagnostics, personal fees from Opgen Inc, personal fees from CosmosID, outside the submitted work; travel funds from Oxford Nanopore Technologies.

Division of Medical Microbiology, Department of Pathology, Johns Hopkins University School of Medicine, Meyer B1-193, 600 North Wolfe Street, Baltimore, MD 21287-7093, USA
* Corresponding author.
E-mail address: psimner1@jhmi.edu

million deaths per year by 2050 [1]. Collective global action is required to face this threat and the promotion of novel, rapid diagnostics to reduce the unnecessary use of antimicrobials needs to be prioritized [1,2].

Next-generation sequencing (NGS) is gaining momentum as a diagnostic tool in Clinical Microbiology Laboratories. Three different applications of NGS have been developed to study antimicrobial resistance (AMR): (1) whole genome sequencing (WGS) with or without assembly of the genome of the pathogen of interest with detection of AMR genes; (2) targeted NGS with different methods for enrichment (ie, polymerase chain reaction amplification of AMR genes followed by NGS); or (3) metagenomic NGS (mNGS) to allow for pan-nucleic acid detection, including AMR genes, directly from patient specimens. These applications have been used to investigate the role of the resistome in tracking antimicrobial resistant organisms [3,4], to define novel mechanisms of resistance [5,6], to study the evolution of resistance within a patient's bacterial isolates [7], and to study the resistome of various microbiomes [8]. The resistome encompasses all the AMR genes in a given organism or microbiome [9].

An exciting development from NGS applications over the past 5 years is its ability to predict phenotypic antimicrobial susceptibility testing (AST) results among bacteria, which is the focus of this review. The resistome can then be translated based on the presence or absence of genes or single nucleotide polymorphisms (SNPs) to predict susceptibility or resistance to antimicrobial agents, using a rule-based approach. Machine learning and statistical models are other novel tools being developed to predict AST using NGS applications (ie, model-based approach).[10] The authors describe the current state of NGS applications to predict AST using both second-generation short-read sequencing and third-generation long-read sequencing methods.

GENOTYPE VERSUS PHENOTYPE DILEMMA

Phenotypic AST methods ask the question "What concentration of the antimicrobial agent inhibits growth of the organism?" Clinicians have grown confident and reliant on phenotypic AST results to guide treatment of patients through many years of experience. Phenotypic AST methods are well-standardized approaches that can provide a minimum inhibitory concentration (MIC) or disk diffusion zone diameter result that can be set up and interpreted following the Clinical and Laboratory Standards Institute (CLSI) or European Committee on Antimicrobial Susceptibility Testing (EUCAST) guidelines [11,12]. The major drawback to this method is the slow turn-around time because it is a growth-dependent method. For nonfastidious organisms, the standard time to result from specimen receipt is 48 to 72 hours (**Fig. 1**). This is further delayed if pure or sufficient growth is not obtained on the first day of isolation, if a slower growing organism is isolated, or if an organism is multidrug-resistant (MDR) requiring the testing of additional antimicrobial agents beyond those present in standard panels. Many new methods have been introduced over the past 10 years to provide more rapid resistance detection such as simplex or multiplex nucleic acid amplification tests (NAT) of AMR genes, chromogenic agars, or rapid phenotypic tests (chromogenic or lateral flow assays) but none have yielded comprehensive results to predict the complete phenotypic AST profile. Nonetheless, these methods have introduced resistance mechanism–guided predictions to pave the way for NGS methodologies.

Contrary to most beliefs, phenotypic AST methods are an imperfect standard, as there can be significant variation in results for certain antimicrobial agent-organism combinations (greater than the standard error of AST ±1 doubling dilution) and subtle testing differences between testers or automated instruments lead to further variability [13]. This variability is not accounted for in the clinical setting, as it is not practical to

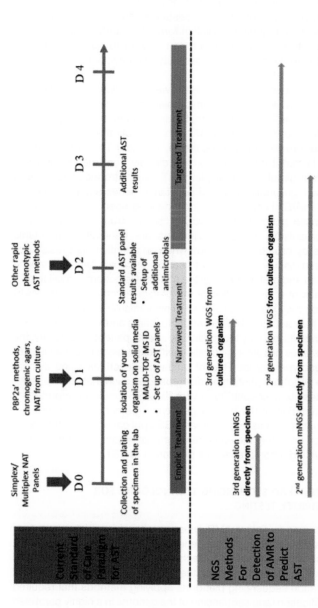

Fig. 1. Summary of current standard of care and NGS methods for antimicrobial susceptibility testing (AST). (*Top half*) The current paradigm for identification and AST in the clinical microbiology laboratory has an average TAT of 2 to 3 days from specimen receipt to finalized AST results. Newer, rapid methods (designated by blue arrows based on TAT) to predict antimicrobial resistance have been introduced for clinical care including nucleic acid amplification tests (NAT), chromogenic agars, and rapid phenotypic tests (eg, chromogenic, lateral flow, and/or agglutination tests). (*Bottom half*) The current TAT based on the literature for second-generation and third-generation next-generation sequencing methods performed directly from specimen using a metagenomic NGS (mNGS) approach or from cultured organism using a whole genome sequencing (WGS) approach.

perform replicate MIC tests for clinical care. Furthermore, the prescribed methods are highly standardized from inoculum density, media, temperature, atmosphere, and incubation period, which do not reflect the variation in the environment and expression of phenotype that can occur during human infections [13]. Interpretation of phenotypic results is independent of the mechanism of resistance and will only detect AMR if expressed in vitro. It is known that expression of resistance can vary based on heteroresistant subpopulations, mixed infections, biofilm formation, further selection, and persistence based on selective pressures, which can all lead to resistance in vivo that were not detected in vitro, leading to the possibility of ineffective antibiotic prescribing [10].

Genotypic methods for detection of resistance answer the following question: "Is there a gene that predicts that a specific antimicrobial agent will not be effective against the pathogen recovered?" Genotypic methods to predict phenotype overcome some major limitations of phenotypic AST, with arguably the most important one being the capability of providing faster results (ie, 1–4 hour TAT). An additional benefit of this approach is that it can be performed directly from the specimen or from cultured growth. Most simplex or multiplex NAT tests introduced for clinical care to date detect a few high-profile acquired resistance genes such as *mecA* in *Staphylococcus aureus*, *vanA/B* in enterococci, and extended-spectrum β-lactamase (*bla*$_{CTX-M}$) or carbapenemase genes (*bla*$_{KPC}$, *bla*$_{NDM}$, *bla*$_{VIM}$, *bla*$_{IMP}$, and *bla*$_{OXA-48}$) among gram-negative organisms. Although clinicians are generally comfortable responding to these tests by broadening therapy when an unanticipated resistance gene is identified, they often display a hesitancy to narrow therapy when a resistance gene has not been identified and prefer to wait till the AST profile becomes available [14]. Furthermore, there is a lack of understanding of the precise function of all the AMR genes (ie, which antibiotics they inactivate) and so clinical microbiology laboratories need to work closely with their antimicrobial stewardship teams and infectious disease colleagues to convey the results in a way that positively affects patient care. Lastly, the detection of an AMR gene does not always correlate with expression and may lead to discordant genotype/phenotype results. Recent guidance describes using a more conservative approach to genotype/phenotype discrepancies such that when a resistance gene is detected despite susceptibility in vitro the AST should be reported as resistant [12]. The major limitation of the current genotypic methods is that they are limited to the specific targets in the assay, whereas NGS applications have the capability of overcoming this by detecting the entire resistome of organisms or the microbiome and therefore providing a comprehensive prediction of AST.

SHORT-READ VERSUS LONG-READ SEQUENCING TECHNOLOGIES FOR ANTIMICROBIAL SUSCEPTIBILITY TESTING

Sequencing technologies used to detect AMR genes can be divided into short-read (ie, second-generation) and long-read (ie, third-generation) sequencing technologies. The advantages and disadvantages of these technologies as they relate to AMR detection are summarized in **Table 1**. Most of the initial studies applying NGS for AMR used second-generation sequencing platforms applying methods that required DNA fragmentation, amplification, and sequencing of the genome in a highly paralleled format that generates short reads (50–600 base pairs) with high accuracy (~0.1% error rate) [15]. Despite its lower cost (~$50–100/per genome in large batches), the genome assemblies using short reads often result in fragmented assemblies especially around repetitive regions often surrounding AMR genes on the chromosome or mobile genetic elements (ie, plasmids), areas with high sequence homology, or

Table 1
Advantages and disadvantages of short-read sequencing versus long-read sequencing for detection of antimicrobial resistance

	Definition	Advantages	Disadvantages

Second-generation short-read sequencing	NGS technologies where nucleic acid is fragmented and amplified followed by sequencing of many different clusters of short reads (50–500 bp) taking place in parallel where base detection is monitored by different methods, including pyrophosphate release (454), hydrogen release (Ion Torrent), release of fluorescent reversible-terminator nucleotides (Illumina), or fluorescent ligated probes (SOLiD)	• High accuracy (~0.1% error rate)
		  ○ Strain typing capability
		  ○ SNP level analysis
		  ○ Detection of chromosomal mutations leading to AMR, entire AMR genes, and distinction of allelic variants
		• Multiplexing capability driving lower costs
			• Long TAT
			• Whole genomes are often difficult to assemble around repetitive regions leading to fragmented assemblies
			• Unable to link AMR genes to genetic context by mNGS methods

Third-generation long-read sequencing	NGS technologies that allow for long-read (1–100kb) single-molecular sequencing by monitoring incorporation of fluorescently labeled nucleotides (Pacific Biosciences, PacBio) or monitoring an electrical signal as nucleic acid is fed through a nano-sized pore (Oxford Nanopore Technology; ONT)	• Real-time analysis
		• Shorter TAT
		• Live streaming capability (ONT)
		• Easier to assemble WGS due to long reads
		• Plasmids are easily assembled and typed
		• AMR genes are easily detected
		• Provides genetic context directly from clinical specimens
			• Lower accuracy (3%–15% error rate)
			  ○ SNP level analysis is not possible
			  ○ Chromosomal mutations leading to AMR or allelic variants are not reliably detected
			• High concentration of input nucleic acid is required

regions with extreme guanine-cytosine content [10,15]. Furthermore, the sequencing run itself generally requires large batches to maintain lower costs and can take 24 to 48 hours depending on the sequencing chemistry resulting in a long TAT, therefore negating any potential benefit as a rapid diagnostic tool to predict AST for clinical care. Illumina has dominated the market with its low-cost sequencing-by-synthesis method driving large-scale projects evaluating WGS to predict AST and evaluating mNGS as an agnostic tool for diagnosing infectious diseases [16].

Newer third-generation sequencing technologies, such as Oxford Nanopore Technologies (ONT) and Pacific Biosciences (PacBio), rely on real-time single-molecule sequencing producing long reads (on average 1–100 kbp) with higher per base error rates (3%–15%) [15]. The lower accuracy of long-read sequencing permits detection of resistance based on the presence or absence of AMR genes but the higher error rate make it difficult to determine a specific allele (eg, bla_{KPC-2} vs bla_{KPC-3}) or identify SNPs in chromosomal genes leading to AMR. On the other hand, the long reads allow for more complete assemblies through repetitive regions, enable complete plasmid assemblies, and provide context to AMR genes detected by mNGS approaches directly from specimens [17].

ONT has perhaps the greatest adaptability compared with other NGS technologies as a diagnostic tool because it allows for real-time base-calling and streaming analysis of results within minutes of starting the sequencing run [18]. Furthermore, it has been demonstrated that a sequencing run of an hour using R9.4 flow cells generates sufficient information to study the entire resistome of an organism to allow for rule-based prediction models [17,19]. The biggest limitation is the high error rate, as chromosomal mutations as small as an SNP can result in drastic changes to prediction models. There are 3 main types of errors produced by ONT sequencing: (1) random errors, (2) homopolymer errors, and (3) methylation errors. Generating sufficient sequencing depth (at least 100x coverage) can overcome most random errors. However, systematic errors in the form of homopolymer indels and methylation errors still result in disagreement compared with Illumina- or hybrid Illumina–corrected assemblies (ie, use of short-reads to correct errors in long-read data) [17,19]. A few different bioinformatics programs have the ability to correct known errors or use lineage-based models to mitigate the low SNP calling accuracy [17,20]. Lastly, the costs of ONT sequencing remain relatively high (~$600–1000). Newer more affordable technologies such as the ONT Flongel disposable flow cells (~$100/flow cell) and more rapid automated protocols will allow more adaptability in the clinical setting.

DIFFERENT PREDICTION MODELS

There are 2 prediction models used to correlate AMR detection with AST phenotype: (1) rule-based approaches using databases of AMR loci and (2) model-based approaches using machine learning and/or statistical models. These approaches are briefly described here to set context. Readers are encouraged to read the more in-depth review by Su and colleagues [10] on this topic. These approaches try to predict AST by correlating the identification of AMR genes to the clinical breakpoints set by CLSI/EUCAST for individual antimicrobial agent/organism combinations or more precisely to the MIC. A report from the EUCAST subcommittee recommended that genotypic-phenotypic concordance from WGS data should primarily be the epidemiologic cut-off value and that a secondary comparator could be the clinical breakpoints to determine clinical impact [21]. However, the US Food and Drug Administration intends to hold molecular-based predictions for phenotypic AST to the same standards as phenotypic qualitative AST devices with broth microdilution as the reference standard where categorical agreement (>89.9%) and error rates would be assessed.

For the rule-based approach, AMR genes or k-mers (small portions of genes, <50 bp) are detected/analyzed using either raw reads or assembled genomes using software that searches databases of AMR loci. For bacteria, common broad AMR pipelines include ResFinder, the Comprehensive Antimicrobial Resistance Database (CARD), Basic Local Alignment Search Tool (BLAST), Antibiotic Resistance Gene-ANNOTation, short read sequencing typing, and National Center for Biotechnology Information's (NCBI) National Database of Antibiotic Resistant Organisms [22,23]. Organism-specific databases have also been generated, such as the *Mycobacterium tuberculosis* (MTB) databases (UVP, Mykrobe, TBDReaMDB, MUBII-TB-DB) [10]. It is important to note that not all databases perform similarly and different results can be obtained using the various databases and bioinformatics pipelines [24].

Detection of AMR genes is the first step; the next step is to correlate the AMR gene or SNP identified to expected phenotypes. Some databases provide correlation to phenotypic results based on genetic studies that link AMR genes to phenotypes. However, caution must be taken as not all predictions have been validated to accurately predict resistance. Moreover, NGS methods may be inadequate in detecting mechanisms of resistance that have not been fully elucidated, such as variations in lipopolysaccharides, alterations of cell membrane permeability, and efflux pump changes, among others [21]. Although detection and acquisition of enzymes known to cleave certain drugs (eg, β-lactamase genes), loss-of-function mutations (eg, porin knockout models), or mutations leading to altered target specificity (eg, *gyrA* and *parC* mutations leading to fluoroquinolone resistance) are relatively easy to interpret, mutations in coding or noncoding regions of the genome that alter the structure, dynamics, and substrate specificity of proteins, enzymes, and cell wall components pose greater challenges [16]. Without a comprehensive understanding of the impact of a mutation or combination of mechanisms on AMR, predicting effects on susceptibility can be difficult and is a noteworthy limitation of WGS [21]. Thus, if considering AMR detection via WGS to forecast AST results for clinical care, specific prediction models need to be further developed and validated. For some mechanisms, prediction is simple such as the presence or absence of *mecA* to predict methicillin susceptibility in *S. aureus*. However, for most cases it is far more complex. For example, fluoroquinolone resistance among *Enterobacterales* is predicted based on single-step or 2-step mutations in the quinolone resistance determining region of *gyrA* and/or *parC* and the presence/absence of plasmid-mediated quinolone resistance genes and different combination thereof. Alternatively, Tamma and colleagues [17] have shown that detection of simply harboring aminoglycoside-modifying (eg, aminoglycoside acetyltransferases, aminoglycoside nucleotidyltransferases, aminoglycoside phosphotransferases) enzyme-encoding genes is not sufficient enough to accurately predict phenotypic AST of aminoglycosides in *Klebsiella pneumoniae*. A 90% to 100% agreement is achieved when an isolate harbored 5 or more aminoglycoside-modifying genes, whereas 2 or less predicted an agreement less than 50%. For studies using rule-based prediction models, the software, database, and prediction algorithms should be specified to the reader.

For model-based approaches, using either machine learning approaches and/or statistical models, the classifier is trained based on a set of genomes with known phenotypes without linking individual AMR genes. Similar to rule-based methods, the models can use k-mers, raw reads, contigs, or assemblies to then predict phenotypic results. The classifier is either provided specific sets of prediction rules or is taught what SNPs, indels, AMR genes, or other genetic features are important to predict phenotype [10]. Rule-based approaches to analyzing WGS data include assumptions about the phenotypes they are trying to predict. Machine learning methods allow the end user to perform analyses without making these assumptions and provide a more unbiased and robust approach [10].

ACCURACY OF WHOLE GENOME SEQUENCING TO PREDICT ANTIMICROBIAL SUSCEPTIBILITY TESTING

WGS is a well-studied and well-adapted method to predict phenotypic AST. A pure culture of an organism of interest is obtained and the genome is sequenced with or without assembly yielding a wealth of information about the epidemiology, virulence, and AMR determinants of the organism. WGS for AST offers the potential to provide rapid, consistent, and accurate predictions of known resistance phenotypes. Studies evaluating both short- and long-read sequencing have been completed and are summarized in the following sections.

SUMMARY OF SHORT-READ WHOLE GENOME SEQUENCING TO PREDICT ANTIMICROBIAL SUSCEPTIBILITY TESTING

Most initial studies applying WGS to predict AST were performed using second-generation sequencing, mostly completed on the Illumina platforms. Performance characteristics of WGS for detection of phenotypic resistance against different mechanisms of action or various antimicrobial agents (cell wall inhibitors, quinolones, protein synthesis inhibitors, antifolate agents, aminoglycosides, and in some cases, RNA synthesis inhibitors) are summarized in **Fig. 2**. Most studies used rule-based approaches but a few groups have used model-based approaches.

For gram-negative organisms, sensitivities greater than 90% among all the agents tested were achieved in *Escherichia coli*, *Campylobacter* species, *Salmonella* spp., *K. pneumoniae,* and *Shigella sonnei* [25–29]. The specificities of all the respective agents tested were greater than 95% with the exception of trimethoprim and streptomycin that had a specificity of 80% and 75%, respectively, in isolates of *S. sonnei*. Despite having a specificity of greater than 90% for the agents tested, variations in the sensitivities suggest that AMR mechanisms are complex and can be specific to a particular agent and organism.

Most studies have focused on the accuracy of AMR gene detection to phenotypic AST without describing the potential impact on patient care. One study by Shelburne and colleagues [30] attempt to address this by performing a proof-of-concept study using WGS to predict empirical therapy with β-lactam agents among patients with febrile neutropenia. They demonstrated that more than 60% of the evaluated *Pseudomonas aeruginosa* and *Enterobacter cloacae* bloodstream isolates had β-lactam resistance due to chromosomal mutations, which traditional β-lactamase NAT methodologies cannot detect. Using the context of their patient population, they demonstrate the feasibility of using WGS as a more comprehensive approach to guide antimicrobial treatment decisions (sensitivity of 87% and specificity of 98%) for patients with life-threatening infections with *E. coli, K. pneumoniae, E. cloacae*, and *P. aeruginosa*.

For gram-positive organisms such as *S. aureus* and *Enterococcus* spp., the detection of resistance against cell wall inhibitors and fluoroquinolones can be achieved with a sensitivity of greater than 90% and 80%, respectively [31–33]. The sensitivities for detection of resistance to protein synthesis inhibitors were less reliable for both organisms at 82% for clindamycin against *S. aureus* and 73% for quinupristin-dalfopristin against *Enterococcus* spp. However, greater than 92% sensitivity was achieved for all other protein synthesis inhibitors. Such discrepancies demonstrate the need for a more comprehensive database of resistance mechanisms. The

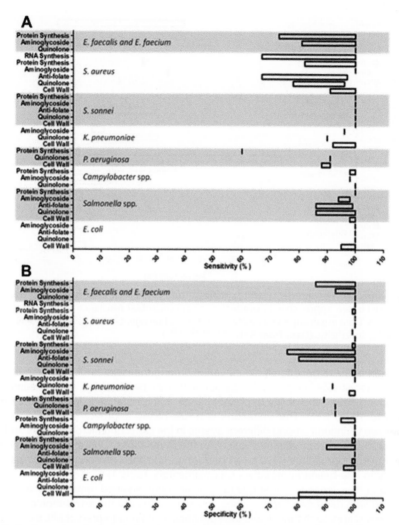

Fig. 2. Performance characteristics of second-generation WGS methods in predicting AST in gram-negative and gram-positive bacteria. (*A*) The sensitivity and (*B*) specificity of rule-based approaches in predicting phenotypic resistance of various antimicrobial agents. Data are grouped by indicated organism, and the specific antimicrobial agents based on mechanisms of action can be found in Supplementary Table 1. (*Data from* Refs [25-29,31-34,59].)

Mykrobe predictor database show low concordance in strains with constitutive clindamycin resistance [31,32]; 8 out of 30 resistant *Enterococcus faecium* lacked known genes [33]. Despite variable sensitivities, all drug classes tested in gram-positive organisms resulted to close to greater than 90% specificity.

Overall, the sensitivities for detection of resistance using WGS is the highest for agents acting on the cell wall and most variable for antifolate agents and protein synthesis inhibitors for both gram-negative and gram-positive bacteria. Based on our literature search, the lowest sensitivity (60%) was achieved in detection for amikacin resistance in *P. aeruginosa* where only 63 of 105 isolates contained a genetic element that predicts resistance and analyses were further complicated when protein

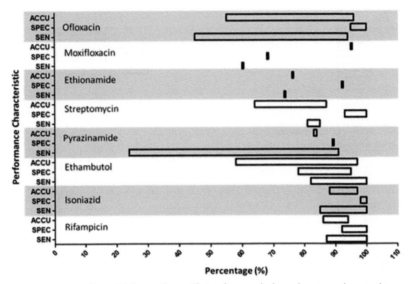

Fig. 3. Comparison of sensitivity and specificity from rule-based approaches and accuracy from model-based approaches in prediction of antimicrobial resistance in *Mycobacterium tuberculosis.* Data are grouped by indicated antimicrobial agent. ACCU, accuracy; SEN, sensitivity; SPEC, specificity. (*Data from* Refs [35,36,42,44–47,60].)

expression of these genetic elements varied among the isolates [34]. Although aminoglycoside resistance, in particular gentamicin, can be detected with a sensitivity approaching 100%, the ability to predict kanamycin resistance is lower, in the range of 81% to 100% [25,33]. The limitations in a rule-based approach may help explain why we see variations among different agents in the same antimicrobial class and using a model-based approach may adjust for these variations. Only a few studies using model-based approaches have been performed and they demonstrate comparable accuracy to rule-based approaches (Supplementary Table 1) [35–39].

Although the limited model-based studies only showed equivalent accuracy compared with rule-based approaches, it is worthy to note the advantage of using a model-based approach that allows the applicability of WGS to predict MICs of antimicrobial agents. It has been shown that with greater than 97% accuracy, the MIC of beta-lactams to +/−1 MIC doubling dilution can be determined for *Streptococcus pneumoniae* using a model-based approach called Random Forest where input data are sequences of penicillin-binding proteins [40]. Similarly, Eyre and colleagues [41] also showed that an overall accuracy of 99% and 95% was achieved when using their linear regression algorithm to determine the MIC for azithromycin and ciprofloxacin, respectively, in *Neisseria gonorrhoeae*. Furthermore, the same group demonstrated an average accuracy of 95% for nontyphoidal *Salmonella* [37] and 92% for *K. pneumoniae* [38] agreement within +/−1 doubling dilution of the MIC.

Using WGS to predict AMR for MTB is extremely useful because WGS data can be generated weeks before phenotypic AST results are available and inform better clinical decision-making processes. This can be particularly helpful for patients infected with MDR or extensively drug-resistant MTB. The overall sensitivity and specificity of WGS to predict first-line MTB agents (rifampicin, isoniazid, and ethambutol) ranges from 80% to 100% (**Fig. 3**; see Supplementary Table 1) [42–47]. Studies evaluating the performance characteristics of detecting resistance of pyrazinamide, another first-line TB agent, have reported more variable sensitivities of 70% to 91% and specificities of 89% to 99%. One study that only included 24 isolates with detectable pyrazinamide resistance by traditional AST reported a sensitivity of 24% when WGS was used to detect resistance [43,44]. The poor sensitivity of WGS methods to detect AMR for the drug pyrazinamide can be attributed to the complex nature of the drug, unknown mechanism of resistance of the drug, and the plethora of genes currently shown to be associated, which would then entail the development of a sophisticated and routinely updated database due to impending research into AMR genes. For similar reasons, when model-based approaches are used to detect for AMR resistance in *M. tuberculosis,* the accuracy is either equivalent or higher than the sensitivities detected by rule-based methods for all antituberculosis agents tested. In the case of pyrazinamide, an accuracy with a range of 89% to 99% has been reported [35,36]. WGS to predict AST for MTB has been widely studied and is likely to be the first WGS-based assay to be available for clinical care.

SUMMARY OF SHORT-READ METAGENOMIC NEXT-GENERATION SEQUENCING TO PREDICT ANTIMICROBIAL SUSCEPTIBILITY TESTING

Most initial efforts applying mNGS directly from specimens as a diagnostic tool for infectious diseases have focused on pathogen detection. However, results from short-read mNGS may also be used to query AMR genes to provide insight into therapeutic management of patients. A proof-of-concept study, evaluating 24 bone and joint infections by mNGS-correlated AMR detection using a mapping approach with the Res-Finder database compared with phenotypic AST, found that correct susceptibilities could be inferred in 94.1% of cases [48]. Of note, they only included culture-positive samples that may have overestimated the predictive power of mNGS in this study. Yan and colleagues [49] recently applied the CosmosID bioinformatics platform to query mNGS results positive for staphylococci for the presence of AMR genes to predict AST to methicillin, clindamycin, trimethoprim-sulfamethoxazole, and vancomycin. They found sensitivities ranging from 65.7% (clindamycin) to 85.0% (trimethoprim-sulfamethoxazole) for predicting resistance with a 77.4% sensitivity for predicting methicillin resistance based on detection of the *mecA* gene. Specificity ranged from 65.7% (TMP-SMX) to 100% for methicillin and vancomycin. The same limitations apply to mNGS for AMR detection as they do for pathogen detection [16,50]. However, the focus to identify specific AMR genes to predict phenotype adds further complexity as the entire genome of the organisms may not be represented in the sequenced reads leading to the possibility of very major errors in prediction models. Thus, the data may only be helpful when detecting an AMR gene rather than the absence for patient care. Also, the presence of the gene in the absence of genetic context may lead to false resistance due to the presence of similar loci occurring in commensal organisms. Further studies are required to assess the ability of mNGS to accurately predict AST and its applicability to patient care.

LONG-READ SEQUENCING TO PREDICT ANTIMICROBIAL SUSCEPTIBILITY TESTING

The use of long-read sequencing to detect AMR for prediction of AST is relatively early in development. Although studies evaluating PacBio sequencing have evolved around AMR detection [51–53], none have specifically tackled the issue of predicting AST and thus the focus here will be on ONT sequencing technologies.

Early studies evaluating ONT for detection of AMR were small proof-of concept and feasibility studies limiting evaluations to acquired resistance genes due to the high per base error rate. These studies demonstrated the potential to live-stream data to detect

AMR. They illustrated how short sequencing times (1–2 hours depending of version of flow cell) could generate sufficient information to study the entire resistome, highlighting their potential role as a diagnostic tool [18,19,54,55]. Only a few studies to date have systematically evaluated the correlation of AMR to phenotypic AST results to draw conclusions on accuracy.

One such study evaluating MinION WGS reads of 14 *N. gonorrhoeae* isolates demonstrated that open access databases were not sufficient to detect AMR in this pathogen and that an in-house developed pipeline with *de novo* assembly and optimized BLAST algorithms were required for accurate prediction of decreased susceptibility in gonococcal isolates. They demonstrated 100% sensitivity of detection to cefixime, ceftriaxone, and ciprofloxacin and 33% sensitivity of azithromycin with 100% specificity for all agents [56]. The investigators concluded that although these results are promising, a larger study with more diverse mechanisms of AMR and strains are required to validate their findings.

A second study evaluated the accuracy of AMR identified by ONT WGS in predicting AST results among carbapenem-resistant *K. pneumoniae* clinical isolates and further assessed the potential impact on patient care [17]. This study evaluated 2 different approaches to analysis using hybrid Illumina and Nanopore assemblies as the reference standard. The 2 approaches included (1) a real-time ONT-only approach without correction or assembly identifying acquired/chromosomal AMR genes using Metrichor's Antimicrobial Resistance Mapping Application (ARMA) and (2) an assembly with correction-based Nanopore-only approach. The real-time approach allowed for full annotation of acquired/chromosomal AMR genes within 8 hours from cultured isolates with 77% (range 30%–100% for various antimicrobial agents) agreement to AST. The assembly with correction-based ONT-only approach allowed for both acquired/chromosomal AMR gene detection and chromosomal SNP analysis of select AMR genes within 14 hours with 92% (range 80%–100% for different antimicrobial agents) agreement (same as the reference hybrid approach). The investigators demonstrated that the correction-based assembly approach, compared with a Nanopore-only real-time approach, enhances the ability to identify chromosomal mutations and allelic variants, increasing the accuracy of predictions for fluoroquinolones, aminoglycosides, and tetracyclines. Moreover, they demonstrated the potential to reduce time to effective antimicrobial therapy by a minimum of 20 hours compared with traditional phenotypic AST [17]. This study highlighted the ability of ONT to accurately predict AST for carbapenem-resistant *K. pneumoniae* clinical isolates ultimately to beneficially affect patient's care, with the use of a bioinformatics approach to overcome the known inaccuracies with this approach. Bioinformatics improvements enabling real-time alignment (without assembly) coupled with rapid extraction, library preparation, and new types of flow cells (ie, Flongel [Oxford Nanopore Technologies]) and automated technologies will further enhance the accuracy and workflow of the Nanopore real-time approach for clinical use.

Two studies evaluated ONT to predict AST directly from specimens using mNGS. A study by Schmidt and colleagues [55] applied ONT sequencing directly from high-burden ($>10^7$ CFU/mL) urinary tract infections/spiked urines to detect the pathogen and predict AST of the predominant pathogen directly from urine using ONT "What's In My Pot?" and ARMA [57] real-time analysis approach [58]. They were able to detect the pathogen and 51 of 55 acquired resistance genes by MinION ONT sequencing but were unable to detect resistance-conferring mutations or allelic variants. The optimized protocol allowed for a 4-hour TAT from sample to results demonstrating the potential to optimize therapy before a second dose of a typical antimicrobial agent (ie, within 8 hours).

A most recent study developed a lineage-based approach to predict AST phenotypes using *S. pneumoniae* and 5 antimicrobials (penicillin, ceftriaxone, trimethoprim-sulfamethoxazole, erythromycin, and tetracycline) as the prototype. To predict resistance in isolates and sputum samples the researchers built a database and generated a K-mer-based (18 bp length) representation of lineages to associate to phenotype. Few samples were tested to draw general limiting confidence in the accuracy of their findings. However, this study does suggest an alternative method to overcome ONT sequencing inaccuracies by associating phylogroup to expected AST phenotype. Caution must be taken although, as some resistance has weak association between lineage and resistance phenotype such as plasmid-mediated resistance genes [20]. Thus, further additions to such an algorithm such as association of plasmids with specific phenotypes could be beneficial.

PROMISES AND HURDLES AHEAD

As we continue to use NGS, we are gaining a better understanding of the correlations between AMR detection and phenotypic AST correlations. However, considerable investigations are still needed to provide a foundation for an accurate alternative for phenotypic AST profiles that are heavily relied on clinically. Model-based approaches seem promising providing an accurate alternative to rule-based prediction models and have the capability to predict an MIC $\pm$ 1 doubling dilution. The use of WGS to predict AST is the most advanced with *M. tuberculosis* complex. Furthermore, although this review focus on bacteria, there has been significant progress for viruses, fungi, and parasites [16].

SUPPLEMENTARY DATA

Supplementary data related to this article can be found online at https://doi.org/10.1016/j.yamp.2019.07.008.

REFERENCES

1. O'Neil J. Tackling drug-resistant infections globally: final report and recommendations, the review on antimicrobial resistance 2016 . Available at: https://amr-review.org/sites/default/files/160518_Final%20paper_with%20cover.pdf.

2. Ardal C, Outterson K, Hoffman SJ, et al. International cooperation to improve access to and sustain effectiveness of antimicrobials. Lancet 2016;387(10015): 296–307.

3. Peacock SJ, Parkhill J, Brown NM. Changing the paradigm for hospital outbreak detection by leading with genomic surveillance of nosocomial pathogens. Microbiology 2018;164(10):1213–9.

4. Schurch AC, van Schaik W. Challenges and opportunities for whole-genome sequencing-based surveillance of antibiotic resistance. Ann N Y Acad Sci 2017;1388(1):108–20.

5. Haidar G, Philips NJ, Shields RK, et al. Ceftolozane-tazobactam for the treatment of multidrug-resistant pseudomonas aeruginosa infections: clinical effectiveness and evolution of resistance. Clin Infect Dis 2017;65(1):110–20.

6. Shields RK, Chen L, Cheng S, et al. Emergence of ceftazidime-avibactam resistance due to plasmid-borne blaKPC-3 mutations during treatment of carbapenem-resistant klebsiella pneumoniae infections. Antimicrob Agents Chemother 2017;61(3) [pii:e02097-16].

7. Simner PJ, Antar AAR, Hao S, et al. Antibiotic pressure on the acquisition and loss of antibiotic resistance genes in Klebsiella pneumoniae. J Antimicrob Chemother 2018;73(7):1796–803.
8. Li J, Rettedal EA, van der Helm E, et al. Antibiotic treatment drives the diversification of the human gut resistome. Genomics Proteomics Bioinformatics 2019; 17(1):39–51.
9. Lanza VF, Baquero F, Martinez JL, et al. In-depth resistome analysis by targeted metagenomics. Microbiome 2018;6(1):11.
10. Su M, Satola SW, Read TD. Genome-based prediction of bacterial antibiotic resistance. J Clin Microbiol 2019;57(3) [pii:e01405-18].
11. EUCAST. Breakpoints tables for interpretation MICs and zone diameter, version 12, 2022. Available at: http://www.eucast.org/clinical_breakpoints/.
12. Clinical and Laboratory Standards Institute. Methods for dilution antimicrobial susceptibility tests for bacteria that grow Aerobically, S29. Wayne (PA): Clinical and Laboratory Standards Institute; 2019.
13. Clinical and Laboratory Standards Institute. Methods for dilution antimicrobial susceptibility tests for bacteria that grow aerobically. 11th edition. Wayne (PA): Clinical and Laboratory Standards Institute; 2018.
14. Banerjee R, Teng CB, Cunningham SA, et al. Randomized trial of rapid multiplex polymerase chain reaction-based blood culture identification and susceptibility testing. Clin Infect Dis 2015;61(7):1071–80.
15. Ameur A, Kloosterman WP, Hestand MS. Single-molecule sequencing: towards clinical applications. Trends Biotechnol 2019;37(1):72–85.
16. Mitchell SL, Simner PJ. Next-Generation Sequencing in Clinical Microbiology: Are We There Yet? Clin Lab Med 2019;39(3):405–18.
17. Tamma PD, Fan Y, Bergman Y, et al. Applying rapid whole-genome sequencing to predict phenotypic antimicrobial susceptibility testing results among carbapenem-resistant klebsiella pneumoniae clinical isolates. Antimicrob Agents Chemother 2019;63(1) [pii:e01923-18].
18. Cao MD, Ganesamoorthy D, Elliott AG, et al. Streaming algorithms for identification of pathogens and antibiotic resistance potential from real-time MinION(TM) sequencing. Gigascience 2016;5(1):32.
19. Lemon JK, Khil PP, Frank KM, et al. Rapid nanopore sequencing of plasmids and resistance gene detection in clinical isolates. J Clin Microbiol 2017;55(12): 3530–43.
20. Břinda K, Callendrello A, Cowley L, et al. Lineage calling can identify antibiotic resistance clones within minutes. Pathog Dis 2018;76(2).
21. Ellington MJ, Ekelund O, Aarestrup FM, et al. The role of whole genome sequencing in antimicrobial susceptibility testing of bacteria: report from the EUCAST Subcommittee. Clin Microbiol Infect 2017;23(1):2–22.
22. Jia B, Raphenya AR, Alcock B, et al. CARD 2017: expansion and model-centric curation of the comprehensive antibiotic resistance database. Nucleic Acids Res 2017;45(D1):D566–73.
23. Zankari E, Hasman H, Cosentino S, et al. Identification of acquired antimicrobial resistance genes. J Antimicrob Chemother 2012;67(11):2640–4.
24. Mason A, Foster D, Bradley P, et al. Accuracy of different bioinformatics methods in detecting antibiotic resistance and virulence factors from staphylococcus aureus whole-genome sequences. J Clin Microbiol 2018;56(9) [pii:e01815-17].
25. Stoesser N, Batty EM, Eyre DW, et al. Predicting antimicrobial susceptibilities for Escherichia coli and Klebsiella pneumoniae isolates using whole genomic sequence data. J Antimicrob Chemother 2013;68(10):2234–44.

26. Zhao S, Tyson GH, Chen Y, et al. Whole-genome sequencing analysis accurately predicts antimicrobial resistance phenotypes in campylobacter spp. Appl Environ Microbiol 2016;82(2):459–66.
27. Sadouki Z, Day MR, Doumith M, et al. Comparison of phenotypic and WGS-derived antimicrobial resistance profiles of Shigella sonnei isolated from cases of diarrhoeal disease in England and Wales, 2015. J Antimicrob Chemother 2017;72(9):2496–502.
28. McDermott PF, Tyson GH, Kabera C, et al. Whole-genome sequencing for detecting antimicrobial resistance in nontyphoidal salmonella. Antimicrob Agents Chemother 2016;60(9):5515–20.
29. Day MR, Doumith M, Do Nascimento V, et al. Comparison of phenotypic and WGS-derived antimicrobial resistance profiles of Salmonella enterica serovars Typhi and Paratyphi. J Antimicrob Chemother 2018;73(2):365–72.
30. Shelburne SA 3rd, Lasky RE, Sahasrabhojane P, et al. Development and validation of a clinical model to predict the presence of beta-lactam resistance in viridans group streptococci causing bacteremia in neutropenic cancer patients. Clin Infect Dis 2014;59(2):223–30.
31. Phaku P, Lebughe M, Strauss L, et al. Unveiling the molecular basis of antimicrobial resistance in Staphylococcus aureus from the Democratic Republic of the Congo using whole genome sequencing. Clin Microbiol Infect 2016;22(7): 644.e1-5.
32. Gordon NC, Price JR, Cole K, et al. Prediction of Staphylococcus aureus antimicrobial resistance by whole-genome sequencing. J Clin Microbiol 2014;52(4): 1182–91.
33. Tyson GH, Sabo JL, Rice-Trujillo C, et al. Whole-genome sequencing based characterization of antimicrobial resistance in Enterococcus. Pathog Dis 2018;76(2).
34. Kos VN, Deraspe M, McLaughlin RE, et al. The resistome of Pseudomonas aeruginosa in relationship to phenotypic susceptibility. Antimicrob Agents Chemother 2015;59(1):427–36.
35. Mahe P, Tournoud M. Predicting bacterial resistance from whole-genome sequences using k-mers and stability selection. BMC Bioinformatics 2018; 19(1):383.
36. Davis JJ, Boisvert S, Brettin T, et al. Antimicrobial resistance prediction in PATRIC and RAST. Sci Rep 2016;6:27930.
37. Nguyen M, Long SW, McDermott PF, et al. Using machine learning to predict antimicrobial mics and associated genomic features for nontyphoidal salmonella. J Clin Microbiol 2019;57(2) [pii:e01260-18].
38. Nguyen M, Brettin T, Long SW, et al. Developing an in silico minimum inhibitory concentration panel test for Klebsiella pneumoniae. Sci Rep 2018;8(1):421.
39. Moradigaravand D, Palm M, Farewell A, et al. Prediction of antibiotic resistance in Escherichia coli from large-scale pan-genome data. PLoS Comput Biol 2018; 14(12):e1006258.
40. Li Y, Metcalf BJ, Chochua S, et al. Validation of beta-lactam minimum inhibitory concentration predictions for pneumococcal isolates with newly encountered penicillin binding protein (PBP) sequences. BMC Genomics 2017;18(1):621.
41. Eyre DW, De Silva D, Cole K, et al. WGS to predict antibiotic MICs for Neisseria gonorrhoeae. J Antimicrob Chemother 2017;72(7):1937–47.
42. Feliciano CS, Namburete EI, Rodrigues Placa J, et al. Accuracy of whole genome sequencing versus phenotypic (MGIT) and commercial molecular tests for detection of drug-resistant Mycobacterium tuberculosis isolated from patients in Brazil and Mozambique. Tuberculosis (Edinb) 2018;110:59–67.

43. Coll F, McNerney R, Preston MD, et al. Rapid determination of anti-tuberculosis drug resistance from whole-genome sequences. Genome Med 2015;7(1):51.

44. Walker TM, Kohl TA, Omar SV, et al. Whole-genome sequencing for prediction of Mycobacterium tuberculosis drug susceptibility and resistance: a retrospective cohort study. Lancet Infect Dis 2015;15(10):1193–202.

45. Chatterjee A, Nilgiriwala K, Saranath D, et al. Whole genome sequencing of clinical strains of Mycobacterium tuberculosis from Mumbai, India: a potential tool for determining drug-resistance and strain lineage. Tuberculosis (Edinb) 2017;107:63–72.

46. Ezewudo M, Borens A, Chiner-Oms A, et al. Integrating standardized whole genome sequence analysis with a global Mycobacterium tuberculosis antibiotic resistance knowledgebase. Sci Rep 2018;8(1):15382.

47. Quan TP, Bawa Z, Foster D, et al. Evaluation of whole-genome sequencing for mycobacterial species identification and drug susceptibility testing in a clinical setting: a large-scale prospective assessment of performance against line probe assays and phenotyping. J Clin Microbiol 2018;56(2) [pii:e01480-17].

48. Ruppe E, Lazarevic V, Girard M, et al. Clinical metagenomics of bone and joint infections: a proof of concept study. Sci Rep 2017;7(1):7718.

49. Yan Q, Wi YM, Thoendel MJ, et al. Evaluation of the CosmosID bioinformatics platform for prosthetic joint-associated sonicate fluid shotgun metagenomic data analysis. J Clin Microbiol 2019;57(2) [pii:e01182-18].

50. Simner PJ, Miller S, Carroll KC. Understanding the promises and hurdles of metagenomic next-generation sequencing as a diagnostic tool for infectious diseases. Clin Infect Dis 2018;66(5):778–88.

51. Carter GP, Schultz MB, Baines SL, et al. Topical antibiotic use coselects for the carriage of mobile genetic elements conferring resistance to unrelated antimicrobials in staphylococcus aureus. Antimicrob Agents Chemother 2018;62(2) [pii:e02000-17].

52. Hoffmann M, Pettengill JB, Gonzalez-Escalona N, et al. Comparative sequence analysis of multidrug-resistant IncA/C plasmids from salmonella enterica. Front Microbiol 2017;8:1459.

53. Hujer AM, Higgins PG, Rudin SD, et al. Nosocomial outbreak of extensively drug-resistant acinetobacter baumannii isolates containing blaOXA-237 carried on a plasmid. Antimicrob Agents Chemother 2017;61(11) [pii:e00797-17].

54. Judge K, Hunt M, Reuter S, et al. Comparison of bacterial genome assembly software for MinION data and their applicability to medical microbiology. Microb Genom 2016;2(9):e000085.

55. Schmidt K, Mwaigwisya S, Crossman LC, et al. Identification of bacterial pathogens and antimicrobial resistance directly from clinical urines by nanopore-based metagenomic sequencing. J Antimicrob Chemother 2017;72(1):104–14.

56. Golparian D, Dona V, Sanchez-Buso L, et al. Antimicrobial resistance prediction and phylogenetic analysis of Neisseria gonorrhoeae isolates using the Oxford Nanopore MinION sequencer. Sci Rep 2018;8(1):17596.

57. Gire SK, Goba A, Andersen KG, et al. Genomic surveillance elucidates Ebola virus origin and transmission during the 2014 outbreak. Science 2014;345(6202):1369–72.

58. de Oliveira WK, Carmo EH, Henriques CM, et al. Zika virus infection and associated neurologic disorders in Brazil. N Engl J Med 2017;376(16):1591–3.

59. Kos VN, McLaughlin RE, Gardner HA. Elucidation of mechanisms of ceftazidime resistance among clinical isolates of pseudomonas aeruginosa by using genomic data. Antimicrob Agents Chemother 2016;60(6):3856–61.

60. Allix-Beguec C, Arandjelovic I, Bi L, et al. Prediction of susceptibility to first-line tuberculosis drugs by DNA sequencing. N Engl J Med 2018;379(15):1403–15.

Utility of Fluorescence *In Situ* Hybridization in Clinical and Research Applications

Gail H. Vance, MD[a,b], Wahab A. Khan, PhD[c,d,*]

KEYWORDS

- Fluorescence *in situ* hybridization (FISH) • Cytogenomics • Microscopy
- Chromosome biology • Medical genetics • Chromosomal microarray
- Copy number alterations • FISH research applications

KEY POINTS

- Fluorescence *in situ* hybridization (FISH) permits nucleic acid sequences to be detected directly on metaphase chromosome or interphase nuclei.
- The FISH assay is a powerful tool in visualizing simple and complex chromosomal rearrangements at single-cell resolution.
- The FISH assay provides cell-based diagnosis and monitoring of abnormal clones in hematological malignancies.
- FISH provides rapid diagnosis in subset of constitutional disorders and complements microarray findings.
- Emerging research applications for FISH are providing novel insights into chromosome biology.

INTRODUCTION

Fluorescence *in situ* hybridization (FISH) has proven to be a key tool in diagnostic molecular cytogenetics along with research applications in chromosome and cell biology. FISH allows the ability to contextually define and localize nucleic acid sequences directly on human metaphase chromosomes and interphase nuclei. From its earliest

This article originally appeared in *Advances in Molecular Pathology*, Volume 3, Issue 1, November 2020.
[a] Department of Medical and Molecular Genetics, Indiana University School of Medicine, 975 West Walnut Street IB 354, Indianapolis, IN 46202, USA; [b] Department of Pathology and Laboratory Medicine, Indiana University School of Medicine, 350 West 11th Street, Indianapolis, IN 46202-5120, USA; [c] Department of Pathology and Laboratory Medicine, Dartmouth-Hitchcock Medical Center, Williamson Translational Research Building–4th Floor, 1 Medical Center Drive, Lebanon, NH 03766, USA; [d] Geisel School of Medicine at Dartmouth College, Hanover, NH, USA
* Corresponding author. Department of Pathology, Dartmouth-Hitchcock Medical Center, Williamson Translational Research Building–4th Floor, 1 Medical Center Drive, Lebanon, NH 03766.
E-mail address: wahab.a.khan@hitchcock.org

Clin Lab Med 42 (2022) 573–586
https://doi.org/10.1016/j.cll.2022.09.020
0272-2712/22/© 2022 Elsevier Inc. All rights reserved.

labmed.theclinics.com

inception in the late 1960s[1] to the first use of nonradioisotopic techniques[2], the impact of FISH has been vast. In particular, in cytogenetics, FISH has provided diagnostic and prognostic information for prenatal and constitutional disorders as well as hematological malignancies, and solid tumors. FISH has also complemented genomic studies, such as chromosomal microarray (CMA)[3]. Research applications in FISH technology have evolved to include the use of superresolution microscopy systems for visualizing intranuclear chromosomal organization, and various methods have been used for improving probe labeling efficiency.

SIGNIFICANCE

As either a stand-alone diagnostic method or a molecular method coupled with standard karyotyping, FISH has significantly improved the resolution and therefore detection of numerical and structural chromosomal abnormalities beyond the light microscope. A distinct advantage of FISH is the application of fluorescent probes to nondividing cells obtained from cell suspension or paraffin-embedded tissues. FISH can detect tumor heterogeneity for both major and minor clonal abnormalities. The use of multicolor probes enables the localization and detection of multiple targets simultaneously.

FISH performed with probes comprising a lymphoma test panel (*BCL2*, *BCL6*, *MYC*) can identify "double-hit" lymphoma in cases with a pathologic diagnosis of diffuse large B-cell lymphoma[4]. FISH is also used to confirm chromosomal rearrangements identified by standard karyotyping or other molecular methods, including CMA. Parental confirmation of copy number gain or loss identified in a proband may be performed with labeled bacterial artificial chromosome DNA probe constructs that capture the copy number abnormality and detect its presence or absence in parental DNA. FISH remains a critical tool for detection and monitoring of genomic abnormalities across the spectrum of prenatal, constitutional, and neoplastic disease.

CLINICAL USE OF FLUORESCENCE *IN SITU* HYBRIDIZATION AND ITS MAJOR AREAS OF ADVANCEMENT

In a clinical context, FISH is typically performed using endpoint analysis because the hybridization kinetics are not observed in real time. However, in order to ensure that hybridization kinetics go to completion, various FISH protocols are validated with respect to probe type (eg, centromeric [repetitive] sequences, single copy unique loci, whole-chromosome paints) and specimen (eg, cell suspension vs tissue blocks). The principles of FISH are analogous to that of Southern blotting whereby single-stranded DNA anneals to its complementary target DNA. The target in FISH is that of DNA (or RNA) within interphase cells or on metaphase chromosomes that are fixed onto a microscope slide. FISH primarily uses DNA fragments that are generated by incorporating fluorophore-coupled nucleotides as probes to examine the absence or presence of complementary sequences with the use of an epifluorescent microscope[5]. This technique may also be performed on fixed and cultured tissue as well as on bone marrow, blood, and cytology smears. Clinical FISH tests that routinely use panels of gene-specific DNA probes targeting pathognomonic deletions, duplications, whole-chromosome gains/losses, and translocations have been widely used in both somatic and constitutional testing.

The major areas of advancement in FISH have seen improvements in probe labeling chemistries and use of high-resolution imaging modalities[6,7]. The former has relied on a range of approaches included but not limited to digoxigenin/biotin labeling of the probe[8], degenerate oligonucleotide primed PCR[9], *cis*-platinum complex-mediated labeling[10], quantum dots, and click chemistry[11,12]. These advances in probe labeling have led to a natural progression in multiplexing and automating the FISH assay.

DIGITIZING AND AUTOMATING FLUORESCENCE *IN SITU* HYBRIDIZATION IMAGING

One of the first automated FISH systems was able to achieve correct segmentation on at least 89% of interphase nuclei; however, it was not designed to count split FISH signals in a given image[13]. Clinical FISH laboratories use various cocktails of DNA probes that are typically prelabeled in different fluorescence spectrums and can be generalized into 2 major categories (**Table 1**). Cytogenetic laboratories are also familiar with nuances in preparing specimen slides using fixed cell suspension or other analysis considerations in which cells may be overlapped or fluorescence signals are present in different focal planes. To accommodate this, technological advancements in FISH imaging modalities and microscopy instrumentation have further enabled automated epifluorescence imaging for more end-user functionality. These advancements allow the user to set thresholds before automated capturing of a FISH microscope slide[14]. Automated capturing parameters can be implemented using neural networks and domain-based algorithms to fine-tune fluorescence signal classification in different focal planes[15,16]. Segmentation of clustered overlapped nuclei can be further refined, and morphologic features resulting from image noise can be removed in order to improve on true signal classification[17].

Presently, several companies have commercialized automated FISH capturing. These companies include MetaSystems, CytoVision, Applied Spectral Imaging, and BioView, among others. All platforms permit automated FISH spot counting with built-in classifiers to generate a gallery of cell images. These images may be triaged and further ranked based on chromosome spreading, nuclei quality, probe signal intensity, and background. The metaphase or interphase cells are scanned from the microscope slide in both Brightfield and fluorescent modes with auto-recorded cell coordinates. These automated platforms are being incorporated into the clinical setting, for example, to provide digital analysis of *HER2* in breast cancer or *ALK* rearrangements in non–small cell lung cancer[18]. As a result, optimizing a given platform's classifiers for proper segmentation of chromosomes and nuclei along with reducing false positive calls is an important consideration for integrating this automation in the laboratory[14,15,17,19]. Despite these advances, however, manual counting and analysis by well-trained technologists remain the predominant procedures in many laboratories; this is in part due to the technologist's ability to quickly determine the quality of an interphase or metaphase cell for further analysis and also to follow unique scanning patterns for specific specimens and probes[20].

Table 1
Categories of Labeled Probes for Fluorescence In Situ Hybridization

Direct-Labeled Nucleotides	Indirect-Labeled Nucleotides
FITC-12-dUTP	Biotin 11-dUTP
AMCA-6-dUTP	Digoxigenin-11-dUTP
Rhodamine-6-dUTP *Cy3-dCTP* *Texas red-12-dUTP*	Dinitrophenyl-11-dUTP

CONSIDERATIONS FOR FLUORESCENCE *IN SITU* HYBRIDIZATION DNA PROBE VALIDATION

As molecular cytogenomics continues to expand because of biomarker discovery, new FISH probes and disease panels are continually developed and commercialized. Therefore, it is important to reiterate the process of validation of FISH probes to be used clinically for quality assurance as put forth by the College of American Pathologists and to ensure excellence in patient care.

The process of establishing the analytical validity of FISH testing is typically divided into 4 major categories. These categories involve, but are not limited to, assessing the accuracy, reproducibility, sensitivity, and specificity of the assay. The series of consensus opinions and expert guidelines have evolved over the years as a resource toward validation of DNA probe-based *in situ* hybridization assays. Mainly, these comprise the American College of Medical Genetics technical document, the Clinical Laboratory Standards Institute guidelines, and the College of American Pathologists checklist items pertaining to FISH[21–23]. It is also important to note that FISH probe validation requirements vary depending on whether the probe has been approved/cleared by the Food and Drug Administration (FDA) or whether it is non-FDA approved, such as an analyte-specific reagent.

Of note, probe sensitivity or frequency of hybridization to an intended genomic target and probe specificity, a measure of a given target detected by the probe, will vary in different sample types. These samples can range from suspension cultures, formalin-fixed paraffin-embedded (FFPE) tissue, or fresh tissue preparations, and therefore, the validation process needs to be established for each. Signal truncation during slide sectioning for FFPE specimens should be carefully considered for probes intended to detect a chromosomal deletion when establishing sensitivity, specificity, and reference ranges[24,25].

Other factors to consider during the probe validation process are cross-hybridization and reproducibility of the assay[25]. Fluorescent signal cross-hybridizations are evaluated on metaphase chromosomes, which also speaks to the specificity of the probe. Instances whereby the FISH probe demonstrates significant cross-hybridizations (eg, recurrent signals at unintended chromosomal bands) may be indicative of probe contamination, which may require further repurification protocols and/or a different lot of FISH probe before clinical use[25]. Alternatively, the probe manufacturer may need to create/design a new version of the probe of interest. Precision or reproducibility of different FISH probes during interphase analysis can be measured in several ways. Blinded interassay (ie, microscope slides hybridized on different days) or intraassay (ie, hybridizations performed on the same day) analysis of FISH probe patterns by multiple microscopists can provide a measurement of reproducibility[26]. Finally, a given FISH probe's performance and overall hybridization efficiency should be periodically monitored as part of an ongoing probe validation and quality control plan. To this end, hybridization performance against a set of internal or external controls can be recorded for each *in situ* hybridization analysis, and periodic reevaluation of normal reference range cutoffs is recommended[21].

ROLE OF *IN SITU* HYBRIDIZATION ASSAYS IN HEMATOLOGICAL MALIGNANCIES WITH A CHROMOSOMAL BASIS

Cytogenetics has contributed significant data to the analysis, prognostication, and risk stratification of hematological malignancies. The Word Health Organization recommends cytogenetic studies at diagnosis and at defined intervals thereafter along with incorporation of morphologic and immunophenotyping data for stratifying leukemias and lymphomas[4,27]. The cytogenetic and/or molecular genetics aberrancies in hematological malignancies are defined by banded karyotype analysis of bone marrow or neoplastic blood metaphase cells as well as FISH and reverse transcriptase polymerase chain reaction studies. The molecular studies, with advancements in absolute chimeric transcript quantification, become especially important in monitoring for minimal residual disease after initial diagnosis[28]. Although not a comprehensive discussion, the following text focuses on FISH diagnosis of some of the recurrent hematological malignancies with a chromosomal basis unique to a particular myeloid or lymphoid lineage.

FLUORESCENCE *IN SITU* HYBRIDIZATION PROBE DESIGN STRATEGIES TO ASSESS CHROMOSOMAL CORRELATES IN ACUTE MYELOID LEUKEMIA

In the more common adult form of acute myeloid leukemia (AML), with prevalence of immature forms of myeloid cells, the genes involved in key rearrangements can be detected by FISH. The principal advantage of an in situ–based approach is that probe signals are localized at single-cell resolution to interphase nuclei without the need to culture cells. Detection of probe signals in these nondividing nuclei uses primarily 2 strategies in DNA probe design. One involves the use of break-apart FISH whereby probes are differentially labeled with fluorophores flanking genomic sequences at known chromosomal breakpoints. The close spatial proximity of the DNA probes that are differentially labeled, typically in the spectrums of green and red fluorescence, appears to the eye as a mixed yellow signal (**Fig. 1**A). As a chromosomal translocation occurs, 1 signal is separated (ie, "split signal") into its independent spectrum components: green or red. The remaining yellow (combined red and green fluorophores) signal indicates the nonrearranged chromosome (**Fig. 1**B).

In a separate fusion strategy of probes labeled with distinct fluorophores, typically dual-color, dual-fusion, FISH probes target specific chromosomal regions that are known to either form chimeric fusion products or close juxtaposition of translocated segments and genes. If a rearrangement occurs, defined by a reciprocal translocation or intrachromosomal event (ie, inversion or deletion), the dual-color probes that otherwise in a wild-type state show distinct copies of a red fluorophore and a green fluorophore for each locus, emitting an RRGG signal pattern (**Fig. 2**A), are brought into close proximity. On exchange of the involved chromosomal segments, yellow (combined

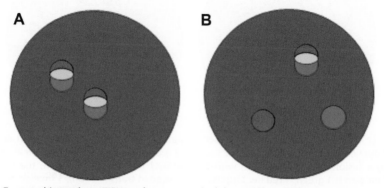

Fig. 1. Expected interphase FISH probe patterns in (*A*) normal and (*B*) rearranged nuclei using a dual-color, break-apart DNA probe strategy. Spectrum yellow is due to juxtaposition of spectrum red and green probe fluorescence.

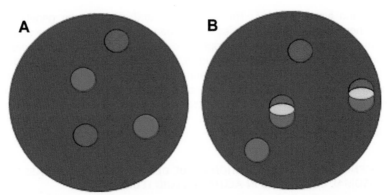

Fig. 2. Expected interphase FISH probe patterns in (*A*) normal nuclei, indicative of the absence of a rearrangement event (translocation/inversion). (*B*) In contrast, a dual-color, dual-fusion DNA probe strategy shows evidence of a reciprocal translocation with fusion signals (*yellow*) on each derivative chromosome. The yellow fluorescence is due to juxtaposition of red and green probe fluorescence.

red and green) signals are visualized (**Fig. 2**B). Either 1 or 2 yellow fusion signals, depending on the probe placement with respect to the breakpoint, will indicate the fusion product on the derivative chromosome. Analogous to a break-apart strategy, the probe signal that is not rearranged, in a fusion strategy, remains as distinct green and red fluorescent signals.

Another FISH probe strategy, similar to the fusion strategy, involves an extra signal probe. This probe set also incorporates the use of a dual-color differentially labeled probe and is often used in detecting a karyotypically cryptic translocation, such as t(12;21)(*ETV6/RUNX1*), common to childhood leukemia (**Fig. 3**A; normal scenario). With this strategy, the fusion produces a yellow signal (combination of red and green) on the derivative (abnormal) chromosome. In the same abnormal cell, there are also

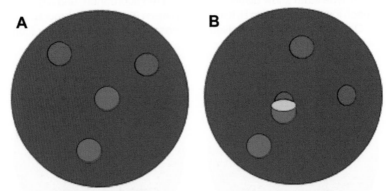

Fig. 3. (*A*) In a normal nucleus, the expected pattern for a cell hybridized with an extra signal dual-color, dual-fusion probe is 2 red and 2 green signals. (*B*) In an abnormal cell containing a fusion event (often seen with *ETV6/RUNX1* using this probe set), the expected signal pattern is 1 green, 1 red (ie, targets not involved in translocation), 1 smaller red signal (ie, residual probe target partially not involved in translocation), and 1 fused yellow signal (translocated product). This strategy increases the sensitivity of the FISH assay in detecting cryptic chromosomal rearrangements.

green and red signals present on chromosomes not involved in the translocation. In addition, there is an "extra" "small" red signal representing a residual portion of one of the involved loci in the translocation on the other derivative chromosome (**Fig. 3**B). This probe strategy has many applications in diagnosis and monitoring of childhood leukemia. FISH provides analysis of a large number of cells because the abnormality is not detectable by trypsin-Giemsa or G-banded metaphases[29]. Multiple FISH strategies designed for the detection of recurrent genetic abnormalities, such as t(8;21)(q22;q22)(*RUNX1/RUNX1T1*), inv(16)(p13.1q22) in AML, or t(15;17)(q24;q21)(*PML/RARA*) in acute promyelocytic leukemia (APL) among others (**Table 2**), allow for rapid analysis and reporting. The FISH strategy to detect the t(15;17) in APL is a STAT test (ie, meaning immediately) in many laboratories with reporting of the result within 24 hours. These cytogenetic markers also serve as prognostic indicators of disease. In addition, the rearrangement of *KTM2A* at 11q23.3, with multiple translocation partners, often is associated with an adverse outcome. FISH analysis has supplemented molecular and traditional cytogenetic testing to define a subset of secondary or therapy-related AML[30]. In these cases, deletion or loss of chromosomes 5/5q or 7/7q and rearrangements of *KMT2A*, *RUNX1* as well as *PML/RARA* may be detected by FISH enumeration or break-apart probe strategies.

FLUORESCENCE *IN SITU* HYBRIDIZATION PROBE STRATEGIES FOR DETECTING MYELOPROLIFERATIVE NEOPLASMS

Among the myeloproliferative disorders, chronic myeloid leukemia (CML) is well known. CML is most commonly a disease of adults with symptomatic findings, including fatigue, malaise, headache, weight loss, and splenomegaly, developing over time. CML was the first malignancy to be associated with a specific chromosome defect, in which patients were found to have the Philadelphia chromosome translocation, t(9;22)(q34;q11.2) by G-banded analysis[31,32]. The Philadelphia chromosome (derivative chromosome 22) is characterized by a balanced translocation between the long arms of chromosomes 9 and 22. Among CML cases, the well-recognized *BCR-ABL1* translocation is pathognomonic and required for the diagnosis. At the molecular level, the gene for *ABL1*, an oncogene on chromosome 9, joins a gene on chromosome 22 named *BCR*. The result of the fusion of these 2 genes is a new fusion

---

Table 2
Abbreviated List of Recurring Cytogenetic Abnormalities and Risk Stratifications in Well-Known Hematological Malignancies

Cytogenetics	Classification	Genes Involved	Outcome
t(8;21)(q22;q22)	AML	*RUNX1/RUNX1T1*	Favorable
inv(16)(p13.1q22) or t(16;16)(p13.1;q22)	AML	*CBFB/MYH11*	Favorable
t(15;17)(q24;q21)	APL	*PML/RARA*	Favorable
t(9;11)(p22;q23)	AML	*MLLT3/KMT2A*	Poor to intermediate
t(6;9)(p23;q34)	AML	*DEK/NUP214*	Poor
−7 or del 7q	MDS	—	Poor
−5 and del 5q	MDS	—	Poor
Isolated del 5q or del 20q	MDS	—	Good
Negative	De novo AML	—	Intermediate

All translocations listed are detectable by interphase and/or metaphase FISH.

protein of about 210 kDa with increased tyrosine kinase signaling that overrides normal cell regulatory mechanism. Cryptic deletions of either distal portion of *BCR* and/or proximal region of *ABL1*, as well as rare cryptic insertions between chromosome 9 and 22, may occur in cases lacking a Philadelphia chromosome and are detected by FISH often using a 3-color, dual-fusion probe strategy[33,34]. Detection of the translocation is especially relevant in an era of tyrosine kinase inhibitors that target the chimeric protein encoded by the *BCR/ABL1* fusion gene.

Another myeloid disorder for which FISH has played a key role at diagnosis is eosinophilia with rearrangements involving *PDGFRA*, *PDGFRB*, and *FGFR1*. FISH breakapart strategies have proved to be useful in detecting *FGFR1* rearrangements with its many translocation partners. With respect to *PDGFRA*, a deletion of *CHIC2* leads to a cryptic fusion of *FIP1L1/PDGFRA* on chromosome 4q12. This abnormality is sensitive to imatinib mesylate and therefore relevant for rapid identification[35]. Similarly, rearrangements of *PDGFRB* at 5q32, such as the translocation t(5;12)(q32;p13.2), may be detected by FISH and is sensitive to tyrosine kinase inhibitors.

FLUORESCENCE *IN SITU* HYBRIDIZATION PROBE STRATEGIES DETECTING CHROMOSOMAL CORRELATES IN MATURE B-CELL NEOPLASMS

For most hematological aberrations in chronic lymphocytic leukemia (CLL) or plasma cell myeloma (PCM, formerly multiple myeloma), FISH is performed in concert with metaphase analysis. Multiple research groups, including the International Myeloma Working Group and the International Workshop on Chronic Lymphocytic Leukemia, recommend the use of FISH as a priority test for diagnostic workup for patients with CLL and PCM[36].

Various probe strategies (eg, break apart, dual color/dual fusion; enumeration) as discussed above may be applied in the context of CLL and/or PCM. These strategies include enumeration probes, especially in PCM, where hyperdiploidy accounts for approximately 45% of cases, and deletions of *TP53* portend an adverse outcome. Translocations involving the immunoglobulin heavy chain (*IGH*) are frequent in PCM and include partner genes *CCND1* (11q13.3), *MAF* (16q23.2), *FGFR3/NSD2* (*FGFR3/MMSET*)(4q16.3), *CCND2* (12p13.32) and *CCND3* (6p21.1), *MAFA* (8q24.3) and *MAFB* (20q12)[4]. It is understood that several of the PCM translocations are cryptic by standard karyotyping and that FISH is a critical component of the PCM diagnostic workup[37–39].

CLL is a disease of older adults with an incidence of ~20 cases/100,000 individuals aged 70 years or older[40]. Often asymptomatic, clinical signs may include lymphadenopathy, splenomegaly, anemia, and thrombocytopenia. Clonal abnormalities are detected in 80% of CLL cases[41,42]. The frequency of these chromosomal abnormalities depends on immunoglobulin heavy chain variable region (IGHV) mutation status. For example, trisomy 12, found in ~20% of cases, overall has an incidence of 15% in mutated IGHV and 19% in unmutated IGHV. Deletions of 11q are seen in 4% of cases with mutated IGHV and ~27% of cases with unmutated IGHV[40]. Recurring chromosomal translocations are less frequent in CLL. The t(14;18)(q32.33;q21.33) *IGH/BCL2* rearrangement, typically associated with follicular and diffuse large B-cell lymphoma, has been identified in ~2% of CLL cases as the sole aberration[40,41].

ROLE OF SINGLE NUCLEOTIDE POLYMORPHISM CHROMOSOMAL MICROARRAYS IN HEMATOLOGICAL MALIGNANCIES

In the constitutional setting, CMA analysis has achieved great success in delineating new genomic disorders and identifying genes with importance in dosage sensitivity. Application of this methodology to neoplasia has further refined assessment of copy number changes on a genomic scale using single nucleotide polymorphism (SNP) arrays. Having the SNP and copy number content on CMA platforms provides additional genotyping information that may not be achieved with FISH or karyotyping, such as the detection of copy-neutral loss of heterozygosity (cn-LOH), along with copy number changes, amplifications, and imbalances involving whole chromosomes (**Fig. 4**). CMA has also uncovered masked hypodiploidy related to poor outcomes. For example, SNP-microarray has proved useful in cases of hypodiploid B-cell acute lymphoblastic leukemia (ALL), whereby detection of the duplication of a hypodiploid clone (see **Fig. 4**) may be limited by traditional cytogenetic methods. In addition, certain focal intragenic deletions can be detected by SNP-microarray and are important for assessing genomic risk in lymphoid malignancies[43]. The detection of intragenic deletions by CMA, such as *IKFZ1*, has also led to changes in treatment protocols in B-cell ALL, especially among the pediatric patient cohort sensitive to relapse[44].

Focal gene amplifications, often associated with features of solid tumors, have also been observed in hematological malignancies by karyotype, FISH, and CMA. For example, the amplification of *RUNX1* (ie, iAMP21), when observed by CMA, revealed in a small number of cases that the amplification was not confined to *RUNX1* but rather spanned a contiguous region encompassing up to ~32 Mb. In these cases, there was also a concomitant deletion of the distal long arm of chromosome 21, including genes *DSCAM*, *AIRE*, and *TSPEAR*[45]. In myeloid malignancies, whole-gene amplifications of *KMT2A*, *MYC* as well as partial tandem duplications of *KMT2A*, sometimes covert by FISH, may be detected by SNP-based CMA[43].

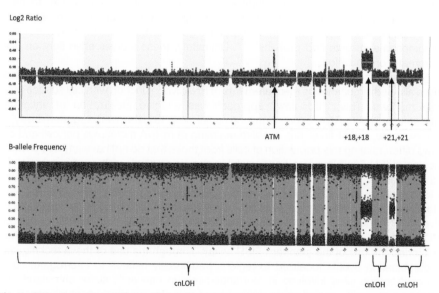

Fig. 4. SNP-microarray performed on a bone marrow specimen from a patient with clinical suspicion of ALL. The top panel indicates the log2 ratio on the y-axis and chromosome number along the x-axis. Gain of *ATM* with 2 additional copies (11q22.3) along with whole-chromosome gains of 18 and 21 are noted. In the bottom panel, the B-allele frequency across the genome suggests cn-LOH for chromosomes 1 to 19, 22, and X. (*From* Berry NK, Scott RJ, Rowlings, et al. Clinical use of SNP-microarrays for the detection of genome-wide changes in haematological malignancies. Crit Rev Oncol Hematol. 2019;142:62; with permission.)

A distinct advantage of SNP-based CMA over karyotyping and FISH is its ability to detect cn-LOH. The presence of cn-LOH can affect prognostication in hematological disease. In myelodysplastic syndrome (MDS), for example, cn-LOH of chromosome 7 has been linked to poor prognostication, similar to deletion of chromosome 7q detected by FISH or karyotype[43,46]. Of particular interest, cn-LOH may lead to loss of tumor suppression transcripts, such as *TP53*, or oncogenes, such as *JAK2* and *FLT3*. The cn-LOH may manifest as a "rescue event" whereby there is loss of the chromosome carrying the wild-type allele with either duplication of the chromosome with the mutated gene or intrachromosomal deletion of the wild-type allele[43]. Currently, detection of balanced chromosomal rearrangements in MDS and other hematological malignancies most frequently requires a metaphase karyotype and/or FISH analysis. However, next-generation sequencing (NGS) -based approaches for translocations with fusion transcript detection are being implemented[47].

EXPANDING TRADITIONAL APPLICATIONS OF FLUORESCENCE *IN SITU* HYBRIDIZATION

FISH in a research context has been applied across broad applications in molecular cytogenetics and genomics. Coupling immunofluorescence with FISH has led to detection of chromosomal abnormalities in cells by their phenotype[48]. Coupling FISH with DNA halo preparations of linearized DNA has aided in visualization of sequences as little as 10 kb apart along with their chromatin interactions[49]. Applying the use of DNA FISH probes in a 3-dimensional (3D) context has contributed to the field of chromosome nanoscience. To this end, superresolution microscopy approaches, such as 3D structured illumination microscopy or single molecule stochastic optical reconstruction microscopy, that are beyond the diffraction limit of light have been applied to the study of short nonrepetitive genomic targets[6,50,51] as well as large chromosomal targets and proteins[52,53]. Ultimately, these studies shed light on 3D-chromatin organization.

Novel applications of FISH performed in suspension rather than in *in situ* cultures have allowed simultaneous measurements of RNA in conjunction with cell surface protein markers. This "FISH-flow" approach has enabled localization of antigens, messenger RNA (mRNA) expression, and nucleic acid targets in an integrated assay[54]. For example, "FISH-flow" has enabled counting of mRNA molecules per cell and allows differentiating this population of cells from those that do not have any mRNA molecules. "FISH-flow" has also been useful in examining single-cell gene expression in rare circulating cancer cells[54]. In more recent efforts, a technique known as Live-FISH exploited the CRISPR-Cas9 editing system to explore movement of DNA-double-strand breaks as well as concomitant viewing of DNA and RNA transcripts in live cells[55]. The use of chromosome orientation or CO-FISH and parent of origin or POD-FISH on homologous targets of mitotic metaphase chromosomes has further extended the use of the standard FISH assay. Through the use of these techniques, recombination events localized to regions traditionally difficult to interrogate, such as centromeric sites involved in rearrangements in cancer[56], sister chromatid exchange patterns[57], as well as discrimination of homologous chromosomes based on copy number changes[58], can be directly visualized. Taken together, research applications of FISH continue to push the limits of the understanding of chromosome biology.

FUTURE CONSIDERATIONS

The future of FISH will be predicated on its ability to provide on demand rapid single-cell resolution of nucleic acids in the genome for a range of targets and tissue types.

Improvements in microscale methods of performing FISH will be important to the success of this approach. Microscale methods will aid in a reduction of FISH probe consumption and time to completion of hybridization reactions for a typical FISH assay[59]. Moreover, diagnostic and prognostic genetic targets in cancer and constitutional disorders will continue to increase with the use of FISH-, CMA-, and NGS-based discovery. Therefore, flexibility in the design of FISH probes as an orthogonal or rapid means of confirmation would be needed in some cases for different targets in the genome. To this end, computational efforts aimed at identifying optimal nucleic acid probe sequences, on demand, instead of relying on collection of preexisting commercial FISH probes will streamline research and clinical applications[60].

SUMMARY

FISH has proven to be a powerful technology with applications in both the clinical and research context. A multitude of FISH probes can be applied in different scenarios ranging from locus-specific targets to whole-chromosome paints. In neoplasia, the utility of FISH has been demonstrated in diagnostics, prognostics, and follow-up studies to monitor abnormal clones. Because the assay is single-cell based, it also provides the ability to rapidly detect low-level clones from uncultured cells. In constitutional studies, FISH serves as a confirmatory assay for microarray-based analysis of copy number variation. Because of its ability to delineate loci directly on chromosome structure, FISH may provide contextual information on gains and losses from metaphase chromosome analysis. Moreover, as a stand-alone test, FISH has enabled the detection of a spectrum of submicroscopic chromosomal abnormalities. As novel genomic targets are discovered, microscopy techniques improve, and genomic science evolves, it is anticipated that molecular cytogenomics will continue to play a key role in cancer and germline diagnostics.

DISCLOSURE

The authors have nothing to disclose.

REFERENCES

1. Pardue ML, Gall JG. Molecular hybridization of radioactive DNA to the DNA of cytological preparations. Proc Natl Acad Sci U S A 1969;64(2):600–4.
2. Manning JE, Hershey ND, Broker TR, et al. A new method of in situ hybridization. Chromosoma 1975;53(2):107–17.
3. Bi W, Borgan C, Pursley AN, et al. Comparison of chromosome analysis and chromosomal microarray analysis: what is the value of chromosome analysis in today's genomic array era? Genet Med 2013;15(6):450–7.
4. Swerdlow S, Campo E, Harris N, et al. 4th edition. WHO classification of tumours of haematopoietic and lymphoid tissues, vol. 2. Lyon (France): WHO Press; 2017.
5. Gozzetti A, Le Beau MM. Fluorescence in situ hybridization: uses and limitations. Semin Hematol 2000;37(4):320–33.
6. Khan WA, Rogan PK, Knoll JH. Localized, non-random differences in chromatin accessibility between homologous metaphase chromosomes. Mol Cytogenet 2014;7(1):70.
7. Yusuf M, Kaneyoshi K, Fukui K, et al. Use of 3D imaging for providing insights into high-order structure of mitotic chromosomes. Chromosoma 2019;128(1):7–13. https://doi.org/10.1007/s00412-018-0678-5.

8. Chen TR. Fluorescence in situ hybridization (FISH): detection of biotin- and digoxigenin-labeled signals on chromosomes. J Tissue Cult Methods 1994; 16(1):39–47.
9. Telenius H, Pelmear AH, Tunnacliffe A, et al. Cytogenetic analysis by chromosome painting using DOP-PCR amplified flow-sorted chromosomes. Genes Chromosomes Cancer 1992;4(3):257–63.
10. Wiegant JC, van Gijlswijk RP, Heetebrij RJ, et al. ULS: a versatile method of labeling nucleic acids for FISH based on a monofunctional reaction of cisplatin derivatives with guanine moieties. Cytogenet Cell Genet 1999;87(1–2):47–52.
11. Knoll JHM. Human metaphase chromosome FISH using quantum dot conjugates. Methods Mol Biol 2007;374:55–66.
12. Müller S, Cremer M, Neusser M, et al. A technical note on quantum dots for multicolor fluorescence in situ hybridization. Cytogenet Genome Res 2009;124(3–4): 351–9.
13. Netten H, Young IT, van Vliet LJ, et al. FISH and chips: automation of fluorescent dot counting in interphase cell nuclei. Cytometry 1997;28(1):1–10.
14. Vrolijk H, Sloos WC, van de Rijke FM, et al. Automation of spot counting in interphase cytogenetics using brightfield microscopy. Cytometry 1996;24(2):158–66.
15. Lerner B, Clocksin WF, Dhanjal S, et al. Automatic signal classification in fluorescence in situ hybridization images. Cytometry 2001;43(2):87–93.
16. Malpica N, de Solórzano CO, Vaquero JJ, et al. Applying watershed algorithms to the segmentation of clustered nuclei. Cytometry 1997;28(4):289–97.
17. Kozubek M, Kozubek S, Lukásová E, et al. High-resolution cytometry of FISH dots in interphase cell nuclei. Cytometry 1999;36(4):279–93.
18. van der Logt EMJ, Kuperus DAJ, van Setten JW, et al. Fully automated fluorescent in situ hybridization (FISH) staining and digital analysis of HER2 in breast cancer: a validation study. PLoS One 2015;10(4):e0123201.
19. Kajtár B, Méhes G, Lörch T, et al. Automated fluorescent in situ hybridization (FISH) analysis of t(9;22)(q34;q11) in interphase nuclei. Cytometry A 2006; 69(6):506–14.
20. Abbott Molecular Inc. UroVysion: Bladder Cancer Kit. Available at: https://www. molecular.abbott/us/en/products/oncology/urovysion-bladder-cancer-kit. Accessed March 14, 2020.
21. Mascarello JT, Hirsch B, Kearney HM, et al. Section E9 of the American College of Medical Genetics technical standards and guidelines: fluorescence in situ hybridization. Genet Med 2011;13(7):667–75.
22. Mascarello JT, Hirsch B, Kearney HM, et al. ADDENDUM: section E9 of the American College of Medical Genetics Technical Standards and Guidelines: fluorescence in situ hybridization. Genet Med 2019;21(10):2405.
23. MM07A2: FISH Methods for Clinical Laboratories - CLSI. Clinical & Laboratory Standards institute. Available at: https://clsi.org/standards/products/moleculardiagnostics/documents/mm07/. Accessed January 6, 2020.
24. Yoshimoto M, Ludkovski O, Good J, et al. Use of multicolor fluorescence in situ hybridization to detect deletions in clinical tissue sections. Lab Invest 2018; 98(4):403–13.
25. Gu J, Smith JL, Dowling PK. Fluorescence in situ hybridization probe validation for clinical use. Methods Mol Biol 2017;1541:101–18.
26. Saxe DF, Persons DL, Wolff DJ, et al. Cytogenetics Resource Committee of the College of American Pathologists. Validation of fluorescence in situ hybridization using an analyte-specific reagent for detection of abnormalities involving the mixed lineage leukemia gene. Arch Pathol Lab Med 2012;136(1):47–52.

27. Sabattini E, Bacci F, Sagramoso C, et al. WHO classification of tumours of haematopoietic and lymphoid tissues in 2008: an overview. Pathologica 2010; 102(3):83–7.

28. Maier J, Lange T, Cross M, et al. Optimized digital droplet PCR for BCR-ABL. J Mol Diagn 2019;21(1):27–37.

29. Wolff DJ, Bagg A, Cooley LD, et al. Guidance for fluorescence in situ hybridization testing in hematologic disorders. J Mol Diagn 2007;9(2):134–43.

30. Bueso-Ramos CE, Kanagal-Shamanna R, Routbort MJ, et al. Therapy-related myeloid neoplasms. Am J Clin Pathol 2015;144(2):207–18.

31. Nowell PC. The minute chromosome (Phl) in chronic granulocytic leukemia. Blut 1962;8:65–6.

32. Rowley JD. Letter: a new consistent chromosomal abnormality in chronic myelogenous leukaemia identified by quinacrine fluorescence and Giemsa staining. Nature 1973;243(5405):290–3.

33. Castagnetti F, Testoni N, Luatti S, et al. Deletions of the derivative chromosome 9 do not influence the response and the outcome of chronic myeloid leukemia in early chronic phase treated with imatinib mesylate: GIMEMA CML Working Party analysis. J Clin Oncol 2010;28(16):2748–54.

34. Luatti S, Baldazzi C, Marzocchi G, et al. Cryptic BCR-ABL fusion gene as variant rearrangement in chronic myeloid leukemia: molecular cytogenetic characterization and influence on TKIs therapy. Oncotarget 2017;8(18):29906–13.

35. Hilal T, Fauble V, Ketterling RP, et al. Myeloid neoplasm with eosinophilia associated with isolated extramedullary FIP1L1/PDGFRA rearrangement. Cancer Genet 2018;220:13–8.

36. Revised International Staging System for Multiple Myeloma: a report from International Myeloma Working Group. - PubMed - NCBI. Available at: https://www.ncbi.nlm.nih.gov/pubmed/?term=26240224. Accessed February 4, 2020.

37. Hu Y, Chen W, Wang J. Progress in the identification of gene mutations involved in multiple myeloma. Oncotargets Ther 2019;12:4075–80.

38. Tan D, Lee JH, Chen W, et al. Recent advances in the management of multiple myeloma: clinical impact based on resource-stratification. Consensus statement of the Asian Myeloma Network at the 16th International Myeloma Workshop. Leuk Lymphoma 2018;59(10):2305–17.

39. Avet-Loiseau H, Brigaudeau C, Morineau N, et al. High incidence of cryptic translocations involving the Ig heavy chain gene in multiple myeloma, as shown by fluorescence in situ hybridization. Genes Chromosomes Cancer 1999;24(1):9–15.

40. Swerdlow SH, Campo E, Pileri SA, et al. The 2016 revision of the World Health Organization classification of lymphoid neoplasms. Blood 2016;127(20):2375–90.

41. Roos-Weil D, Nguyen-Khac F, Chevret S, et al. Mutational and cytogenetic analyses of 188 CLL patients with trisomy 12: a retrospective study from the French Innovative Leukemia Organization (FILO) working group. Genes Chromosomes Cancer 2018;57(11):533–40.

42. Chastain EC, Duncavage EJ. Clinical prognostic biomarkers in chronic lymphocytic leukemia and diffuse large B-cell lymphoma. Arch Pathol Lab Med 2015; 139(5):602–7.

43. Berry NK, Scott RJ, Rowlings P, et al. Clinical use of SNP-microarrays for the detection of genome-wide changes in haematological malignancies. Crit Rev Oncol Hematol 2019;142:58–67.

44. Sutton R, Venn NC, Law T, et al. A risk score including microdeletions improves relapse prediction for standard and medium risk precursor B-cell acute lymphoblastic leukaemia in children. Br J Haematol 2018;180(4):550–62.

45. Baughn LB, Biegel JA, South ST, et al. Integration of cytogenomic data for furthering the characterization of pediatric B-cell acute lymphoblastic leukemia: a multi-institution, multi-platform microarray study. Cancer Genet 2015; 208(1–2):1–18.

46. da Silva FB, Machado-Neto JA, Bertini VHLL, et al. Single-nucleotide polymorphism array (SNP-A) improves the identification of chromosomal abnormalities by metaphase cytogenetics in myelodysplastic syndrome. J Clin Pathol 2017; 70(5):435–42.

47. Zhong Y, Beimnet K, Alli Z, et al. Multiplexed digital detection of B-cell acute lymphoblastic leukemia fusion transcripts using the nanoString nCounter System. J Mol Diagn 2020;22(1):72–80.

48. Fuller KA, Bennett S, Hui H, et al. Development of a robust immuno-S-FISH protocol using imaging flow cytometry. Cytometry A 2016;89(8):720–30.

49. Elcock LS, Bridger JM. Fluorescence in situ hybridization on DNA halo preparations and extended chromatin fibres. Methods Mol Biol 2010;659:21–31.

50. Knoll JHM, Rogan PK. Sequence-based, in situ detection of chromosomal abnormalities at high resolution. Am J Med Genet A 2003;121A(3):245–57.

51. Ni Y, Cao B, Ma T, et al. Super-resolution imaging of a 2.5 kb non-repetitive DNA in situ in the nuclear genome using molecular beacon probes. eLife 2017;6: e21660.

52. Khan WA, Chisholm R, Tadayyon S, et al. Relating centromeric topography in fixed human chromosomes to α-satellite DNA and CENP-B distribution. Cytogenet Genome Res 2013;139(4):234–42.

53. Kyriacou E, Heun P. High-resolution mapping of centromeric protein association using APEX-chromatin fibers. Epigenetics Chromatin 2018;11(1):68.

54. Arrigucci R, Bushkin Y, Radford F, et al. FISH-Flow, a protocol for the concurrent detection of mRNA and protein in single cells using fluorescence in situ hybridization and flow cytometry. Nat Protoc 2017;12(6):1245–60.

55. Wang H, Nakamura M, Abbott TR, et al. CRISPR-mediated live imaging of genome editing and transcription. Science 2019;365(6459):1301–5.

56. Giunta S. Centromere chromosome orientation fluorescent in situ hybridization (Cen-CO-FISH) detects sister chromatid exchange at the centromere in human cells. Bio Protoc 2018;8(7):e2792.

57. Williams ES, Cornforth MN, Goodwin EH, et al. CO-FISH, COD-FISH, ReD-FISH, SKY-FISH. Methods Mol Biol 2011;735:113–24.

58. Weise A, Gross M, Hinreiner S, et al. POD-FISH: a new technique for parental origin determination based on copy number variation polymorphism. Methods Mol Biol 2010;659:291–8.

59. Huber D, Kaigala GV. Rapid micro fluorescence in situ hybridization in tissue sections. Biomicrofluidics 2018;12(4):042212.

60. Beliveau BJ, Kishi JY, Nir G, et al. OligoMiner provides a rapid, flexible environment for the design of genome-scale oligonucleotide in situ hybridization probes. Proc Natl Acad Sci U S A 2018;115(10):E2183–92.

Precision Medicine Using Pharmacogenomic Panel-Testing

Current Status and Future Perspectives

Cathelijne H. van der Wouden, PharmD[a,b],
Henk-Jan Guchelaar, PharmD, PhD[a,b], Jesse J. Swen, PharmD, PhD[a,b,*]

KEYWORDS

• Pharmacogenomics • Panel-testing • Implementation • Adverse drug reactions

KEY POINTS

• Logistics and cost-effectiveness of pharmacogenomics (PGx)-guided prescribing may be optimized when delivered in a preemptive panel approach.
• Barriers impeding implementation of a preemptive PGx-panel approach include the lack of evidence of (cost-)effectiveness, the undetermined optimal target population and timing for delivering PGx, and the lack of tools supporting implementation.
• Developments in sequencing and artificial intelligence will further improve the predictive utility of genetic variation to predict drug response.

INTRODUCTION

Although drug treatment is often successful, adverse drug reactions (ADRs) and lack of efficacy present a significant burden for individual patients and society as a whole. ADRs are an important cause of emergency department visits and hospital admissions. A study in 2 large UK hospitals showed that 6.5% of hospital admissions were attributable to ADRs[1]. In the United States, ADR-related morbidity and mortality have been estimated at $30 billion to $136 billion annually[2]. In parallel, lack of efficacy also results in a significant burden. Its magnitude can be estimated by inspecting the number needed to treat of commonly used drugs[3], which are commonly more than 10.

This article originally appeared in *Advances in Molecular Pathology*, Volume 3, Issue 1, November 2020.

Funding: The research leading to these results has received funding from the European Community's Horizon 2020 Program under grant agreement no. 668353 (U-PGx).

[a] Department of Clinical Pharmacy & Toxicology, Leiden University Medical Center, Albinusdreef 2, Leiden 2333ZA, The Netherlands; [b] Leiden Network for Personalised Therapeutics, Leiden, The Netherlands
* Corresponding author. Albinusdreef 2, Postzone L0-P, Leiden 2333ZA, The Netherlands.
E-mail address: j.j.swen@lumc.nl

0272-2712/22/© 2022 The Author(s). Published by Elsevier Inc. All rights reserved.

As a result, most patients will not benefit from drug treatment and, in contrast, may experience harm from unsuccessfully treated disease. It has been estimated that $100 billion a year is wasted on ineffective drug treatment[4].

Precision medicine aims to individualize or stratify application of pharmacotherapy, as opposed to the current population-based application, in an effort to optimize the benefit/risk ratio[5,6]. By enabling identification of individuals who are at higher risk for ADRs or lack of efficacy, before drug initiation and potential harm, an individualized dose and drug selection may be applied to reduce this risk. An individual's germline genetic variation is a particularly promising predictive factor that can enable drug response prediction. This notion is supported by its pharmacologic plausibility and has been demonstrated in various studies[7–10]. Drug-gene interactions (DGIs) can be categorized into 3 groups (**Fig. 1A–C**): pharmacokinetic-dependent ADRs (see **Fig. 1A**), pharmacodynamic-dependent ADRs (see **Fig. 1B**), and idiosyncratic ADRs (see **Fig. 1C**).

Pharmacogenomics (PGx) uses an individual's germline genetic profile to identify those who are at higher risk for ADRs or lack of efficacy (see **Fig. 1D**)[11–13]. This information can be used by health care professionals (HCPs) to guide dose and drug selection before drug initiation in an effort to optimize drug therapy[14]. Within germline PGx, the focus lies on inherited variation in genes, which play a role in drug absorption, distribution, metabolism, and elimination (ADME). To date, several randomized controlled trials (RCT) support the clinical utility of individual DGIs to either optimize dosing[15–18] or drug selection[19,20]. Following the completion of the Human Genome Project, the Royal Dutch Pharmacists Association anticipated a proximate future where patients would present themselves in the pharmacy with their genetic information. In anticipation, the Dutch Pharmacogenetics Working Group (DPWG) was established in 2005 with the objective to develop clear guidelines for HCPs on how to interpret and apply PGx test results[21,22]. In parallel, the Clinical Pharmacogenetics Implementation Consortium was initiated in 2008 and devises similar guidelines[23].

Significant debate persists regarding the optimal timing and methodology of testing for delivering PGx testing in clinical care[24]. Some support a pretherapeutic single gene–drug approach, in which a PGx test of a single relevant gene is ordered once a target drug is prescribed, while others advocate for a preemptive panel-based strategy, in which multiple genes are tested simultaneously and saved for later use in preparation of future prescriptions throughout a patient's lifetime[25]. When combined with a clinical decision support system (CDSS), the corresponding PGx guideline can be deployed by the CDSS at the point of care, thereby providing clinicians with the necessary information to optimize drug prescribing, when a target drug is prescribed. A CDSS is deemed useful because patients will receive multiple drug prescriptions with potential DGIs within their lifetime[24,26]. It has been estimated that half of the patients older than 65 years will use at least one of the drugs for which PGx guidelines are available during a 4-year period, and one-fourth to one-third will use 2 or more of these drugs[27]. Logistics and cost-effectiveness are therefore optimized when delivered in a preemptive panel-based approach; pharmacotherapy does not have to be delayed, in awaiting single-gene testing results, and costs for genotyping are minimized, because marginal acquisition costs of testing and interpreting additional pharmacogenes is near zero[28]. When PGx is adopted in such a model, it has been estimated that 23.6% of all indecent prescriptions will have a relevant DGI[29]. To date, a small number of individual genes are tested pretherapeutically to guide pharmacotherapy of high-risk drugs. For example, *DPYD*-guided initial drug and dose selection of fluoropyridines to reduce risk of severe toxicity has been widely implemented in the Netherlands[30]. Despite the progress in application of PGx in single-gene scenarios,

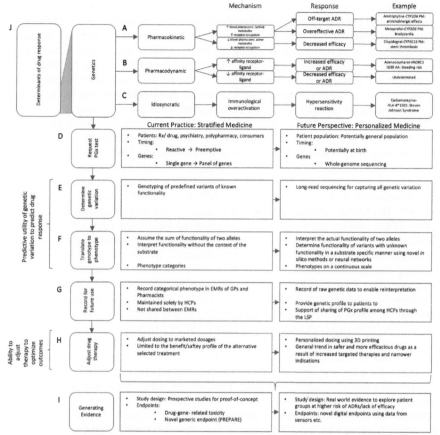

Fig. 1. Precision medicine using pharmacogenomic panel testing: current status and future perspectives. conc., concentration; PM, poor metabolizers; Rx, prescription.

a preemptive PGx-panel approach is still not routinely applied. As such, several barriers preventing the implementation of preemptive panel testing have been identified[31–33]. Remaining barriers include the lack of evidence of (cost-)effectiveness supporting a PGx-panel approach, the undetermined optimal target population, and timing for delivering a PGx panel and the lack of tools supporting implementation. These remaining barriers and steps to overcome them are discussed in this review. Furthermore, the authors discuss future perspectives of these domains.

THE LACK OF EVIDENCE OF (COST-) EFFECTIVENESS SUPPORTING A PHARMACOGENOMICS-PANEL APPROACH

Several of the reported hurdles obstructing the implementation of PGx-panel testing are currently being addressed by various initiatives, in both the United States and the European Union. Overviews of these initiatives have previously been published[24,34]. Despite these initiatives, a major hurdle preventing implementation is the absence of evidence presenting the collective clinical utility of a panel of PGx markers for preemptive PGx testing. Although several RCT support the clinical utility of individual gene-drug pairs, delivered in a single-gene reactive approach[15–20], evidence supporting clinical utility of the remaining DGIs for which recommendations are available when delivered in a preemptive panel approach is lacking. Significant debate persists regarding both the nature and the strength of evidence required for the clinical application of these remaining DGIs. Some argue an RCT is required for each individual DGI before clinical implementation is substantiated[35]. Others argue that a mandatory requirement for prospective evidence to support the clinical validity for each PGx interaction is incongruous and excessive[36–39]. Generating gold-standard evidence for each individual DGI for which PGx guidelines are available separately would require unrealistically large amounts of funds. On the other hand, extrapolating efficacy of all of these DGIs based on the conclusions of the previously mentioned RCTs, supporting clinical utility for a subset of individual DGIs, is also not substantiated.

Regardless of the inconvenience, there is still a demand for evidence substantiating patient benefit and cost-effectiveness, to enable stakeholders to practice evidence-based medicine. The Ubiquitous Pharmacogenomics Consortium (U-PGx), a European Consortium funded by the Horizon 2020 program, aims to generate such evidence[34]. The U-PGx consortium set out to quantify the collective clinical utility of a panel of PGx markers (50 variants in 13 pharmacogenes) within a single trial (the PREPARE study, ClinicalTrials.gov: NCT03093818) as a proof-of-concept across multiple potentially clinically relevant DGIs[34,40]. It is a block RCT aiming to enroll 8100 patients across 7 European countries. Additional outcomes include cost-effectiveness, process indicators for implementation, and provider adoption of PGx.

In the meantime, several smaller randomized and observational studies indicate the cost-effectiveness of PGx panel–based testing in psychiatry and polypharmacy patients[41–44]. Observed cost savings ranged from $218[42] to $2778[45] per patient. Others have modeled the cost-effectiveness of one-time genetic testing to minimize a lifetime of ADRs and concluded an incremental cost-effectiveness ratio (ICER) of $43,165 per additional life-year and $53,680 per additional quality-adjusted life-year, therefore considered cost-effective[46]. However, cost-effectiveness may vary across ethnic populations, as a result of differences in allele frequencies, differences in prescription patterns, and differences in health care costs and ICER cost-effectiveness thresholds. The study designed by the U-PGx consortium (the PREPARE Study) will enable the quantification of the cost-effectiveness over a 12-week time horizon.

Clinical trials and prospective cohorts typically measure short-term benefits of PGx testing, whereas the time horizon for the benefits and risks of PGx testing is over a lifetime and therefore unable to be captured within regular trials. As such, the life-long cost-effectiveness of one-time preemptive panel-based testing to prevent ADRs is yet undetermined. Other methodologies, such as Markov models, can be deployed to simulate effectiveness over longer time horizons. The results of such models will be of interest to reimbursement policymakers, who require evidence that panel-based testing will yield downstream improved health outcomes at acceptable costs. Therefore, once the effectiveness of PGx-panel testing has been established, future research should model the cost-effectiveness of preemptive PGx testing to prevent a lifetime of ADRs. Optimally, such an analysis could be run on a longitudinal cohort of patients for which both prescription data and PGx results are available. Furthermore, such a data set could be used to explore the optimal timing and subgroup application of testing to optimize cost-effectiveness.

FINDING THE OPTIMAL TARGET POPULATION AND TIMING FOR DELIVERING PHARMACOGENOMICS

The optimal target population and time at which panel-based testing should be performed remain to be determined. In the most progressive application of PGx panel-testing could be performed when no drug initiation is indicated, in anticipation of future drug prescriptions. However, if no drug is initiated in the near future, PGx testing would be a waste of resources. Alternatively, in a more efficient scenario, panel testing could be performed once a patient plans to initiate a drug for which PGx testing may be useful and reuse these results when future DGIs are encountered. Such a model was deployed in a pilot study[47], whereby pharmacists requested a PGx-panel test when patients planned to initiate one of 10 drugs for which PGx guidelines are available. Here, 97% of patients (re)used PGx-panel results for at least one, and 33% for up to 4 newly initiated prescriptions with possible DGIs within a 2.5-year follow-up. In this case, 24% were actionable DGIs, requiring pharmacotherapy adjustment. This high rate of reuse indicates that such a model may be promising for delivering PGx panel-based testing. As an alternative model, another initiative at Vanderbilt University Medical Center has used a prediction model to select patients who may benefit from PGx testing in the near future algorithmically and using prescription data[48,49].

In addition to undetermined timing and methodology, the most optimal target group for testing is also yet undetermined. Current studies have identified potential patient subgroups for which preemptive PGx-panel testing may be most useful. Some initiatives have selected patients with particular indications in psychiatry[43,44,50,51]. Others have selected patients with particular characteristics, such as polypharmacy and elderly patients[41,42].

Alternatively, consumers who have an interest in their PGx profile may also obtain their PGx test results outside the realm of health care and without the intervention of an HCP. In 2018, direct-to-consumer (DTC) PGx testing for specific DGIs was approved by the Food and Drug Administration (FDA). However, in contrast to DTC tests provided before 2013, the FDA has approved only a limited scope of 33 variants in 8 genes, and providers have mandated the need to retest. Concerns of DTC PGx testing have been reported to relate to patient actions (eg, to stop taking a prescribed medication or adjusting the regimen based on genotype without consultation with a health provider)[52]. However, a longitudinal study of DTC consumers showed that only 5.6% of consumers reported changing a medication they were taking or starting a new medication because of their PGx results. Of these, 45 (83.3%) reported consulting with an HCP regarding the change[53]. Nonetheless, the involvement of HCPs will optimize the use of PGx results when delivered in a DTC setting. In the same longitudinal study, the authors found that 63% of consumers planned to share their results with a primary care provider. However, at 6-month follow-up, only 27% reported having done so, and 8% reported sharing with another HCP. Among participants who discussed results with their PCP, 35% were very satisfied with the encounter, and 18% were not at all satisfied. These results indicate that PGx testing in a DTC model may be a safe model for obtaining PGx testing.

THE LACK OF TOOLS SUPPORTING IMPLEMENTATION OF PHARMACOGENOMICS-PANEL TESTING
Development of a Pharmacogenomics Panel to Facilitate Implementation

Another important challenge hampering adoption of preemptive panel testing is the lack of standardization regarding variants included in such panels. Standardization would enable clinicians to understand PGx test results without extensive scrutiny of the alleles included in the panel. Despite the identification of standardization as a potential accelerator for PGx adoption, exchange, and continuity[54], there are currently no standards defining which variants should be tested[55,56]. Although some initiatives have developed standardized panels of relevant variants within individual genes[57], and other initiatives across multiple genes[58], a panel covering widely accepted genetic variants reflecting an entire set of guidelines is not yet available. Thus, in order to facilitate the clinical implementation of PGx testing, the U-PGx consortium set out to develop a pan-European panel based on actionable DPWG guidelines, called the "PGx-Passport"[59]. Here, germline variant alleles were systematically selected using predefined criteria regarding allele population frequencies, effect on protein functionality, and association with drug response. A "PGx-Passport" of 58 germline variant alleles, located within 14 genes (CYP2B6, CYP2C9, CYP2C19, CYP2D6, CYP3A5, DPYD, F5, HLA-A, HLA-B, NUDT15, SLCO1B1, TPMT, UGT1A1 and VKORC1), was composed. This "PGx-Passport" can be used in combination with the DPWG guidelines to optimize drug prescribing for 49 commonly prescribed drugs. An advantage of the approach is that the number of clinically interpretable results within their "PGx-Passport" is maximized, while costs remain reasonable.

Importantly, the presented panel will not be able to fully identify those at risk for unwanted drug response. The overall ability of a panel to predict drug response is dependent on, first, the predictive utility of genetic variation to predict drug response and, second, the ability to adjust pharmacotherapy to reduce the risk of unwanted effects among high-risk individuals. In the following sections, the current limitations of both domains are further elaborated.

Current predictive utility of genetic variation to predict drug response

Even though multiple genetic variants have been discovered, the authors currently restrict testing to a subset of these variants. However, restricting testing to individual variants disregards untested or undiscovered variants that may also influence the functionality of the gene product. Therefore, the functionality of the gene product cannot be fully predicted (see **Fig. 1E**). Reasons for restriction of testing are twofold. First, technical limitations regarding the sequencing of complex loci prevent complete determination of both the gene of interest and other areas in the genome, which may have an effect on the gene product. Determining genetic variation is specifically difficult in highly polymorphic genes, such as the HLA genes, or genes located near pseudogenes, such as CYP2D6. Although sequencing of these loci is technically possible, it are costly and time-consuming. Second, even if one were to determine all genetic variation, the downstream effect on protein functionality may be unknown and therefore impossible to interpret clinically[60].

However, progress in the interpretation of functional consequences of such uncharacterized variations may support future interpretation in silico[61], in vitro, or in vivo[62]. Importantly, a study has shown that 92.9% of genetic variation in ADME genes is rare, and an estimated 30% to 40% of functional variability in pharmacogenes can be attributed to these variants[63]. In addition to the downstream functionality, the penetrance (ie, the potential of a variant to accurately predict the genetic component of drug response) is also unknown. The penetrance is a function of both the variant's effect on protein functionality and the extent to which the protein functionality is associated with clinical outcome. Significant debate persists regarding both the nature and the strength of evidence required for the clinical application of variant alleles of unknown functionality. Because the strength of these functions differs across genes and DGIs, the authors do not foresee a one-size-fits-all consensus regarding and evidence threshold across all DGIs, but rather a different evidence threshold per individual DGI based on the genetics and pharmacology of the interaction. For example, in the case of the TPMT-thiopurine interaction, the effect of TPMT variation on protein functionality has been firmly established because it exhibits behavior similar to monogenetic codominant traits[64]. Therefore, identified variants in TPMT (*3A/*3B/*3C) are considered to have sufficient evidence to be applied in the clinic. The clinical interpretation has been clinically validated in a study specifically investigating clinical effects in patients carrying these variants[18]. On the other hand, clinically relevant variant alleles in *CYP2D6* are based on the pharmacology of the interaction. For example, the flecainide-*CYP2D6* interaction is based on the associations between decreasing *CYP2D6* activity leading to increasing flecainide plasma levels, which in turn leads to increased risk for flecainide intoxication. Therefore, all identified variants in *CYP2D6*, shown to have a significant effect on CYP2D6 enzyme activity, are considered clinically applicable. As such, both the functional effects and the penetrance of many rare variants are yet unknown. As an additional complication, these may also differ across substrates and drug responses. Even more fundamentally, variants may impact each other's functionality, and therefore, individual variants may have different functionalities depending on the absence or presence of other variants.

Another significant limitation, which is applicable to PGx testing and interpretation as it is performed today, is that predicted phenotypes are interpreted as categories rather than continuous scores, and it is assumed the sum of both alleles equals total metabolic capacity (see **Fig. 1**F). For example, for *CYP2D6*, patients are categorized into normal metabolizers, intermediate metabolizers, poor metabolizers, or ultrarapid metabolizers. However, the actual *CYP2D6* phenotype is likely normally distributed[65,66]. Imposing categorization, as opposed to the interpretation of the actual diplotype, therefore sacrifices information in order to simplify clinical interpretation. In the process, the functionality of each allele is interpreted individually, and it is assumed that the sum of these activity scores equals the total activity of the diplotype. Furthermore, these categorizations are currently substrate independent, even though the effects on metabolic capacity are known to differ between substrates[67].

Current ability to adjust pharmacotherapy to optimize outcomes
In addition to the ability of genetic variation to predict drug response, the second component determining the utility of PGx-guided pharmacotherapy is the ability to adjust pharmacotherapy to the specific genetic variants. Currently, there are 2 options to reduce the risk of ADRs and lack of efficacy: (1) selecting another drug and (2) adjusting the dose (see **Fig. 1**H).

A successful example of choosing an alternative therapy to avoid an ADR is preemptive testing for *HLA-B*57:01* to guide drug selection for abacavir or another antiretroviral. Here, 0% of the prospectively screened group versus 2.7% of the control group experienced immunologically confirmed hypersensitivity[19]. In this example, the PGx intervention and subsequent adjustment completely eliminated the risk of hypersensitivity.

An example of adjusting the dose to reduce the risk of ADRs is preemptive testing for *TPMT* to guide dose selection of thiopurines to reduce the risk of severe hematologic ADRs[18]. In contrast to the previously described abacavir/*HLA-B*57:01* example, this intervention has a smaller effect size. Here, severe hematologic ADRs still occurred in 2.6% of *TPMT* variant carriers who received an adjusted dose, compared with 22.9% of *TPMT* variant carriers treated with a normal dose. Although dose adjustment prevented ~89% of severe hematologic ADRs, the remaining ~11% could not be prevented by this intervention. Indeed, this could partially be a result of the sensitivity of *TPMT* testing not reaching 100%, but could also be due to the fact that dose reduction was not sufficient for avoiding this ADR. Furthermore, the incidence of severe hematological ADRs among noncarriers of *TPMT* variants was 7.3%, indicating that other (genetic) factors, such as *NUDT15*, may play a role in the risk of severe hematological ADRs.

Enable Recording of Pharmacogenomics-Panel Results for Future Use

To enable preemptive PGx testing, it is imperative that the PGx test results are recorded in the electronic medical records (EMRs) for future use (see **Fig. 1**G). Within a pilot study, the authors found that both pharmacists and general practitioners (GPs) are able to record PGx results in their EMRs as contraindications (96% and 33% of pharmacists and GPs, respectively), enabling the deployment of relevant guidelines by the CDSS when a DGI is encountered at both prescribing and dispensing[47]. In contrast, a recent study showed that genotyping results were sparsely communicated and recorded correctly; only 3.1% and 5.9% of reported genotyping results were recorded by GPs and pharmacists, respectively, within a similar follow-up time of 2.36 years[68].

FUTURE PERSPECTIVES
Generating Evidence for Effectiveness of Precision Medicine Approaches

In an era where digitalization is driving data accumulation and a concomitant increase in stratification of patient groups and a more precise diagnosis, we are moving toward the utilization of real-world data to support precision medicine (see **Fig. 1**I). Several investigators have pointed out that precision medicine, and genomic medicine, in particular, would benefit from a convergence of implementation science and a learning health system to measure outcomes and generate evidence across a large population[69,70]. However, this requires standardization of outcomes in EMRs to enable aggregation of phenotype data across large populations for both discovery and outcomes assessment within a genomic medicine implementation[71]. Many nationwide, large-scale initiatives are generating prospective longitudinal evidence supporting precision medicine approaches[72–74]. For example, a landmark project specifically generating evidence for PGx is the All of Us project[75]. Alternatively, pragmatic clinical trials offer researchers a means to study precision medicine interventions in real-world settings[76,77]. In contrast to traditional clinical trials that are performed in ideal conditions, these pragmatic trials are conducted in the context of usual care[77]. Pragmatic clinical trials easily transition into existing health care infrastructures and therefore make them particularly appealing to comparative effectiveness research and the evidence-based mission of learning health care systems[78,79]. An example of such a pragmatic trial for generating evidence for preemptive PGx testing is the I-PICC study[80].

In parallel, evolving digital health technologies are driving data accumulation. Data collected by sensors (in smartphones, wearables, and ingestibles), mobile apps, and social media can be processed by machine learning to support medical decision making[81]. Raw sensor data can also be processed into digital biomarkers and endpoints[82]. This development may be particularly useful for endpoint definition in disease areas where biological endpoints are lacking, such as in psychiatry and neurology, to enable quantification of disease progression and drug response. For example, novel digital endpoints are being developed to stratify mental health conditions and predict remission using passively collected smartphone data[83]. Another example is the development of a digital biomarker for Parkinson disease using motor active tests and passive monitoring through a smartphone[84]. For precision medicine, in particular, we may also be more able to stratify patient groups into responders and nonresponders with improved endpoint development in these disease areas. Increased stratification of patient groups on the basis of genetic, (digital) biomarker, phenotypic, of psychosocial characteristics will drive more precise diagnoses and pharmacotherapy optimization[85,86]. This trend will drive demand for innovations for more efficient study designs because of increasing numbers of indications, whereas resources to fund these trials remain constant[87].

Determining Optimal Timing and Target Group for Pharmacogenomics-Panel Testing

Consensus regarding who should be tested, and when it is most cost-effective to perform preemptive panel-testing, remains undetermined[28]. Moreover, the most cost-effective technique to determine the PGx profile is also undetermined. As novel DGIs are discovered, it may be more efficient to sequence whole genomes, to avoid testing of additional variants through genotyping over time. Clinically relevant PGx variants can successfully be extracted from sequencing data using bioinformatics pipelines[88,89]. As the cost of sequencing techniques decrease, genotype-based testing will become obsolete. In this case, it may be more cost-effective to perform population-wide sequencing at birth, to ensure the maximization of instances in which a PGx result is available when a DGI is encountered. However, whole-exome sequencing and whole-genome sequencing are increasingly applied for other medical indications and objectives[90,91]. As this development expands, determining the cost-effectiveness of implementing PGx testing may become redundant, because the information on PGx variants becomes secondary findings, free of additional costs.

Improving Predictive Utility of Genetic Variation to Predict Drug Response

Recent advances have been made to improve the ability to determine an individual's genetic variation. Technical limitations regarding the sequencing of complex loci may be overcome by advances in long-read sequencing technologies and synthetic long-read assembly[92]. As a result, an increasing number of variants with unknown functionality will need to be interpreted. Because of the vast increasing number of rare variants, it is impossible to determine functionality in traditional expression systems. To overcome this challenge, advances have been made in the development of in silico methods to predict functionality. However, these methods are based on genes that are evolutionarily highly conserved. Because many ADME genes are only poorly conserved, steps have been taken to calibrate in silico models on data sets. For example, recently investigators developed a novel computational functionality prediction model optimized for pharmacogenetic assessments, which substantially outperformed standard algorithms[62].

Nonetheless, these models still do not enable prediction of the functionality of synonymous mutations, intronic variants, or variants in noncoding regions of the genome. Recent initiatives have provided an alternative method for the interpretation of variants with unknown functionality using machine learning[65,93], one using an existing data set for model training and the other using a mock data set. In the first, the investigators trained a neural network model on the long-read sequencing profiles of CYP2D6 of 561 patients and used the metabolic ratio between tamoxifen and endoxifen as an outcome measure. The model explains 79% of the interindividual variability in CYP2D6 activity compared with 55% with the conventional categorization approach. In addition, this model is capable of assigning accurate enzyme activity to alleles containing previously uncharacterized combinations of variants. The suggested model has provided a method to determine predicted phenotype on a continuous scale. Indeed, enzyme activity may be expected to be normally distributed within a population and therefore better described by such a scale. A future is envisioned where phenotypes can be predicted more precisely by using all of an individual's genetic variation, as opposed to limiting the view only to those variants included in a tested panel.

Following a further understanding of the effects of individual variants to inform phenotype prediction on a continuous scale, one can imagine that this phenotype prediction will ultimately become substrate specific on top of gene specific. More fundamentally, in PGx, the view is currently limited to a single DGI, whereas multiple genes may be involved in the metabolism of drugs and their metabolites. If one were to expand their view to multiple genes involved to predict drug response, the predictive utility will further improve. To incorporate genetic variations of multiple genes, polygenic risk scores may prove useful[94].

Although genetics is considered the causal anchor of biological processes[95], the biological mechanism underlying drug response may be downstream of a genetic variant. In these cases, genetics will have no predictive utility for drug response (see **Fig. 1**J, top left). Therefore, incorporating processes downstream of the genome, such as the epigenome[96], transcriptome, microbiome[97], and metabolome[98], may further optimize the ability to predict drug response to enable more accurate stratification of patient populations. Combining these profiles in a systems medicine approach may have a synergistic effect.

Improving Ability to Adjust Pharmacotherapy to Optimize Outcomes

In the future, pharmacotherapy adjustment may be further improved by imminent technologies, such as 3-dimensional (3D) printing to enable personalized dosing and delivery[99]. Currently, the DPWG calculates specific dose adjustments based on pharmacokinetic studies and rounds the recommended dose to the nearest corresponding marketed dose for clinical feasibility. The utilization of 3D-printing technologies may enable rapid compounding of tablets with a specific dose based on an individual's genetic profile. In any case, adjustment of the pharmacotherapy will always be limited by the safety profile of available drugs. Opportunely, over the last decades, newly developed drugs have been shifting from unspecific small molecules to more targeted drugs in the form of humanized monoclonal antibodies[100], cell therapies[101], and gene therapies[102] with fewer off-target ADRs.

Recording Pharmacogenomics-Panel Results for Future Use

Future initiatives should focus on the development of automated sharing of PGx results across EMRs. In the Netherlands, such an initiative has been launched but requires patient consent before it can be used. The National Exchange Point ("Landelijk Schakel Punt" [LSP]) is a nationwide secured EMR infrastructure to which nearly all HCPs can access[103]. Only when a patient has provided written consent for the LSP can a professional summary of the local pharmacy or GP EMR, including PGx results, be downloaded by another treating HCP in the same region, unless the patient chose to shield this information. Alternatively, providing the PGx results directly to patients may resolve the issue in terms of communicating and recording PGx results; for example, using the MSC safety-code card as used in the PREPARE study[104,105].

SUMMARY

In conclusion, developments in evidence generation and in genetic sequencing and interpretation will revolutionize current stratified medicine to enable true precision medicine, whereby multiple -omics profiles of an individual are combined to predict drug response and optimize pharmacotherapy accordingly.

DISCLOSURE

The authors have nothing to disclose.

REFERENCES

1. Pirmohamed M, James S, Meakin S, et al. Adverse drug reactions as cause of admission to hospital: prospective analysis of 18 820 patients. BMJ 2004; 329(7456):15-9.
2. Johnson JA, Bootman JL. Drug-related morbidity and mortality. A cost-of-illness model. Arch Intern Med 1995;155(18):1949-56.
3. Therapy (NNT) Reviews. Available at: https://www.thennt.com/home-nnt/#nntblack. Accessed November 11, 2019.
4. Harper AR, Topol EJ. Pharmacogenomics in clinical practice and drug development. Nat Biotechnol 2012;30(11):1117-24.
5. Jameson JL, Longo DL. Precision medicine–personalized, problematic, and promising. N Engl J Med 2015;372(23):2229-34.
6. Peck RW. Precision medicine is not just genomics: the right dose for every patient. Annu Rev Pharmacol Toxicol 2018;58:105-22.
7. Matthaei J, Brockmoller J, Tzvetkov MV, et al. Heritability of metoprolol and torsemide pharmacokinetics. Clin Pharmacol Ther 2015;98(6):611-21.
8. Alexanderson B, Evans DA, Sjoqvist F. Steady-state plasma levels of nortriptyline in twins: influence of genetic factors and drug therapy. Br Med J 1969; 4(5686):764-8.
9. Vesell ES, Page JG. Genetic control of drug levels in man: phenylbutazone. Science 1968;159(3822):1479-80.
10. Stage TB, Damkier P, Pedersen RS, et al. A twin study of the trough plasma steady-state concentration of metformin. Pharmacogenet Genomics 2015; 25(5):259-62.
11. Relling MV, Evans WE. Pharmacogenomics in the clinic. Nature 2015;526(7573): 343-50.
12. Weinshilboum R, Wang L. Pharmacogenomics: bench to bedside. Nat Rev Drug Discov 2004;3(9):739-48.
13. Roden DM, McLeod HL, Relling MV, et al. Pharmacogenomics. Lancet 2019; 394(10197):521-32.
14. Pirmohamed M. Personalized pharmacogenomics: predicting efficacy and adverse drug reactions. Annu Rev Genomics Hum Genet 2014;15:349-70.
15. Pirmohamed M, Burnside G, Eriksson N, et al. A randomized trial of genotype-guided dosing of warfarin. N Engl J Med 2013;369(24):2294-303.
16. Wu AH. Pharmacogenomic testing and response to warfarin. Lancet 2015; 385(9984):2231-2.
17. Verhoef TI, Ragia G, de Boer A, et al. A randomized trial of genotype-guided dosing of acenocoumarol and phenprocoumon. New Engl J Med 2013; 369(24):2304-12.
18. Coenen MJ, de Jong DJ, van Marrewijk CJ, et al. Identification of patients with variants in TPMT and dose reduction reduces hematologic events during thiopurine treatment of inflammatory bowel disease. Gastroenterology 2015; 149(4):907-17.e7.
19. Mallal S, Phillips E, Carosi G, et al. HLA-B*5701 screening for hypersensitivity to abacavir. N Engl J Med 2008;358(6):568-79.
20. Claassens DMF, Vos GJA, Bergmeijer TO, et al. A genotype-guided strategy for oral P2Y12 inhibitors in primary PCI. N Engl J Med 2019;381(17):1621-31.
21. Swen JJ, Nijenhuis M, de Boer A, et al. Pharmacogenetics: from bench to byte–an update of guidelines. Clin Pharmacol Ther 2011;89(5):662-73.

22. Swen JJ, Wilting I, de Goede AL, et al. Pharmacogenetics: from bench to byte. Clin Pharmacol Ther 2008;83(5):781–7.

23. Relling MV, Klein TE. CPIC: clinical pharmacogenetics implementation consortium of the pharmacogenomics research network. Clin Pharmacol Ther 2011;89(3):464–7.

24. Dunnenberger HM, Crews KR, Hoffman JM, et al. Preemptive clinical pharmacogenetics implementation: current programs in five US medical centers. Annu Rev Pharmacol Toxicol 2015;55:89–106.

25. Weitzel KW, Cavallari LH, Lesko LJ. Preemptive panel-based pharmacogenetic testing: the time is now. Pharm Res 2017;34(8):1551–5.

26. Driest VSL, Shi Y, Bowton EA, et al. Clinically actionable genotypes among 10,000 patients with preemptive pharmacogenomic testing. Clin Pharmacol Ther 2014;95(4):423–31.

27. Samwald M, Xu H, Blagec K, et al. Incidence of exposure of patients in the United States to multiple drugs for which pharmacogenomic guidelines are available. PLoS One 2016;11(10):e0164972.

28. Roden DM, Van Driest SL, Mosley JD, et al. Benefit of preemptive pharmacogenetic information on clinical outcome. Clin Pharmacol Ther 2018;103(5):787–94.

29. Bank PCD, Swen JJ, Guchelaar HJ. Estimated nationwide impact of implementing a preemptive pharmacogenetic panel approach to guide drug prescribing in primary care in The Netherlands. BMC Med 2019;17(1):110.

30. Lunenburg CA, van Staveren MC, Gelderblom H, et al. Evaluation of clinical implementation of prospective DPYD genotyping in 5-fluorouracil- or capecitabine-treated patients. Pharmacogenomics 2016;17(7):721–9.

31. Abbasi J. Getting pharmacogenomics into the clinic. JAMA 2016;316(15): 1533–5.

32. Haga SB, Burke W. Pharmacogenetic testing: not as simple as it seems. Genet Med 2008;10(6):391–5.

33. Swen JJ, Huizinga TW, Gelderblom H, et al. Translating pharmacogenomics: challenges on the road to the clinic. PLoS Med 2007;4(8):e209.

34. van der Wouden CH, Cambon-Thomsen A, Cecchin E, et al. Implementing pharmacogenomics in Europe: design and implementation strategy of the Ubiquitous Pharmacogenomics consortium. Clin Pharmacol Ther 2017;101(3):341–58.

35. Janssens AC, Deverka PA. Useless until proven effective: the clinical utility of preemptive pharmacogenetic testing. Clin Pharmacol Ther 2014;96(6):652–4.

36. Altman RB. Pharmacogenomics: "noninferiority" is sufficient for initial implementation. Clin Pharmacol Ther 2011;89(3):348–50.

37. van der Wouden CH, Swen JJ, Schwab M, et al. A brighter future for the implementation of pharmacogenomic testing. Eur J Hum Genet 2016;24(12):1658–60.

38. Pirmohamed M, Hughes DA. Pharmacogenetic tests: the need for a level playing field. Nat Rev Drug Discov 2013;12(1):3–4.

39. Khoury MJ. Dealing with the evidence dilemma in genomics and personalized medicine. Clin Pharmacol Ther 2010;87(6):635–8.

40. Manson LE, van der Wouden CH, Swen JJ, et al. The Ubiquitous Pharmacogenomics Consortium: making effective treatment optimization accessible to every European citizen. Pharmacogenomics 2017;18(11):1041–5.

41. Elliott LS, Henderson JC, Neradilek MB, et al. Clinical impact of pharmacogenetic profiling with a clinical decision support tool in polypharmacy home health patients: a prospective pilot randomized controlled trial. PLoS One 2017;12(2): e0170905.

42. Brixner D, Biltaji E, Bress A, et al. The effect of pharmacogenetic profiling with a clinical decision support tool on healthcare resource utilization and estimated costs in the elderly exposed to polypharmacy. J Med Econ 2016;19(3):213–28.

43. Pérez V, Salavert A, Espadaler J, et al. Efficacy of prospective pharmacogenetic testing in the treatment of major depressive disorder: results of a randomized, double-blind clinical trial. BMC Psychiatry 2017;17(1):250.

44. Espadaler J, Tuson M, Lopez-Ibor JM, et al. Pharmacogenetic testing for the guidance of psychiatric treatment: a multicenter retrospective analysis. CNS Spectr 2017;22(4):315–24.

45. Winner JG, Carhart JM, Altar CA, et al. Combinatorial pharmacogenomic guidance for psychiatric medications reduces overall pharmacy costs in a 1 year prospective evaluation. Curr Med Res Opin 2015;31(9):1633–43.

46. Alagoz O, Durham D, Kasirajan K. Cost-effectiveness of one-time genetic testing to minimize lifetime adverse drug reactions. Pharmacogenomics J 2015;16(2):129–36.

47. van der Wouden CH, Bank PCD, Ozokcu K, et al. Pharmacist-initiated preemptive pharmacogenetic panel testing with clinical decision support in primary care: record of PGx results and real-world impact. Genes (Basel) 2019; 10(6):416.

48. Pulley JM, Denny JC, Peterson JF, et al. Operational implementation of prospective genotyping for personalized medicine: the design of the Vanderbilt PREDICT project. Clin Pharmacol Ther 2012;92(1):87–95.

49. Grice GR, Seaton TL, Woodland AM, et al. Defining the opportunity for pharmacogenetic intervention in primary care. Pharmacogenomics 2006;7(1):61–5.

50. Bradley P, Shiekh M, Mehra V, et al. Improved efficacy with targeted pharmacogenetic-guided treatment of patients with depression and anxiety: a randomized clinical trial demonstrating clinical utility. J Psychiatr Res 2018;96: 100–7.

51. Walden LM, Brandl EJ, Tiwari AK, et al. Genetic testing for CYP2D6 and CYP2C19 suggests improved outcome for antidepressant and antipsychotic medication. Psychiatry Res 2018;279:111–5.

52. Haga SB. Managing increased accessibility to pharmacogenomic data. Clin Pharmacol Ther 2019;106(5):922–4.

53. Carere DA, VanderWeele TJ, Vassy JL, et al. Prescription medication changes following direct-to-consumer personal genomic testing: findings from the Impact of Personal Genomics (PGen) Study. Genet Med 2017;19(5):537–45.

54. Caudle KE, Keeling NJ, Klein TE, et al. Standardization can accelerate the adoption of pharmacogenomics: current status and the path forward. Pharmacogenomics 2018;19(10):847–60.

55. Pratt VM, Everts RE, Aggarwal P, et al. Characterization of 137 genomic DNA reference materials for 28 pharmacogenetic genes: a GeT-RM collaborative project. J Mol Diagn 2016;18(1):109–23.

56. Pratt VM, Zehnbauer B, Wilson J, et al. Characterization of 107 genomic DNA reference materials for CYP2D6, CYP2C19, CYP2C9, VKORC1, and UGT1A1: a GeT-RM and Association for Molecular Pathology collaborative project. J Mol Diagn 2010;12(6):835–46.

57. Pratt VM, Del Tredici AL, Hachad H, et al. Recommendations for clinical CYP2C19 genotyping allele selection: a report of the association for molecular pathology. J Mol Diagn 2018;20(3):269–76.

58. Bush WS, Crosslin DR, Owusu-Obeng A, et al. Genetic variation among 82 pharmacogenes: the PGRNseq data from the eMERGE network. Clin Pharmacol Ther 2016;100(2):160–9.

59. Van der Wouden CH, Van Rhenen MH, Jama W, et al. Development of the PGx-passport: a panel of actionable germline genetic variants for pre-emptive pharmacogenetic testing. Clin Pharmacol Ther 2019;106(4):866–73.

60. Drogemoller BI, Wright GE, Warnich L. Considerations for rare variants in drug metabolism genes and the clinical implications. Expert Opin Drug Metab Toxicol 2014;10(6):873–84.

61. Li B, Seligman C, Thusberg J, et al. In silico comparative characterization of pharmacogenomic missense variants. BMC Genomics 2014;15(Suppl 4):S4.

62. Zhou Y, Mkrtchian S, Kumondai M, et al. An optimized prediction framework to assess the functional impact of pharmacogenetic variants. Pharmacogenomics J 2019;19(2):115–26.

63. Kozyra M, Ingelman-Sundberg M, Lauschke VM. Rare genetic variants in cellular transporters, metabolic enzymes, and nuclear receptors can be important determinants of interindividual differences in drug response. Genet Med 2016;19(1):20–9.

64. Weinshilboum RM, Sladek SL. Mercaptopurine pharmacogenetics: monogenic inheritance of erythrocyte thiopurine methyltransferase activity. Am J Hum Genet 1980;32(5):651–62.

65. van der Lee M, Allard WG, Vossen RHAM, et al. A unifying model to predict variable drug response for personalised medicine. Biorxiv. 2020:2020.2003.2002.967554.

66. Hertz DL, Rae J. Pharmacogenetics of cancer drugs. Annu Rev Med 2015;66: 65–81.

67. Hicks JK, Swen JJ, Gaedigk A. Challenges in CYP2D6 phenotype assignment from genotype data: a critical assessment and call for standardization. Curr Drug Metab 2014;15(2):218–32.

68. Simoons M, Mulder H, Schoevers RA, et al. Availability of CYP2D6 genotyping results in general practitioner and community pharmacy medical records. Pharmacogenomics 2017;18(9):843–51.

69. Chambers DA, Feero WG, Khoury MJ. Convergence of implementation science, precision medicine, and the learning health care system: a new model for biomedical research. JAMA 2016;315(18):1941–2.

70. Lu CY, Williams MS, Ginsburg GS, et al. A proposed approach to accelerate evidence generation for genomic-based technologies in the context of a learning health system. Genet Med 2018;20(4):390–6.

71. Peterson JF, Roden DM, Orlando LA, et al. Building evidence and measuring clinical outcomes for genomic medicine. Lancet 2019;394(10198):604–10.

72. Turnbull C, Scott RH, Thomas E, et al. The 100 000 Genomes Project: bringing whole genome sequencing to the NHS. BMJ 2018;361:k1687.

73. Gottesman O, Scott SA, Ellis SB, et al. The CLIPMERGE PGx Program: clinical implementation of personalized medicine through electronic health records and genomics-pharmacogenomics. Clin Pharmacol Ther 2013;94(2):214–7.

74. Leitsalu L, Haller T, Esko T, et al. Cohort profile: estonian biobank of the Estonian Genome Center, University of Tartu. Int J Epidemiol 2015;44(4):1137–47.

75. Collins FS, Varmus H. A new initiative on precision medicine. N Engl J Med 2015;372(9):793–5.

76. Khoury MJ, Rich EC, Randhawa G, et al. Comparative effectiveness research and genomic medicine: an evolving partnership for 21st century medicine. Genet Med 2009;11(10):707–11.
77. Ford I, Norrie J. Pragmatic trials. N Engl J Med 2016;375(5):454–63.
78. Fiore LD, Lavori PW. Integrating randomized comparative effectiveness research with patient care. N Engl J Med 2016;374(22):2152–8.
79. Weinfurt KP, Hernandez AF, Coronado GD, et al. Pragmatic clinical trials embedded in healthcare systems: generalizable lessons from the NIH Collaboratory. BMC Med Res Methodol 2017;17(1):144.
80. Brunette CA, Miller SJ, Majahalme N, et al. Pragmatic trials in genomic medicine: the Integrating Pharmacogenetics in Clinical Care (I-PICC) study. Clin Transl Sci 2019. https://doi.org/10.1111/cts.12723.
81. Sim I. Mobile devices and health. N Engl J Med 2019;381(10):956–68.
82. Coravos A, Khozin S, Mandl KD. Developing and adopting safe and effective digital biomarkers to improve patient outcomes. NPJ Digit Med 2019;2(1):14.
83. Mindstrong health and Takeda partner to explore development of digital biomarkers for mental health conditions. Available at: https://www.prnewswire.com/news-releases/mindstrong-health-and-takeda-partner-to-explore-development-of-digital-biomarkers-for-mental-health-conditions-300604553.html. Accessed December 10, 2020.
84. Lipsmeier F, Taylor KI, Kilchenmann T, et al. Evaluation of smartphone-based testing to generate exploratory outcome measures in a phase 1 Parkinson's disease clinical trial. Mov Disord 2018;33(8):1287–97.
85. Clay I. Impact of digital technologies on novel endpoint capture in clinical trials. Clin Pharmacol Ther 2017;102(6):912–3.
86. Haendel MA, Chute CG, Robinson PN. Classification, ontology, and precision medicine. N Engl J Med 2018;379(15):1452–62.
87. Miksad RA, Samant MK, Sarkar S, et al. Small but mighty: the use of real-world evidence to inform precision medicine. Clin Pharmacol Ther 2019;106(1):87–90.
88. Yang W, Wu G, Broeckel U, et al. Comparison of genome sequencing and clinical genotyping for pharmacogenes. Clin Pharmacol Ther 2016;100(4):380–8.
89. van der Lee M, Allard WG, Bollen S, et al. Repurposing of diagnostic whole exome sequencing data of 1,583 individuals for clinical pharmacogenetics. Clin Pharmacol Ther 2019. https://doi.org/10.1002/cpt.1665.
90. Holm IA, Agrawal PB, Ceyhan-Birsoy O, et al. The BabySeq project: implementing genomic sequencing in newborns. BMC Pediatr 2018;18(1):225.
91. Kalia SS, Adelman K, Bale SJ, et al. Recommendations for reporting of secondary findings in clinical exome and genome sequencing, 2016 update (ACMG SF v2.0): a policy statement of the American College of Medical Genetics and Genomics. Genet Med 2017;19(2):249–55.
92. Lauschke VM, Ingelman-Sundberg M. How to consider rare genetic variants in personalized drug therapy. Clin Pharmacol Ther 2018;103(5):745–8.
93. McInnes G, Dalton R, Sangkuhl K, et al. Transfer learning enables prediction of CYP2D6 haplotype function. Biorxiv 2020:684357.
94. Gibson G. On the utilization of polygenic risk scores for therapeutic targeting. PLoS Genet 2019;15(4):e1008060.
95. Watson JD, Crick FH. Genetical implications of the structure of deoxyribonucleic acid. Nature 1953;171(4361):964–7.
96. Lauschke VM, Zhou Y, Ingelman-Sundberg M. Novel genetic an epigenetic factors of importance for inter-individual differences in drug disposition, response and toxicity. Pharmacol Ther 2019;197:122–52.

97. Sun L, Xie C, Wang G, et al. Gut microbiota and intestinal FXR mediate the clinical benefits of metformin. Nat Med 2018;24(12):1919–29.
98. Kaddurah-Daouk R, Weinshilboum R. Metabolomic signatures for drug response phenotypes: pharmacometabolomics enables precision medicine. Clin Pharmacol Ther 2015;98(1):71–5.
99. Afsana, Jain V, Haider N, et al. 3D printing in personalized drug delivery. Curr Pharm Des 2018;24(42):5062–71.
100. Hansel TT, Kropshofer H, Singer T, et al. The safety and side effects of monoclonal antibodies. Nat Rev Drug Discov 2010;9(4):325–38.
101. Jackson HJ, Rafiq S, Brentjens RJ. Driving CAR T-cells forward. Nat Rev Clin Oncol 2016;13(6):370–83.
102. Naldini L. Gene therapy returns to centre stage. Nature 2015;526(7573):351–60.
103. Track your own healthcare with 'Volgjezorg. Available at: https://www.volgjezorg.nl/en. Accessed January 18, 2019.
104. Samwald M, Minarro-Giménez JAA, Blagec K, et al. Towards a global IT system for personalized medicine: the Medicine Safety Code initiative. Stud Health Technol Inform 2014;205:261–5.
105. Blagec K, Koopmann R, Crommentuijn-van Rhenen M, et al. Implementing pharmacogenomics decision support across seven European countries: the Ubiquitous Pharmacogenomics (U-PGx) project. J Am Med Inform Assoc 2018;25(7): 893–8.

HLA Typing by Next-Generation Sequencing
Lessons Learned and Future Applications

Caleb Cornaby, PhD[a], Eric T. Weimer, PhD[a,b,*]

KEYWORDS

- HLA • Next-generation sequencing • Nanopore • HLA regulation
- Transplant diagnostics

KEY POINTS

- HLA typing by molecular methods have evolved from sequence-specific oligonucleotide probes to next-generation sequencing (NGS).
- Introduction of NGS-based HLA typing significantly reduced the number of ambiguities observed through full HLA gene sequencing.
- HLA enrichment methods will continue to improve the speed of HLA typing and enable additional content to be evaluated for hematopoietic cell transplant patients as well as solid organ transplant patients.
- Application of NGS to the HLA region will further the study of HLA regulation and expression as it has an impact on transplant outcomes.
- Long-read HLA sequencing will enhance understanding of HLA haplotypes and alter how laboratories perform high-resolution HLA typing.

INTRODUCTION

The HLA region on chromosome 6p21 covers more than 224 annotated genes, covering a span of more than 3.6 megabases. Although that may seem large, it comprises less than 0.15% of the whole human genome[1]. This region has been one of the most studied regions of the human genome since its discovery[2] and contains a plethora of genes that are crucial for immune cell function and regulation[3,4]. The major histocompatibility complex (MHC) class I molecules, encoded by *HLA-A*, *HLA-B*, and

This article originally appeared in Advances in Molecular Pathology, Volume 3, Issue 1, November 2020.
[a] McLendon Clinical Laboratories, UNC Hospitals, 101 Manning Drive, Chapel Hill, NC 27514, USA; [b] Department of Pathology and Laboratory Medicine, University of North Carolina at Chapel Hill School of Medicine, Chapel Hill, NC 27514, USA
* Corresponding author. 101 Manning Drive, Room 1032 East Wing, Chapel Hill, NC 27514.
E-mail address: eric.weimer@med.unc.edu
Twitter: @ericweimer (E.T.W.)

0272-2712/22/© 2022 Elsevier Inc. All rights reserved.

HLA-C, are used by nearly all cells in the human body to express endogenous proteins on their surface for immune cell surveillance[5]. Through this mechanism the immune system can identify defective and pathogen infected cells[6]. MHC class II molecules, encoded by HLA loci *DPB1, DM, DO, DQB1, DQA1, DRB1*, and *DRA* among others, are used by antigen-presenting leukocytes to exhibit pathogenic peptides for T-lymphocyte examination and recruitment[7]. Additionally, the HLA region encodes the complement system proteins vital for the innate immune response, which is responsible for opsonization and neutralization of pathogens[8].

HLA typing is essential for assessment and treatment of a variety of medical conditions, including hematologic, rheumatologic, autoimmune, and cardiologic, among other diseases. The prevalence of hematologic malignancy in the general population has been observed to be greater than 63 per 100,000 people[9]. Although there are a variety of treatment regimens for these malignancies, hematopoietic cell transplant (HCT) often is the treatment. Some patients can benefit from an autologous transplant; however, a large portion of patients need an HCT allotransplant. HLA typing is required to find an appropriate HLA match even if the HCT allotransplant donor is a sibling or other blood relative[10]. In patients receiving a solid organ transplant, HLA typing has been observed to be most beneficial, particularly in cases where sensitized transplant patients have developed allele specific antibodies[11]. Lack of appropriate typing, particularly at the *HLA-A, HLA-B*, and *HLA-DRB1* loci, puts these patients at risk of transplant rejection and possible chronic systemic disease.

Typing of HLA allele variants is associated with a diverse array of human diseases. There are a host of autoimmune diseases associated with HLA variants, including systemic lupus erythematosus, psoriasis, multiple sclerosis, and sarcoidosis, among others. For some of these autoimmune diseases, HLA-associated risk alleles have been identified as strong genetic predictors of disease development. Other diseases associated with HLA alleles include type II diabetes, schizophrenia, Parkinson disease, and coronary artery disease[12]. Furthermore, there are HLA alleles correlated with adverse drug reactions. Some examples include abacavir in patients with the HLA-B*57:01 allele and carbamazepine and oxcarbazepine in patients with the HLA-B*15:02, HLA-B15:11, or HLA-A*31:01 allele[13]. From the numerous examples available in the literature to date, typing of the HLA region has become a crucial part for diagnosing disease as well as a vital component of transplant medicine and treatment regimen implementation[14,15].

HLA TYPING IN THE BEGINNING

One of the first, and for decades considered the gold standard of, HLA typing is serologic typing[16]. This approach uses serologic and deductive methods to identify the patient HLA type. To perform this type of HLA typing, isolated recipient lymphocytes are placed in wells with dye, complement, and different sera with affinity for characterized HLA alleles. If the recipient lymphocytes display the HLA type that the sera are characterized for, then complement is able to bind to the cells and compromise the cell membrane. This permeabilization allows the cells to take up the dye. Cells in each well with the different sera are inspected under a microscope for dye. By identifying which combination of sera caused cell lysis, the HLA type for the recipient can be determined.

The advantage of this method in the past was the speed at which typing could be achieved. In several hours, a basic HLA typing could be assigned. The disadvantage to this method was that serologic typing has poor sensitivity for the detection of small amino acid differences in HLA proteins, which can elicit a significant immune response. Also, a laboratory could use only previously characterized sera for known HLA alleles. This becomes increasingly difficult as novel alleles are continuing to be identified and largely has been abandoned with the adoption of molecular typing techniques.

MOLECULAR-BASED HLA TYPING ERA

As molecular methods for HLA typing became available, they soon began to be employed in HLA typing laboratories. One of the earliest molecular typing techniques utilized was restriction fragment length polymorphism[17,18]. This technique uses DNA restriction endonucleases to cleave isolated genomic DNA, which then is run on an agarose gel and transferred to a membrane for probing with HLA locus unique primers. Although having continual problems with cross-hybridization issues, another disadvantage was that not all alleles could be differentiated using this technique alone[18]. Later, when polymerase chain reaction (PCR) technology became available, the 2 techniques were utilized together. PCR-amplified HLA alleles could be digested with restriction enzymes to ascertain appropriate HLA typing. This was used for many years to help resolve ambiguous HLA typing results[19].

A variety of other typing methodologies became available with the advent of PCR. With the ability to amplify DNA, probes for specific HLA alleles could be developed. This technique was referred to as sequence-specific oligonucleotide probe (SSOP) typing. Key to SSOP is immobilization of amplified DNA, typically to a paper or membrane; then the probes can be applied. Visualization of the bound primers can be done by chemiluminescence or fluorescence. By observing the developed blots, an HLA typing then could be established[18,20,21].

Another PCR-based method using HLA allele–specific primers during amplification of genomic DNA commonly was used for typing, referred to as sequence-specific primer typing[22,23]. This method was useful because 1 of the primers could be used universally for many different alleles of a single HLA loci, whereas the second primer of the set could be variable, sometimes by just 1 nucleotide, to allow the specific amplification of only certain alleles. These reactions could be validated in house or purchased in kits of varying complexities, depending on the resolution of results that needed to be achieved[24]. Depending on the locus of interest for typing, a laboratory could have results after only a couple hours[25].

Direct sequencing of the alleles of interest, or sequence-based typing (SBT), involves identifying the nucleotide sequence at specific HLA loci and comparing it to a database of allele sequences confirmed by SBT to identify the patient HLA type. For several years, SBT was performed exclusively using Sanger dideoxynucleotide sequencing[26]. Although there are different platforms that perform Sanger sequencing, the principle of identifying the nucleotide sequence of interest is similar. Depending on the protocol, the isolated genomic DNA is PCR amplified using HLA loci–specific primers. Postamplification, the DNA is amplified again, using only 1 primer and dideoxynucleotides. Dideoxynucleotides act to terminate the PCR process for that strand. The resultant solution contains partially amplified fragments of all lengths that then can be length separated using a gel system or capillary electrophoresis. The termination labeled nucleotides then are read for each separated band and the nucleotides are identified and placed in sequence[27].

As can be imagined, SBT has many advantages over previous molecular methods. Although PCR methods can be faster, be less labor intensive, and work as a closed system, confirmatory testing often is required, and results often can still be ambiguous. In many cases, typing never is resolved fully. Sanger sequencing, on the other hand, can query every base pair. This ability allowed for more rapid discovery of novel HLA alleles than at any time previous. Typing also could be done with a new level of confidence because bases could be matched to show the differences between alleles. The ability to judge how well a transplant candidate was for a match could be weighed against the mismatch of the donor HLA loci. Setting the scene for this terminology and field of HLA research that still is of great import today. Sanger sequencing also has its disadvantages. Compared with some of the previous methods, it was both time consuming and labor intensive to obtain typing by SBT.

SBT has become virtually synonymous with Sanger sequencing, which has been the standard for providing high-resolution typing. There are many laboratories that continue to use Sanger sequencing as the method of choice for high-resolution typing due to instrumentation costs, implementation costs, and low volumes. Although those are valid reasons for continuing with Sanger sequencing, the declining costs of next-generation sequencing (NGS) coupled with the higher resolution, phasing, and elimination of ambiguities will result in continued expansion of these new sequence-based methods within clinical laboratories.

NEXT-GENERATION SEQUENCING–BASED HLA TYPING

With the advent of NGS technologies for sequencing, it did not take long for these methodologies to be applied to HLA typing. Almost as soon as NGS technology became more economically feasible for research, some of the earlier studies of the HLA locus were done using NGS methods, such as pyrosequencing[1,28]. Soon thereafter, several clinical HLA laboratories received American Society of Histocompatibility and Immunogenetics approval to utilize NGS-based HLA typing methods[29]. Since that time, the number of clinical HLA laboratories that use NGS for HLA typing has only increased. With the rising use of NGS in HLA typing, there has been a proportional expansion of NGS HLA typing assays, novel allele discoveries, and disease associations with HLA alleles[30,31].

Although the technique used for massive parallel sequencing might be slightly different, depending on the platform and assay used for HLA typing, the fundamentals of NGS are very similar and can be divided into several major steps. The first step requires the amplification or targeted concentration of isolated genomic DNA from the patient. This is followed by DNA clean up, fragmentation, adapter and index ligation, normalization, and sample pooling. The order and operation of these steps depends on the NGS protocol and technique used for library preparation[32]. Once the samples are loaded onto the NGS platform of choice and sequencing is performed, the final step in the process is the bioinformatic analysis to compile and parse reads to obtain the actual base pair sequence[33].

Of the methodologies utilized in target enrichment, HLA laboratories currently using NGS-based HLA typing typically employ either short-range PCR[34,35], long-range PCR[36–38], or hybrid capture-based methods[39,40]. These approaches enable HLA enrichment so that a depth of coverage adequate for high-resolution HLA typing can be achieved. Short-range PCR generally has the advantage of speed and higher depth of coverage compared with long-range PCR. A disadvantage of short-range PCR is the potential loss of phasing over longer stretches of DNA/RNA. Long-range PCR uses HLA loci primers to specifically amplify the HLA regions of interest, most commonly whole-gene amplification. Sometimes primer sets used can amplify sequences that include the introns, andmany untranslated regions. The major advantage of long-range PCR is amplification of the entire HLA gene at the expense of time. There now are commercial long-range PCR products, however, that amplify the HLA genes within 3 hours[41,42]. For practicality in the clinical HLA laboratory, assays often use multiplexed primers that amplify only regions of interest. These HLA loci of interest often include *HLA-A*, *HLA-B*, *HLA-C*, *HLA-DPA1*, *HLA-DPB1*, *HLA-DQA1*, and *HLA-DRB1*[43,44].

Short-range and long-range PCR-based HLA enrichment methods have been used for years in the clinical HLA setting with reliable performance. There is greater opportunity and reliability in identifying novel alleles during HLA typing, with substantially fewer ambiguities. With NGS-based typing methods, laboratories also can perform better quality control. Minor allele fractions can be calculated to ensure that there is no allele bias and provide a haplotype estimate. There are potential drawbacks, however, with PCR-based enrichment. As with all PCR-based strategies, there is potential for allele bias amplification and, importantly for HLA typing, PCR can contribute to allele dropout or allele imbalance[1,32,45]. Typically, allele dropout is due to sequence variation at primer binding sites or preferential allele amplification. Allele dropout (approximately 1%) is a rare observation within clinical HLA laboratories due to quality assurance practices and the high-quality assays available for HLA typing[46,47].

An alternative HLA enrichment method to PCR-based approaches is hybridization of a probe to specific HLA loci during library preparation. In short, complementary nucleic acid sequences, RNA or DNA, for HLA loci bound to magnetic beads are used to specifically select for these regions during DNA purification. Using this method, hybridization probes can target capture class I and class II HLA loci with lower-risk allele dropout or allele imbalance compared with PCR amplification methods[48,49]. Also, removing the majority of nonspecific reads that otherwise would be discarded during bioinformatic analysis ensures a larger portion of the DNA used for sequencing will be from HLA loci of interest for typing. A beneficial byproduct of this method is that it also allows for sequencing coverage of other HLA loci besides the traditional loci targeted using PCR. Furthermore, hybrid capture NGS assays can be done in significantly less time than some long-range PCR-based NGS because there is no need for PCR amplification prior to library preparation.

FUTURE FOR CLINICAL NEXT-GENERATION SEQUENCING HLA TYPING

Adoption of NGS for HLA typing in the clinical setting has continued to rise, typically in laboratories evaluating solid organ transplant patients and donors, and these laboratories have realized several benefits of HLA typing by NGS. Transplanted recipients benefit from NGS HLA typing by having high-resolution HLA typing available on donors to improve donor-specific antibody assessments[41,50]. In addition, NGS HLA typing can enhance virtual crossmatch assessment and aid in interpretation of physical crossmatch results by providing the level HLA expression[41,51]. For example, rs9277534, a single-nucleotide polymorphism within HLA-DPB1 that has regulatory function and impact on HCT outcomes, has been suggested to have an impact on B-cell flow cytometric cross-matches[52]. Additionally, rs9267649 has been associated with DNA methylation of *HLA-DRB*1 and reduced expression of *HLA-DRB1*[53]. Taken together, the application of NGS to HLA typing has demonstrated the importance of HLA regulation and expression and the subsequent impact on clinical outcomes. The continued expansion of HLA typing by NGS will serve to increase this growing field of study.

The future of clinical HLA (or immunogenetics in general) relies on connection of the vast amount of data captured by NGS to clinical outcomes. The current standard of care for HCT patients requires only a particular group of HLA loci to be typed. Additionally, the standard of care requires only the antigen-binding domain (ABD) to be sequenced. Although there are some reports that indicate that sequencing the ABD is sufficient[54] there also are reports that the information beyond the ABD influence clinical outcomes[55–57]. There is increasing evidence that other regions, beyond the antigen recognition domain, may influence patient outcomes. For example, Petersdorf and colleagues[58], found that exon 1 (leader peptide) of HLA-B informed graft-versus-host disease risk and permits risk stratification–based HLA matching for HCT patients. Additionally, Petersdorf and colleagues[59] found that HLA-DRB1 amino acid repertoire influenced transplant survivorship. These studies and others demonstrate there is still much to learn out of traditional HLA typing for improved transplant outcomes.

An area of continued exploration is extending the IMGT/HLA reference sequences. The lack of full-length reference sequences is a substantial roadblock in establishing unambiguous HLA genotypes. Recently, the Anthony Nolan Research Institute has addressed this issue by extending reference sequences for 95 HLA class I alleles[60]. In addition, the HLA Informatics Group at Anthony Nolan Research Institute, who maintain the IMGT/HLA database, now are receiving more full-length HLA class I submission than partial gene sequences with the continued adoption of HLA typing by NGS[61].

With the advent of the third-generation sequencing methods, including Pacific Biosciences' Single-Molecule Real-Time (SMRT) DNA sequencing and Oxford Nanopore Technologies (ONT), sequencing laboratories have begun long-read sequencing. Long-read sequencing enables laboratories to sequence DNA/RNA sequences beyond the capability of traditional Illumina or Ion Torrent platforms. There is a growing list of clinical laboratories employing third-generation sequencing technologies to provide single-molecule HLA typing. The main advantage is single-molecular sequencing generates long reads, often greater than 20 kilobases, which enables the entire HLA class I and II genes to be sequenced[62]. At the moment, there are several clinical laboratories using SMRT methodologies for HLA genotyping, there are fewer laboratories using ONT sequencing, particularly for HLA class II genotyping. A recent publication by De Santis and colleagues[42], however, demonstrated the feasibility of rapid, high-resolution HLA genotyping using ONT sequencing within 4 hours.

The potential application of ONT sequencing for HLA genotyping may enable true epitope-based matching algorithms. The current approach has been inferenced HLA genotypes based on ethnicity and haplotype information. Although inference-based HLA genotype has an accuracy ranging from 80% to 100%, depending on ethnicity and bioinformatics approach[63–66], optimal epitope determination is based on high-resolution HLA genotyping data. Advancements, such as rapid, high-resolution HLA genotyping for deceased donors, will have a significant impact on patient outcomes[50].

By combining rapid, high-resolution HLA genotyping, HLA expression, and virtual crossmatch, HLA laboratories may improve recipient and donor matching along with patient outcomes for solid organ recipients. The HLA community continues to make significant strides in expanding knowledge of the HLA region beyond ABD and the implications for patients.

DISCLOSURE

Dr E.T. Weimer reports a grant from Omixon and personal fees from CareDx during the conduct of this review. Dr C. Cornaby has nothing to disclose.

REFERENCES

1. Hosomichi K, Shiina T, Tajima A, et al. The impact of next-generation sequencing technologies on HLA research. J Hum Genet 2015;60:665–73.

2. Horton R, Wilming L, Rand V, et al. Gene map of the extended human MHC. Nat Rev Genet 2004;5:889–99.
3. Crux NB, Elahi S. Human Leukocyte Antigen (HLA) and immune regulation: How do classical and non-classical HLA alleles modulate immune response to human immunodeficiency virus and hepatitis C virus infections? Front Immunol 2017; 8:832.
4. Reeves E, James E. Antigen processing and immune regulation in the response to tumours. Immunology 2017;150:16–24.
5. Dendrou CA, Petersen J, Rossjohn J, et al. HLA variation and disease. Nat Rev Immunol 2018;18. https://doi.org/10.1038/nri.2017.143.
6. Montgomery RA, Tatapudi VS, Leffell MS, et al. HLA in transplantation. Nat Rev Nephrol 2018;14. https://doi.org/10.1038/s41581-018-0039-x.
7. Miles JJ, Mccluskey J, Rossjohn J, et al. Understanding the complexity and malleability of T-cell recognition. Immunol Cell Biol 2015;93:433–41.
8. Kulski JK, Shiina T, Inoko H, et al. An update of the HLA genomic region, locus information and disease associations: 2004. Tissue Antigens 2019;64:631–49.
9. Li J, Smith A, Crouch S, et al. Estimating the prevalence of hematological malignancies and precursor conditions using data from Haematological Malignancy Research Network (HMRN). Cancer Causes Control 2016;27:1019–26.
10. Edgerly CH, Weimer ET. The past, present, and future of HLA typing in transplantation. Methods Mol Biol 1802;(2018):1–10.
11. Duquesnoy RJ, Kamoun M, Baxter-Lowe LA, et al. Should HLA mismatch acceptability for sensitized transplant candidates be determined at the high-resolution rather than the antigen level? Am J Transplant 2015;15:923–30.
12. Trowsdale J, Knight JC. Major histocompatibility complex genomics and human disease. Annu Rev Genomics Hum Genet 2013;14:301–23.
13. Fan W-L, Shiao M-S, Hui RC-Y, et al. Review Article HLA association with drug-induced adverse reactions. J Immunol Res 2017. https://doi.org/10.1155/2017/3186328.
14. Kawai T, Cosimi AB, Spitzer TR, et al. HLA-mismatched renal transplantation without maintenance immunosuppression from the transplantation unit. N Engl J Med 2008;358(4):353–61.
15. Kamburova EG, Wisse BW, Joosten I, et al. Differential effects of donor-specific HLA antibodies in living versus deceased donor transplant. Am J Transplant 2018;18:2274–84.
16. Althaf MM, El Kossi M, Jin JK, et al. Human leukocyte antigen typing and cross-match: A comprehensive review. World J Transplant 2017;7:339–48.
17. Bidwell JL, Bidwell EA, Savage DA, et al. A DNA-RFLP typing system that positively identifies serologically well-defined and ill-defined HLA-DR and DQ alleles, including DRw10. Transplantation 1988;45:640–6.
18. Gerlach JA. Human lymphocyte antigen molecular typing how to identify the 1250 alleles out there. Arch Pathol Lab Med 2002;126(3):281–4.
19. Hui KM, Bidwell JL. Handbook of HLA Typing Techniques. Boca Raton, FL: Google Books, CRC Press; 1993. (n.d.).
20. Wordsworth P. Techniques used to define human MHC antigens: polymerase chain reaction and oligonucleotide probes. Immunolog Letters 1991; 29(1-2):37–9.
21. Suberbielle-Boissel C, Chapuis E, D.C.-T. Comparative study of two methods of HLA-DR typing: serology and PCR/dot blot reverse. Transplant Proceedings 1997;29(5):2335–6.

22. Metcalfe P, Waters AH. HPA-1 typing by PCR amplification with sequence-specific primers (PCR-SSP): a rapid and simple technique. Br J Haematol 1993;85:227–9.
23. Bunce M, Taylor CJ, Welsh KI. Rapid HLA-DQB typing by eight polymerase chain reaction amplifications with sequence-specific primers (PCR-SSP). Hum Immunol 1993;37:201–6.
24. Bunce M, O'Neill CM, Barnardo MCNM, et al. Phototyping: comprehensive DNA typing for HLA-A, B, C, DRB1, DRB3, DRB4, DRB5 & DQB1 by PCR with 144 primer mixes utilizing sequence-specific primers (PCR-SSP). Tissue Antigens 1995;46:355–67.
25. Olerup O, Zetterquist H. HLA-DR typing by PCR amplification with sequence-specific primers (PCR-SSP) in 2 hours: an alternative to serological DR typing in clinical practice including donor-recipient matching in cadaveric transplantation. Tissue Antigens 1992;39. https://doi.org/10.1111/j.1399-0039.1992.tb01940.x.
26. Sanger F, Nicklen S, Coulson AR. DNA sequencing with chain-terminating inhibitors. Proc Natl Acad Sci U S A. 1977;74(12):5463-7.
27. Dunn PPJ. Human leucocyte antigen typing: techniques and technology, a critical appraisal. Int J Immunogenet 2011;38:463–73.
28. Bentley G, Higuchi R, Hoglund B, et al. High-resolution, high-throughput HLA genotyping by next-generation sequencing. Tissue Antigens 2009;74:393–403.
29. Montgomery MC, Petraroia R, Weimer ET. Buccal swab genomic DNA fragmentation predicts likelihood of successful HLA genotyping by next-generation sequencing. Hum Immunol 2017;78:634–41.
30. Ingram KJ, O'Shields EF, Kiger DF, et al. NGS and HLA: The long road ahead. Hum Immunol 2020. https://doi.org/10.1016/j.humimm.2020.03.001.
31. Shieh M, Chitnis N, Monos D. Human Leukocyte Antigen and Disease Associations: A Broader Perspective. Clin Lab Med 2018;38(4):679-93.
32. Profaizer T, Kumánovics A. Human Leukocyte Antigen Typing by Next-Generation Sequencing. Clin Lab Med 2018;38(4):565-78.
33. Klasberg S, Surendranath V, Lange V, et al. Bioinformatics strategies, challenges, and opportunities for next generation sequencing-based HLA genotyping. Transfus Med Hemother 2019;46:312–25.
34. Nelson WC, Pyo CW, Vogan D, et al. An integrated genotyping approach for HLA and other complex genetic systems. Hum Immunol 2015;76:928–38.
35. Smith AG, Pyo CW, Nelson W, et al. Next generation sequencing to determine HLA class II genotypes in a cohort of hematopoietic cell transplant patients and donors. Hum Immunol 2014;75:1040–6.
36. Holcomb CL, Hoglund B, Anderson MW, et al. A multi-site study using high-resolution HLA genotyping by next generation sequencing. Tissue Antigens 2011;77:206–17.
37. Ehrenberg PK, Geretz A, Sindhu RK, et al. High-throughput next-generation sequencing to genotype six classical HLA loci from 96 donors in a single MiSeq run. HLA 2017;90:284–91.
38. Weimer ET, Montgomery M, Petraroia R, et al. Performance characteristics and validation of next-generation sequencing for human leucocyte antigen typing. J Mol Diagn 2016;18:668–75.
39. Wittig M, Anmarkrud JA, Kassens JC, et al. Development of a high-resolution NGS-based HLA-typing and analysis pipeline. Nucleic Acids Res 2015;43:e70.

40. Lank SM, Golbach BA, Creager HM, et al. Ultra-high resolution HLA genotyping and allele discovery by highly multiplexed cDNA amplicon pyrosequencing. BMC Genomics 2012;13:378.

41. Liu C, Duffy BF, Weimer ET, et al. Performance of a multiplexed amplicon-based next-generation sequencing assay for HLA typing. PLoS One 2020;15:e0232050.

42. De Santis D, Truong L, Martinez P, et al. Rapid high-resolution HLA genotyping by MinION Oxford nanopore sequencing for deceased donor organ allocation. HLA 2020. https://doi.org/10.1111/tan.13901.

43. Montgomery M, Berka J, immunology EW-H, et al. Suitability of dried DNA for long-range PCR amplification and HLA typing by next-generation sequencing. Hum Immunol 2019;80(2):135–9.

44. Ehrenberg PK, Geretz A, Baldwin KM, et al. High-throughput multiplex HLA genotyping by next-generation sequencing using multi-locus individual tagging. BMC Genomics 2014;15:864.

45. Walsh PS, Erlich HA, Higuchi R. Preferential PCR amplification of alleles: mechanisms and solutions. PCR Methods Appl 1992;1(4):241-50.

46. Osoegawa K, Vayntrub TA, Wenda S, et al. Quality Control Project of NGS HLA Genotyping for the 17th International HLA and Immunogenetics Workshop. Hum Immunol 2019. https://doi.org/10.1016/j.humimm.2019.01.009.

47. Montgomery MC, Weimer ET. Clinical validation of next generation sequencing for HLA typing using trusight HLA. Hum Immunol 2015;76:139.

48. Gandhi MJ, Ferriola D, Huang Y, et al. Targeted next-generation sequencing for human leukocyte antigen typing in a clinical laboratory: metrics of relevance and considerations for its successful implementation. Arch Pathol Lab Med 2017;141:806–12.

49. Wittig M, Juzenas S, Vollstedt M, et al. High-resolution HLA-typing by next-generation sequencing of randomly fragmented target DNA. Methods Mol Biol 2018;63–88.

50. Senev A, Emonds M, Van Sandt V, et al. The clinical importance of extended 2nd field high-resolution HLA genotyping for kidney transplantation. Am J Transplant 2020. https://doi.org/10.1111/ajt.15938.

51. Badders JL, Jones JA, Jeresano ME, et al. Variable HLA expression on deceased donor lymphocytes: Not all crossmatches are created equal. Hum Immunol 2015; 76:795–800.

52. Soe NN, Yin Y, Valenzuela NM, et al. OR3 HLA-DPB1 single nucleotide polymorphism determines DP molecule expression and B lymphocyte crossmatch results. Hum Immunol 2017;78:3.

53. Kular L, Liu Y, Ruhrmann S, et al. DNA methylation as a mediator of HLA-DRB1 15:01 and a protective variant in multiple sclerosis. Nat Commun 2018;9:1–15.

54. Hurley CK, Ng J. Continue to focus clinical decision-making on the antigen recognition domain for the present. Hum Immunol 2019;80:79–84.

55. Mayor NP, Hayhurst JD, Turner TR, et al. Recipients receiving better hla-matched hematopoietic cell transplantation grafts, uncovered by a novel hla typing method, have superior survival: a retrospective study. Biol Blood Marrow Transplant 2019;25:443–50.

56. Shieh M, Chitnis N, Clark P, et al. Computational assessment of miRNA binding to low and high expression HLA-DPB1 allelic sequences. Hum Immunol 2019;80: 53–61.

57. Thibodeau J, Moulefera MA, Balthazard R. On the structure–function of MHC class II molecules and how single amino acid polymorphisms could alter intracellular trafficking. Hum Immunol 2019;80:15–31.

58. Petersdorf EW, Carrington M, O'hUigin C, et al. Role of HLA-B exon 1 in graft-versus-host disease after unrelated haemopoietic cell transplantation: a retrospective cohort study. Lancet Haematol 2020;7:e50–60.

59. Petersdorf EW, Stevenson P, Malkki M, et al. Patient HLA germline variation and transplant survivorship. J Clin Oncol 2018;36:2524–31.

60. Hassall KB, Latham K, Robinson J, et al. Extending the sequences of HLA class I alleles without full-length genomic coverage using single molecule real-time DNA sequencing. HLA 2020;95:196–9.

61. Robinson J, Barker DJ, Georgiou X, et al. IPD-IMGT/HLA Database. Nucleic Acids Res 2019;48:D948–55.

62. Mayor NP, Robinson J, McWhinnie AJ, et al. HLA Typing for the Next Generation. PLoS One 2015;10:e0127153.

63. Dilthey AT, Gourraud PA, Mentzer AJ, et al. High-accuracy hla type inference from whole-genome sequencing data using population reference graphs. PLoS Comput Biol 2016;12:e1005151.

64. Xie C, Yeo ZX, Wong M, et al. Fast and accurate HLA typing from short-read next-generation sequence data with xHLA. Proc Natl Acad Sci U S A 2017;114:8059–64.

65. Xie M, Li J, Jiang T. Accurate HLA type inference using a weighted similarity graph. BMC Bioinformatics 2010;11:S10.

66. Huang Y, Dinh A, Heron S, et al. Assessing the utilization of high-resolution 2-field HLA typing in solid organ transplantation. Am J Transplant 2019;19:1955–63.

Applications of Noninvasive Prenatal Testing for Subchromosomal Copy Number Variations Using Cell-Free DNA

Jiale Xiang, MS[a,b], Zhiyu Peng, PhD[a,b,*]

KEYWORDS

- Noninvasive prenatal testing • Copy number variation
- Subchromosomal abnormalities • Microdeletion • Microduplication
- Prenatal screening

KEY POINTS

- Noninvasive prenatal testing (NIPT) is now clinically available for screening fetal subchromosomal copy number variations (CNVs).
- The sensitivity of NIPT for CNVs is challenging to calculate in clinical settings because the number of the missed cases is unknown. This is attributable to the fact that CNV phenotypes can be invisible, mild, or progressive at birth, meaning that some cases require longitudinal follow-up to be identified.
- The positive predictive value (PPV) of NIPT for genome-wide CNVs is 32% to 47%, which is comparable with the PPV for trisomy 13 (43.9%–53%).
- Four critical factors affect the clinical validity of NIPT for detecting subchromosomal CNVs: fetal fraction, sequencing depth, CNV size, and technical variability of the CNV region. Increasing the fetal fraction and sequencing depth improves the NIPT detection rate of subchromosomal CNVs.

INTRODUCTION

In 1997, the detection of male DNA in peripheral blood samples from women bearing male fetuses proved that fetal DNA circulates in maternal plasma and serum[1]. Circulating "fetal" cell-free DNA (cfDNA), which is mainly released from the placenta into maternal circulation, is used in noninvasive prenatal testing (NIPT). Currently, NIPT

This article originally appeared in *Advances in Molecular Pathology*, Volume 4, Issue 1, November 2021.
[a] BGI Genomics, BGI-Shenzhen, Shenzhen 518083, China; [b] College of Life Sciences, University of Chinese Academy of Sciences, Beijing 100049, China
* Corresponding author.
E-mail address: pengzhiyu@bgi.com

is primarily used to screen for 3 fetal aneuploidies, trisomy 21, trisomy 18, and trisomy 13, and its performance in detecting these has been well studied in both high-risk and low-risk populations[2]. The high sensitivity, low false-positive rate, and high positive predictive value (PPV) of NIPT have led to its widespread clinical adoption. In recent years, NIPT has revolutionized the prenatal screening landscape and become a routine test in Belgium and the Netherlands[3,4].

Researchers and clinicians have great interest in applying NIPT to screen subchromosomal copy number variations (CNVs) in addition to the 3 traditionally screened aneuploidies. In this review, the authors focus on the current status, development, and challenges of using NIPT to screen fetal subchromosomal CNVs in pregnancies.

Subchromosomal Copy Number Variations

Subchromosomal CNVs are abnormalities in which sections of the genome are deleted (loss) or duplicated (gain). They are relatively common in prenatal diagnosis. Wapner and coauthors[5] used chromosomal microarray analysis (CMA) to reveal that 2.5% of samples with normal karyotypes had a microdeletion or microduplication of clinical significance. Based on low-coverage genome sequencing, Wang and colleagues[6] reported that 5.3% of pregnant women undergoing prenatal diagnosis had pathogenic/likely pathogenic CNVs.

Subchromosomal CNVs are associated with severe phenotypes, including structural anomalies, intellectual disability, developmental delay, and autism spectrum disorders[7]. Some presentations, such as structural anomalies, are detectable by ultrasound scans; however, neurologic or neurocognitive features are undetectable via prenatal ultrasound scans. Currently, there are no screening options to identify CNVs at the prenatal stage[8]. To fill this gap, the use of NIPT to screen subchromosomal CNVs is becoming more popular in clinics[4,9,10].

Noninvasive Prenatal Testing for Subchromosomal Copy Number Variations

NIPT can detect aneuploidies through either targeted or random (genome-wide) sequencing, both of which are also technically feasible approaches for detecting subchromosomal CNVs[2]. The targeted approach relies on the amplification of informative single-nucleotide polymorphisms (SNPs)[11]; that is, a targeted SNP-based NIPT is designed to detect a preselected region. In comparison, genome-wide NIPT randomly sequences and analyzes all chromosomes, which has the inherent advantage of detecting CNVs anywhere in the genome instead of only in targeted regions[12].

Selected Copy Number Variations

A handful of selected CNVs with well-defined, severe phenotypes is included in the NIPT screening panel (**Table 1**), including DiGeorge syndrome (22q11.2 deletion), Prader-Willi and Angelman syndromes (15q11.2-q13 deletion), 1p36 deletion syndrome, Cri-du-chat syndrome (terminal 5p deletion), Jacobsen syndrome (terminal 11q deletion), Wolf-Hirschhorn syndrome (terminal 4p deletion), and Langer-Giedion syndrome (8q24 deletion)[2]. Five of these conditions (DiGeorge syndrome, Prader-Willi/Angelman syndromes, 1p36 deletion syndrome, and Cri-du-chat syndrome) are the best validated and most reported[9,13,14]. The remaining conditions, including Jacobsen syndrome, Wolf-Hirschhorn syndrome, and Langer-Giedion syndrome, are rarely reported[13].

More specifically, Wapner and colleagues[14] validated the use of SNP-based NIPT for CNVs by testing 469 samples (358 plasma samples from pregnant women, 111 artificial plasma mixtures). The results demonstrated that the sensitivity was 97.8% (45/46) for DiGeorge syndrome and 100% for Prader-Willi syndrome (15/15),

Table 1
Characteristics of Selected Subchromosomal Copy Number Variations

No.	Syndrome	Cytoband	Origin	Size	Prevalence	Reference
1	DiGeorge syndrome	22q11.2	90% de novo; 10% inherited	The majority of affected individuals (85%) has a 3-Mb deletion	1/3800–1/6000	53
2	Prader-Willi syndrome	15q11-q13	de novo	65%–75% cases have interstitial 5- to 6-Mb deletion	1/10,000–1/30,000	54
3	Angelman syndrome	15q11-q13	de novo	65%–75% cases have interstitial 5- to 7-Mb deletion	1/12,000–1/24,000	55
4	Cri-du-chat syndrome	5p	~80% de novo; 10% result of a parental translocation; 10% an unusual cytogenetic aberration	Variable, ~5–40 Mb	1/15,000–1/50,000	56,57
5	1p36 deletion syndrome	1p36	de novo	Variable, ~1.5 to >10 Mb	1/5000–1/10,000	57,58
6	Wolf-Hirschhorn syndrome	4p	55% de novo; 40%–45% inherited from a parent with a balanced rearrangement	Variable, 0.5–2.0 Mb critical region in 4p16.3	1/50,000	59,60
7	Jacobsen syndrome	11q23-q25	de novo	Variable, 5–20 Mb	1/100,000	61
8	Langer-Giedion syndrome	8q24	de novo	Critical region for the disorder q24.11-q24.13	Unknown	62

Angelman syndrome (21/21), 1p36 deletion syndrome (1/1), and Cri-du-chat syndrome (24/24). Later, the same team retrospectively analyzed SNP-based NIPT data (≥3.2 million reads per sample) from 80,449 referrals for DiGeorge syndrome and 42,326 referrals for the other 4 conditions. The PPV was 15.7% (24/153) for DiGeorge syndrome, 0% (0/1) for Prader-Willi syndrome, 1.5% (1/68) for Angelman syndrome, 20% (2/10) for 1p36 deletion syndrome, and 8.9% (4/45) for Cri-du-chat syndrome[15].

Genome-wide NIPT can also be used to identify specific, selected CNVs. Using genome-wide NIPT in 175,393 high-risk pregnancies, Helgeson and colleagues[13] reported the PPV was 100% (23/23) for DiGeorge syndrome, 100% (8/8) for Prader-Willi/Angelman syndromes, 75% (3/4) for 1p36 deletion syndrome, and 66.7% (4/6) for Cri-du-chat syndrome. However, it is worth noting that this study also counted CNVs that were in the maternal genome as true positives; thus, the PPV is likely overestimated. In addition, a prospective study using genome-wide NIPT in 94,085 pregnancies demonstrated that the PPV was 92.9% (13/14) for DiGeorge syndrome, 75% (3/4) for Prader-Willi/Angelman syndromes, 0% (0/2) for 1p36 deletion syndrome, and 50% (3/6) for Cri-du-chat syndrome[9].

Genome-Wide Copy Number Variations

In genome-wide NIPT, all of the chromosomes are randomly sequenced and analyzed, allowing the detection of CNVs in each chromosome[12]. Three studies investigated the analytical validity of genome-wide NIPT for detecting CNVs[16–18]. These studies chose different CNV reporting strategies based on CNV size. In one study, the sensitivity was 97.7% (42/43) for CNVs ≥7 Mb[16], 90.9% (10/11) for CNVs greater than 5 Mb[17], and 14.3% (1/7) for CNVs less than 5 Mb[17]. In another study, sensitivity was 88.9% (24/27) for CNVs greater than 10 Mb[18], and 72.7% (8/11) for CNVs less than 10 Mb[18].

Recently, 3 teams prospectively investigated the PPV of genome-wide NIPT for CNVs in large populations. The first study, reported in 2019, was in the Netherlands, where NIPT is now a routine prenatal test. The researchers recruited 73,239 low-risk pregnancies, accounting for 42% of all pregnancies in the Netherlands at the time. An NIPT with 0.2× genome coverage identified 29 true-positive and 62 false-positive subchromosomal CNVs ranging from 10 to 100 Mb. The overall PPV was 32%. However, the overall sensitivity cannot be calculated because data on missed cases are not available[10].

The second study, reported by Liang and colleagues[9] in 2019, recruited 94,085 pregnancies. As a result of maternal age, 40.41% of the participants were high-risk pregnancies, whereas 59.58% were low-risk pregnancies. An NIPT with 10 to 19 million uniquely mapped reads and 36 bp per read (translated to 0.12–0.23× genome coverage) identified 49 true-positive and 71 false-positive subchromosomal CNVs. The overall PPV was 40.8%, including 92.9% for DiGeorge syndrome, 66.7% for 22q duplication syndrome, 50.0% for Cri-du-chat syndrome, 75.0% for Prader-Willi syndrome, 31.9% for CNVs greater than 10 Mb, and 18.8% for CNVs less than 10 Mb. The investigators reported an overall sensitivity of 90.74%.

The final study, reported in 2021, was carried out in Belgium, the first country to implement and fully reimburse NIPT as a first-tier screening test. Van Den Bogaert and colleagues[4] analyzed genome-wide NIPT data from 153,575 pregnancies in the first 2 years (2018–2019) of the national implementation of NIPT. The mean maternal age in 2018 and 2019 was 30.7 years and 30.8 years, respectively. The PPV was calculated to be 47% (43/92). The reported CNV size ranged from 2 to 100 Mb.

To sum up, the sensitivity of NIPT for either selected CNVs or genome-wide CNVs varied between different validation studies[14,16–18]. In clinical settings, however, the sensitivity is challenging to calculate because the number of the missed cases is unknown. This is attributable to the fact that the phenotypes of CNVs could be invisible, mild, or progressive at birth, requiring longitudinal follow-up to identify some cases. The PPV of NIPT for genome-wide CNVs ranges from 32% to 47%, which is comparable with the PPV for trisomy 13 (43.9%–53%), one of the commonly screened chromosome aneuploidies[4,9,10].

Confirmatory Test for Subchromosomal Copy Number Variations

A confirmatory test should be offered when an NIPT identifies a CNV[8]. Karyotyping, fluorescence in situ hybridization (FISH), CMA, and low-coverage genome sequencing can be used to confirm subchromosomal CNVs[19,20]. Briefly, karyotyping is a method using staining procedures to visualize chromosomes in banding patterns with a microscope. Standard banding techniques produce approximately 400 to 500 bands per haploid genome, so karyotyping can normally only detect CNVs larger than 10 Mb. However, a higher-resolution technique achieving approximately 1000 bands per haploid genome can extend the resolution to 3 Mb[20].

FISH is a method for detecting the presence or absence of a particular DNA sequence in situ in a cell. FISH technology relies on DNA probes and provides much higher resolution. A disadvantage of FISH is that it requires prior knowledge of the region of interest in order to design DNA probes[21].

CMA is a method that tests for matches against an array of genomic segments on a microscope slide. Two CMA techniques are used for identifying chromosomal imbalance: comparative genomic hybridization and SNP-based arrays[22]. The resolution of CMA depends on probe density, which varies between CMA platforms. For routine clinical testing, probe spacing on the array provides a resolution of 100 to 250 kb in nontargeted regions and 20 to 50 kb in targeted regions[23]. This resolution is high enough to confirm subchromosomal CNVs that are identified by NIPT.

With the advance of massively parallel sequencing techniques in recent years, low-coverage genome sequencing ($\sim 0.25\times$ of the human genome) has been validated to detect genome-wide subchromosomal CNVs greater than 50 kb[24]. In a prenatal diagnosis cohort with 1023 pregnancies, Wang and colleagues[6] compared the performance of low-coverage genome sequencing and CMA. The results demonstrated that low-coverage genome sequencing not only detected all of the pathogenic/likely pathogenic CNVs detected by CMA but also defined 17 additional and clinically relevant pathogenic/likely pathogenic CNVs. These CNVs were missed by CMA because of insufficient probe coverage in the targeted regions.

Opinions of Professional Societies

Although NIPT for subchromosomal CNVs is now clinically available, most professional societies do not recommend its clinical use. In 2020, the American College of Obstetrics and Gynecology recommended that cell-free DNA screening for microdeletion syndromes should not be performed because it has not been validated clinically[25]. In 2016, the American College of Medical Genetics and Genomics recommended informing all pregnant women of the availability of NIPT's expanded use to screen for clinically relevant CNVs when many criteria are met. However, it did not recommend screening for genome-wide CNVs[8]. In 2015, the European Society of Human Genetics and the American Society of Human Genetics did not recommend the expanded use of NIPT for subchromosomal CNVs because of ethical concerns, counseling challenges, and an increase in invasive diagnostic testing[26]. With the availability of prospective studies in large populations in recent years[4,9,10], these recommendations could be reevaluated and discussed further.

FACTORS AFFECTING NONINVASIVE PRENATAL TESTING SCREENING SUBCHROMOSOMAL COPY NUMBER VARIATION

Irrespective of the approach used (targeted or genome-wide), 4 critical factors affect the clinical validity and utility of NIPT for subchromosomal CNVs. These factors are fetal fraction, sequencing depth, CNV size, and biological and technical variability of the CNV region[27].

Fetal Fraction

The ratio of placental to total cfDNA in maternal plasma is known as the "fetal fraction." The average fetal fraction is 10% to 15%, ranging from less than 3% to more than 30%[28]. Using simulated samples, the detection rate of subchromosomal CNVs was shown to increase with fetal fraction[29]. In clinical plasma samples, increased fetal fraction improved the sensitivity for CNVs[30] and reduced maternal background interference[31]. Although NIPT with an increased fetal fraction was reported to have high specificity for CNVs[30], its impact on the false-positive rate was not systematically compared. It is worth noting that there is controversy about the effect of fetal fraction on the detection of aneuploidies. Hu and colleagues[32] demonstrated that an increase in fetal fraction (from 11.3% to 22.6%) increased the number of false-positive cases from 8 to 10. In contrast, He and colleagues[33] reported that an increase in fetal fraction (from 12.6% to 30.6%) decreased the number of false-positive cases from 11 to 3. Further studies are needed to clarify the impact of increased fetal fraction on NIPT's clinical validity for subchromosomal CNVs.

The fetal fraction can be enriched via different approaches, including **size selection**[34] and **DNA repair**[35]. The enrichment of fetal DNA via size selection relies on the fact that the size profile of fetal and maternal cfDNA is different. In general, fetal cfDNA is shorter than maternal cfDNA[36,37]. To date, magnetic nanoparticles[32,38], E-gel[39,40], and BluePippin[30] have been used for size selection of cfDNA in maternal plasma.

In 2019, Hu and colleagues[32] used magnetic nanoparticles to enrich the fetal fraction. As a result, the fetal fraction increased from 11.3% to 22.6%. In 2020, Zhang and colleagues[38] used 2 types of magnetic nanoparticles (carboxyl-nanoparticles and hydroxyl-nanoparticles) to increase the fetal fraction from 13% to 20%. One caveat was that the enrichment significantly reduced the total amount of cfDNA. The reduction in these 2 studies was 91.76% and 78.41%, respectively[32,38]. This reduction in turn resulted in higher duplicate reads in sequencing and finally a decreased number of unique mapped reads (sequencing depth) for bioinformatic analysis.

Agarose gel electrophoresis is another approach used for size selection in NIPT. Instead of manual gel electrophoresis, which tends to be labor- and time-consuming, there are 2 well-established semiautomatic systems for preparative gel electrophoresis and size selection, the E-gel system and the Pippin serial products.

The E-gel system generally uses precast agarose gels to separate DNA of different sizes and premade holes in the middle of the gel to collect DNA within a specific size range. Since 2018, several studies performed by Wang's group have demonstrated a similar and remarkable increase in fetal fraction by E-gel electrophoresis, which further reduced the "no-call" rate of NIPT for chromosomal aneuploidies in both singleton and twin pregnancies[31,39,40]. For example, Liang and colleagues[31] reported a 2.16-fold increase in fetal fraction and 1.3-fold reduction in maternal background interference in 1004 plasma samples after E-gel–based size selection of 100 to 150 bp. For subjects with high body mass index, E-gel electrophoresis significantly increased the average fetal fraction from 3.4% to 15.48%[40]. Similarly, in 86 plasma samples with dizygotic twin pregnancies, E-gel–based size selection of shorter fragments (107–145 bp) elevated the fetal fraction by around 3.2-fold, strongly enhancing the detection performance of NIPT for chromosomal aneuploidies[39].

Similar to the E-gel system, Pippin series products, including Pippin Prep, BluePippin, and PippinHT, use a precast agarose gel cassette. The systems collect target DNA by switching the channel to Elution Port upon the optical detection of a marker. As early as 2012, Quail and colleagues[34,41] demonstrated that size selection by Pippin Prep was more precise than other methods, capturing a tighter range of DNA size than manual gel electrophoresis or magnetic beads. Recently, Bluepippin was shown to dramatically increase fetal fraction by 2.3-fold in 1264 samples undergoing NIPT, resulting in a 2.2-fold increase in Z scores of positive samples and a substantial gain in sensitivity and specificity for the detection of microdeletions[30]. The analytical sensitivity and specificity were 95.6% and 99.95%, respectively, for the detection of DiGeorge syndrome after size selection[30].

DNA repair
Based on the hypothesis that fetal DNA has more damage than maternal cfDNA, Vong and colleagues[35] used a PreCR repair mix (a commercial DNA repair kit) to repair cfDNA in maternal plasma in pregnant women. The fetal fraction was increased slightly, by 4%, which was attributable to the recovery of a subset of long (>250 bp) cfDNA molecules.

Sequencing Depth

It is clear that a higher sequencing depth is better for accuracy in detecting subchromosomal CNVs. The read depth used for aneuploidies (4–10 million reads per sample) achieved a sensitivity of 83% for CNVs larger than 6 Mb. A higher read depth (up to 120 million reads per sample) increased the sensitivity to 94%[42]. Rampasek and colleagues[43] presented a probabilistic method for detecting fetal CNVs from maternal plasma. With the use of deep sequencing, CNVs greater than 400 kb could be detected with 90% sensitivity and CNVs of 50 to 400 kb with 40% sensitivity if the fetal fraction is sufficiently high (13%). Srinivasan and colleagues[44] estimated that NIPT could detect fetal CNVs as small as 300 kb using one billion reads.

Deeper sequencing improves the resolution and accuracy but substantially increases the cost per test, which precludes its routine use. To balance these factors, studies tend to increase sequencing depth in a limited manner, which has proven to improve the performance of NIPT in detecting subchromosomal CNVs. For example, sensitivity increased from 71.8% to 94.5% for CNVs larger than 1 Mb when the sequencing depth was increased from 3.5 million to 10 million reads[29]. Martin and colleagues[15] increased the sequencing reads from 3.2 million to 6 million for SNP-based NIPT, resulting in an increase in PPV from 15.7% to 44.2% for 22q11.2 and from 5.2% to 31.7% for Prader-Willi/Angelman syndromes, 1p36 deletion syndrome, and Cri-du-chat syndrome. A recent study recommended using 16 to 17 million reads (approximately 0.35× genome coverage) because the detection rate reached a plateau for CNVs larger than 3 Mb at a fetal fraction of 10%[45].

Copy Number Variation Size

In principle, larger CNVs in the fetus are easier to detect against a background of normal maternal DNA. Lo and colleagues[42] reported that NIPT with 4 to 10 million sequence reads and 50 bp per read (approximately 0.07–0.17× coverage) detected 15/18 (83%) samples with pathogenic CNVs greater than 6 Mb but only 2/10 samples with CNVs less than 6 Mb. Similarly, Liao and colleagues[46] used NIPT for common aneuploidies (approximate $0.1\times$ human genome) to detect the CNVs. The detection rate of fetal CNVs greater than 5 Mb and CNVs less than 5 Mb was 90.9% and 14.3%, respectively[17].

Copy Number Variation Region

The CNV region is the fourth factor affecting NIPT detection of subchromosomal CNVs. Biological and technical variability in the CNV region includes GC bias, repetitive elements, and ease of mapping[27], all of which can affect performance.

CHALLENGES

Although the use of NIPT for subchromosomal CNVs has progressed quickly in the past 3 years and become clinically available[4,9,10], many challenges remain in terms of its clinical application, including the selection of CNVs for screening, the presence of maternal CNVs, and the need for counseling. CNVs selected for screening should have severe and well-defined phenotypes with high penetrance. A low penetrance CNV alone does not seem to contribute to developmental, intellectual, and structural anomalies in a prenatal setting[47]. However, screening for such CNVs, for example, 22q11.2 duplication syndrome with a low penetrance of 21.9%[48], was reported[9,49]. This could cause considerable anxiety to couples, especially when the fetus has no ultrasound anomalies. The screening of genome-wide CNVs presents even more challenges. One critical step is to interpret the clinical relevance when CNVs are identified. This cannot be an easy task given the lack, limited, or conflicting phenotypic associations in prenatal setting. Although technical standards for the interpretation and reporting of CNVs were recently published[50], interpretation in the prenatal setting still poses several challenges given the lack of prenatal genotype-phenotype databases, and the penetrance issues described above.

The presence of maternal CNVs is another emerging challenge for screening fetal CNVs. Theoretically, maternal CNVs are easier to identify because around 90% of the cfDNA mixture is maternal in origin[28]. Statistically, maternal CNVs are not as rare as expected. Girirajan and colleagues[51] investigated the inheritance of CNVs using parental data that were available for 653 affected probands. Of 66 CNVs, there were 18 that were exclusively de novo; that is, the majority (48/66) were inherited. Another example is the report by Helgeson and coauthors[13] that identified 55 microdeletions from a randomly selected population of 175,393 pregnancies via NIPT, 25 of which had a maternal contribution. Technically, NIPT can identify maternal CNVs but cannot distinguish whether a CNV is a maternal-only or a maternal-and-fetal abnormality. Prenatal diagnosis is required to determine the status of the fetus when a maternal CNV is suspected, which leads to more invasive testing. However, with knowledge of the fetal fraction and a higher read depth, it is technically possible to determine whether the fetus has inherited the CNVs or not[42]. Further studies are thus warranted.

The last challenge is counseling. Counseling about CNVs is confounded by issues around penetrance[48], variable expressivity[51], CNV size being screened, and genes in the detected CNV[2]. Counseling should be personalized and should provide sufficient information. This is to ensure that patients make autonomous decisions with a full understanding of the benefits and limitations of the test[52]. However, counselors who can discuss prenatal testing options are not always accessible. More importantly, some critical test metrics are currently unavailable for NIPT in CNVs detection. For example, it is challenging to determine the number of missed CNVs in large-scale population studies[10] because subchromosomal CNVs may have variable expressivity, which cannot be identified by a physical check at birth. Long-term follow-up of negative cases has not been done and may not be feasible. As a result, sensitivity and negative predictive value cannot be calculated. When a positive screening result is confirmed, appropriate counseling is important for informed decision making, especially for those with novel CNVs. The American College of Medical Genetics and Genomics recommends providing accurate, balanced, up-to-date information at an appropriate literacy level when a fetus is diagnosed with a CNV[8].

SUMMARY

The application of NIPT for subchromosomal CNVs has been clinically available for several years. Although the sensitivity is unknown in clinical settings, the PPV for genome-wide CNV is clear. It ranges from 32% to 47%, which is comparable with the PPV for trisomy 13 (43.9%–53%), one of the commonly screened chromosome aneuploidies[4,9,10]. Four key factors affect the clinical validity of NIPT for subchromosomal CNVs: fetal fraction, sequencing depth, CNV size, and CNV region. Increasing the fetal fraction and sequencing depth can substantially improve the detection rate of subchromosomal CNVs. However, clinical application of NIPT for CNVs still presents several challenges, including the selection of CNVs for screening, the interpretation of genome-wide CNVs, false positives from maternal CNVs, and the need for appropriate counseling.

DISCLOSURE

J. Xiang and Z. Peng were employed at BGI Genomics at the time of submission.

REFERENCES

1. Lo YM, Corbetta N, Chamberlain PF, et al. Presence of fetal DNA in maternal plasma and serum. Lancet 1997;350(9076):485–7.
2. Bianchi DW, Chiu RWK. Sequencing of circulating cell-free DNA during pregnancy. N Engl J Med 2018;379(5):464–73.
3. Gadsboll K, Petersen OB, Gatinois V, et al. Current use of noninvasive prenatal testing in Europe, Australia and the USA: a graphical presentation. Acta Obstet Gynecol Scand 2020;99(6):722–30.
4. Van Den Bogaert K, Lannoo L, Brison N, et al. Outcome of publicly funded nationwide first-tier noninvasive prenatal screening. Genet Med 2021;23(6):1137–42.
5. Wapner RJ, Martin CL, Levy B, et al. Chromosomal microarray versus karyotyping for prenatal diagnosis. N Engl J Med 2012;367(23):2175–84.
6. Wang H, Dong Z, Zhang R, et al. Low-pass genome sequencing versus chromosomal microarray analysis: implementation in prenatal diagnosis. Genet Med 2020;22(3):500–10.
7. Capalbo A, Rienzi L, Ubaldi FM. Diagnosis and clinical management of duplications and deletions. Fertil Steril 2017;107(1):12–8.
8. Gregg AR, Skotko BG, Benkendorf JL, et al. Noninvasive prenatal screening for fetal aneuploidy, 2016 update: a position statement of the American College of Medical Genetics and Genomics. Genet Med 2016;18(10):1056–65.
9. Liang D, Cram DS, Tan H, et al. Clinical utility of noninvasive prenatal screening for expanded chromosome disease syndromes. Genet Med 2019;21(9): 1998–2006.

10. van der Meij KRM, Sistermans EA, Macville MVE, et al. TRIDENT-2: national implementation of genome-wide non-invasive prenatal testing as a first-tier screening test in the Netherlands. Am J Hum Genet 2019;105(6):1091–101.

11. Liao GJ, Chan KC, Jiang P, et al. Noninvasive prenatal diagnosis of fetal trisomy 21 by allelic ratio analysis using targeted massively parallel sequencing of maternal plasma DNA. PLoS One 2012;7(5):e38154.

12. Chiu RW, Chan KC, Gao Y, et al. Noninvasive prenatal diagnosis of fetal chromosomal aneuploidy by massively parallel genomic sequencing of DNA in maternal plasma. Proc Natl Acad Sci U S A 2008;105(51):20458–63.

13. Helgeson J, Wardrop J, Boomer T, et al. Clinical outcome of subchromosomal events detected by whole-genome noninvasive prenatal testing. Prenat Diagn 2015;35(10):999–1004.

14. Wapner RJ, Babiarz JE, Levy B, et al. Expanding the scope of noninvasive prenatal testing: detection of fetal microdeletion syndromes. Am J Obstet Gynecol 2015;212(3):332 e1–9.

15. Martin K, Iyengar S, Kalyan A, et al. Clinical experience with a single-nucleotide polymorphism-based non-invasive prenatal test for five clinically significant microdeletions. Clin Genet 2018;93(2):293–300.

16. Lefkowitz RB, Tynan JA, Liu T, et al. Clinical validation of a noninvasive prenatal test for genomewide detection of fetal copy number variants. Am J Obstet Gynecol 2016;215(2):227.e1–16.

17. Li R, Wan J, Zhang Y, et al. Detection of fetal copy number variants by noninvasive prenatal testing for common aneuploidies. Ultrasound Obstet Gynecol 2016;47(1):53–7.

18. Liu H, Gao Y, Hu Z, et al. Performance evaluation of NIPT in detection of chromosomal copy number variants using low-coverage whole-genome sequencing of plasma DNA. PLoS One 2016;11(7):e0159233.

19. Dong Z, Yan J, Xu F, et al. Genome sequencing explores complexity of chromosomal abnormalities in recurrent miscarriage. Am J Hum Genet 2019;105(6): 1102–11.

20. Shaffer LG, Bejjani BA. A cytogeneticist's perspective on genomic microarrays. Hum Reprod Update 2004;10(3):221–6.

21. Huber D, Voith von Voithenberg L, Kaigala GV. Fluorescence in situ hybridization (FISH): history, limitations and what to expect from micro-scale FISH? Micro Nano Eng 2018;1:15–24.

22. Levy B, Burnside RD. Are all chromosome microarrays the same? What clinicians need to know. Prenat Diagn 2019;39(3):157–64.

23. Miller DT, Adam MP, Aradhya S, et al. Consensus statement: chromosomal microarray is a first-tier clinical diagnostic test for individuals with developmental disabilities or congenital anomalies. Am J Hum Genet 2010;86(5):749–64.

24. Dong Z, Zhang J, Hu P, et al. Low-pass whole-genome sequencing in clinical cytogenetics: a validated approach. Genet Med 2016;18(9):940–8.

25. Rose NC, Kaimal AJ, Dugoff L, et al. Screening for fetal chromosomal abnormalities: ACOG Practice Bulletin, Number 226. Obstet Gynecol 2020;136(4):e48–69.

26. Dondorp W, de Wert G, Bombard Y, et al. Non-invasive prenatal testing for aneuploidy and beyond: challenges of responsible innovation in prenatal screening. Eur J Hum Genet 2015;23(11):1438–50.

27. Zhao C, Tynan J, Ehrich M, et al. Detection of fetal subchromosomal abnormalities by sequencing circulating cell-free DNA from maternal plasma. Clin Chem 2015;61(4):608–16.

28. Canick JA, Palomaki GE, Kloza EM, et al. The impact of maternal plasma DNA fetal fraction on next generation sequencing tests for common fetal aneuploidies. Prenat Diagn 2013;33(7):667–74.

29. Yin AH, Peng CF, Zhao X, et al. Noninvasive detection of fetal subchromosomal abnormalities by semiconductor sequencing of maternal plasma DNA. Proc Natl Acad Sci U S A 2015;112(47):14670–5.

30. Welker NC, Lee AK, Kjolby RAS, et al. High-throughput fetal fraction amplification increases analytical performance of noninvasive prenatal screening. Genet Med 2021;23(3):443–50.

31. Liang B, Li H, He Q, et al. Enrichment of the fetal fraction in non-invasive pre-natal screening reduces maternal background interference. Sci Rep 2018;8(1): 17675.

32. Hu P, Liang D, Chen Y, et al. An enrichment method to increase cell-free fetal DNA fraction and significantly reduce false negatives and test failures for non-invasive prenatal screening: a feasibility study. J Transl Med 2019; 17(1):124.

33. He QZ, Wu XJ, He QY, et al. A method for improving the accuracy of non-invasive prenatal screening by cell-free foetal DNA size selection. Br J Biomed Sci 2018; 75(3):133–8.

34. Quail MA, Gu Y, Swerdlow H, et al. Evaluation and optimisation of preparative semi-automated electrophoresis systems for Illumina library preparation. Electro-phoresis 2012;33(23):3521–8.

35. Vong JSL, Jiang P, Cheng SH, et al. Enrichment of fetal and maternal long cell-free DNA fragments from maternal plasma following DNA repair. Prenat Diagn 2019;39(2):88–99.

36. Lo YM, Chan KC, Sun H, et al. Maternal plasma DNA sequencing reveals the genome-wide genetic and mutational profile of the fetus. Sci Transl Med 2010; 2(61):61ra91.

37. Fan HC, Blumenfeld YJ, Chitkara U, et al. Analysis of the size distributions of fetal and maternal cell-free DNA by paired-end sequencing. Clin Chem 2010;56(8): 1279–86.

38. Zhang B, Zhao S, Wan H, et al. High-resolution DNA size enrichment using a magnetic nano-platform and application in non-invasive prenatal testing. Analyst 2020;145(17):5733–9.

39. Qiao L, Yu B, Liang Y, et al. Sequencing shorter cfDNA fragments improves the fetal DNA fraction in noninvasive prenatal testing. Am J Obstet Gynecol 2019; 221(4):345.e1–11.

40. Qiao L, Zhang Q, Liang Y, et al. Sequencing of short cfDNA fragments in NIPT improves fetal fraction with higher maternal BMI and early gestational age. Am J Transl Res 2019;11(7):4450–9.

41. Quail MA, Swerdlow H, Turner DJ. Improved protocols for the Illumina genome analyzer sequencing system. Curr Protoc Hum Genet 2009. Chapter 18:Unit 18 2.

42. Lo KK, Karampetsou E, Boustred C, et al. Limited clinical utility of non-invasive prenatal testing for subchromosomal abnormalities. Am J Hum Genet 2016; 98(1):34–44.

43. Rampasek L, Arbabi A, Brudno M. Probabilistic method for detecting copy num-ber variation in a fetal genome using maternal plasma sequencing. Bioinformat-ics 2014;30(12):i212–8.

44. Srinivasan A, Bianchi DW, Huang H, et al. Noninvasive detection of fetal subchromosome abnormalities via deep sequencing of maternal plasma. Am J Hum Genet 2013;92(2):167–76.
45. Kucharik M, Gnip A, Hyblova M, et al. Non-invasive prenatal testing (NIPT) by low coverage genomic sequencing: detection limits of screened chromosomal microdeletions. PLoS One 2020;15(8):e0238245.
46. Liao C, Yin AH, Peng CF, et al. Noninvasive prenatal diagnosis of common aneuploidies by semiconductor sequencing. Proc Natl Acad Sci U S A 2014;111(20):7415–20.
47. Maya I, Sharony R, Yacobson S, et al. When genotype is not predictive of phenotype: implications for genetic counseling based on 21,594 chromosomal microarray analysis examinations. Genet Med 2018;20(1):128–31.
48. Rosenfeld JA, Coe BP, Eichler EE, et al. Estimates of penetrance for recurrent pathogenic copy-number variations. Genet Med 2013;15(6):478–81.
49. Hu H, Wang L, Wu J, et al. Noninvasive prenatal testing for chromosome aneuploidies and subchromosomal microdeletions/microduplications in a cohort of 8141 single pregnancies. Hum Genomics 2019;13(1):14.
50. Riggs ER, Andersen EF, Cherry AM, et al. Technical standards for the interpretation and reporting of constitutional copy-number variants: a joint consensus recommendation of the American College of Medical Genetics and Genomics (ACMG) and the Clinical Genome Resource (ClinGen). Genet Med 2020;22(2):245–57.
51. Girirajan S, Rosenfeld JA, Coe BP, et al. Phenotypic heterogeneity of genomic disorders and rare copy-number variants. N Engl J Med 2012;367(14):1321–31.
52. Sachs A, Blanchard L, Buchanan A, et al. Recommended pre-test counseling points for noninvasive prenatal testing using cell-free DNA: a 2015 perspective. Prenat Diagn 2015;35(10):968–71.
53. McDonald-McGinn DM, Hain HS, Emanuel BS, et al. 22q11.2 deletion syndrome. In: Adam MP, Ardinger HH, Pagon RA, et al, editors. GeneReviews® [Internet]. Seattle (WA): University of Washington, Seattle; 2020. p. 1993–2021. Available at: https://www.ncbi.nlm.nih.gov/books/NBK1523/.
54. Driscoll DJ, Miller JL, Schwartz S, et al. Prader-Willi syndrome. In: Adam MP, Ardinger HH, Pagon RA, et al, editors. GeneReviews® [Internet]. Seattle (WA): University of Washington, Seattle; 1998. p. 1993–2021. Available at: https://www.ncbi.nlm.nih.gov/books/NBK1330/.
55. Dagli AI, Mueller J, CA W. Angelman syndrome. In: Adam MP, Ardinger HH, Pagon RA, et al, editors. GeneReviews® [Internet]. Seattle (WA): University of Washington, Seattle; 1998. 1993-2021. Available at: https://www.ncbi.nlm.nih.gov/books/NBK1144/.
56. Cerruti Mainardi P. Cri du chat syndrome. Orphanet J Rare Dis 2006;1:33.
57. Firth HV, Richards SM, Bevan AP, et al. DECIPHER: Database of Chromosomal Imbalance and Phenotype in Humans Using Ensembl Resources. Am J Hum Genet 2009;84(4):524–33.
58. Jordan VK, Zaveri HP, Scott DA. 1p36 deletion syndrome: an update. Appl Clin Genet 2015;8:189–200.
59. Battaglia A, Carey JC, ST S. Wolf-Hirschhorn syndrome – RETIRED CHAPTER, FOR HISTORICAL REFERENCE ONLY [Updated 2015 Aug 20]. In: Adam MP, Ardinger HH, Pagon RA, et al, editors. GeneReviews® [Internet]. Seattle (WA): University of Washington, Seattle; 2002. 1993-2021. Available at: https://www.ncbi.nlm.nih.gov/books/NBK1183/.

60. Battaglia A, Carey JC, South ST. Wolf-Hirschhorn syndrome: a review and update. Am J Med Genet C Semin Med Genet 2015;169(3):216–23.
61. Mattina T, Perrotta CS, Grossfeld P. Jacobsen syndrome. Orphanet J Rare Dis 2009;4:9.
62. Maas S, Shaw A, Bikker H, et al. Trichorhinophalangeal syndrome. In: Adam MP, Ardinger HH, Pagon RA, et al, editors. GeneReviews® [Internet]. Seattle (WA): University of Washington, Seattle; 2017. p. 1993–2021. Available at: https://www.ncbi.nlm.nih.gov/books/NBK425926/.

The Role of the Human Gutome on Chronic Disease
A Review of the Microbiome and Nutrigenomics

Carrie C. Hoefer, PhD, MBA[a],*, Leah K. Hollon, ND, MPH[b,1],
Jennifer A. Campbell, PharmD[c]

KEYWORDS

- Nutrigenomics • Microbiome • Nutrition • Diabetes • Cardiovascular • Obesity
- Breast cancer • Colon cancer

KEY POINTS

- The microbiome and optimal nutrition vary among individuals and may be used along with pharmacogenomics to further improve individualized treatment strategies.
- Common genetic variants associated with chronic disease and the therapeutic effects of nutrition and human microbiome are summarized.
- The gut microbiome and nutrigenomics modify chronic disease and acute disease progression and outcomes.
- The gut microbiome and nutrigenomics influence obesity, diabetes, cardiovascular disease, and cancer treatment.

INTRODUCTION

The human gutome is a mosaic of nutrients, gut flora/bacteria, and genomic biomarkers that play a role in human health and disease[1,2]. One can look at the gutome in 2 distinct ways: the human gut microbiome and nutrigenomics. Nutrigenomics studies the influence and interaction of nutrition and genes and can facilitate understanding of nutrient consumption and genomic biomarkers that may lead to the

This article originally appeared in Advances in Molecular Pathology, Volume 4, Issue 1, November 2021.

C.C. Hoefer and L.K. Hollon: contributing first author.

[a] James L. Winkle College of Pharmacy, University of Cincinnati, 231 Albert Sabin Way, MSB 3005, Cincinnati, OH 45267, USA; [b] Richmond Natural Medicine, National University of Natural Medicine Residency, 9211 Forest Hill Avenue, Richmond, VA 23235, USA; [c] Manchester University, College of Pharmacy, Natural, and Health Sciences, 10627 Diebold Road, Fort Wayne, IN 46845, USA

[1] Present address: 9211 Forest Hill Avenue, Richmond, VA 23235.

* Corresponding author. 45 Arcadia Pl., Cincinnati OH, 45208.

E-mail address: hoefercc@ucmail.uc.edu

development of nutrition-related diseases and metabolic syndromes[1,3]. The human gut microbiome is defined as the totality of microorganisms, bacteria, viruses, protozoa, and fungi, including their collective genetic material inhabiting the gastrointestinal system[4]. Therefore, the gut microbiome is a notably diverse habitat that provides a collective and historical picture of the environmental exposures throughout one's life. Although it is colonized throughout life, it is initially seeded during fetal development and thus imprinted from our ancestors. It has been noted that "Homeostasis of the intestinal microbial environment is likely to be affected multiple times across the lifespan of the average individual due to antibiotic usage, inflammation, aging, psychological stress, nutrition and lifestyle choices, as well as other environmental factors"[5].

The gut microbiome plays a significant role in health as well as the development of chronic disease owing to its ability to regulate the immune, endocrine, and neurologic systems[5,6]. This role of the human gut microbiome is a more recently recognized determinant in human disease; little research has assessed the interaction of the gut microbiome and genomic biomarkers in disease[1]. Furthermore, the gut microbiome, which varies throughout the lifetime, may begin to metabolize orally administered medications and lead to variability in medication response. Additionally, this collaborative community of organisms is constantly communicating within the microbiome and requires key nutrients for effective function[7]. Deficiencies of certain nutrients including vitamins A, D, and E, calcium, and magnesium are associated with fewer healthy bacterial populations and can also promote harmful populations within the microbiome[8]. The purpose of this review is to bring together the 2 concepts of the human gut microbiome and nutrigenomic factors that impact nutrition related diseases.

SIGNIFICANCE
Gut Microbiome

The human gut microbiome has been an evolving source of information in the quest to understand ongoing health and disease. Similarities as well as differences exist from person to person relating to microbiome diversity. Yet, within each individual, these organisms can be symbiotic, commensal, therapeutic, and even pathogenic. Inherently, some species are pathogenic and others are beneficial. Certain species that are inherently commensal or neutral can become pathogenic. In these cases, the role of the organism can be based on the amount found within the gut and the balance of other flora. In general, the greater the diversity of flora the more protective against chronic disease. This diversity of flora leads to greater stability of the mucosal barrier facilitating appropriate production of carbohydrate and protein fuel for the gut. Yet, if only a few species are found in excess and are inherently pathogenic or excess of commensal bacteria exist, microbial metabolism of intestinal contents is altered because these species have the ability to hijack the functions at the mucosal lining, altering the carbohydrates made to promote their own food for consumption and leading to overpopulation[9]. This influence on the health and variability of the gut have led some investigators to believe that the human gut microbiome should be considered its own organ system, in addition to seeing it as a collection of our external environmental experiences over life.

This variability begins in utero and continues into childbirth where genetic and nongenetic material are passed from mother to child[10,11]. As such, some individuals are seeded early with pathogenic microbes or may lack commensal flora owing to determinants of their mother's health, including her diet, pharmacotherapy, immune (infections), and endocrine functions[12,13]. Throughout life, this variability compounds; some individuals are more likely to retain beneficial microbes fostering health, whereas others may adopt pathogenic growth. The human gut microbiome changes throughout one's life as well as throughout various times of the year[14]. This demonstrates the microbiome is modifiable and can therefore be altered to improve or worsen health.

If the microbiome contains overpopulated dysbiosis, there can be an increased risk of chronic disease, specifically autoimmune disease. One of the earliest and most notable findings within the literature demonstrated *Klebsiella* fostered the development of rheumatoid arthritis and inflammatory bowel disease (IBD)[13,15]. In some cases, bacteria had been laid years before their presentation of autoimmune disease. This knowledge of autoimmune disease now extends to include *Bifidobacterium*, *Staphylococcus*, *Enterococcus*, *Salmonella*, *Lactobacillus*, *Pseudomonas*, and *Proteus*[5]. Additionally, deficient amounts of *Faecalibacterium* and *Roseburia* lead to an increased risk of rheumatoid arthritis and IBD[16,17]. As discussed elsewhere in this article, gut flora balance is a significant determinant of whether or not disease presents itself. In cases where pathogenic bacteria play a role, a key mechanism remains at the lining of the gut. Secretory IgA serves as a protective lining, but can be altered under stress, poor food choices (eg, inflammatory foods), and even pharmacotherapy. This factor impacts the permeability of the lining, leading pathogens and food particulates to cross over outside of the gut. At this point, immune proteins including IL-23 alert additional inflammatory pathways including tumor necrosis factor-alpha, which become systemic and cross-reactive with other parts of the body, causing peripheral symptoms such as pain[17]. Thus, excessive, or insufficient microbes can contribute to autoimmune disease.

Nutrigenomics and Disease

To fully understand the human gutome, one must be able to identify the molecular level at which metabolic syndromes can be exacerbated. As much as diet can have beneficial effects on overall health, there is a wide range of interindividual variability in response to specific diets[3]. Just as pharmacogenomics can be used to predict drug response, nutrigenomics assesses the genetic predictability in diseases relevant to diet and nutrition[2]. The intestinal tract in which drug and food absorption occurs contains numerous phase I and II drug-metabolizing enzymes. The alteration of pharmacokinetics via microbial activity is an additional level of interindividual drug response altering the disposition and toxicity of drugs and their metabolites[18,19]. With both enzymes and microbial activity altering drug therapy and nutrition, it should be concerning that obesity has increased by more than 10% in the last 20 years, because obesity is linked to poor gut health[20]. Obesity is one of the leading risk factors in developing metabolic syndromes, which can lead to diseases such as type 2 diabetes (T2DM) and cardiovascular disease (CVD)[21]. **Table 1** is a representative example of genes linked to obesity that frequently appear in the literature.

The World Health Organization estimates that 422 million people worldwide have diabetes. Diabetes is considered one of the largest health burdens globally, especially those in low- and middle-income countries[22]. T2DM is a complex disease owing to the numerous biomarkers, such as insulin secretion and resistance, environmental factors including diet and nutrition, and genes associated with T2DM. Gene–nutrient interactions play a crucial role in the pathogenesis of T2DM; therefore, a better understanding of the nutrigenomics of diabetes is essential to the development of prevention, detection, and treatment of the disease[23]. **Table 2** is a representative example of genes linked to T2DM that frequently appear in the literature.

Table 1
Genes and Polymorphisms Related to Obesity and/or Fat Gain

Gene	Prominent SNPs (Minor Allele; Frequency)	Evidence Associations	References
APOA Family	rs5082 (MA:G; 0.24)	Associated with higher intake of PUFAs (T-allele), and BMI (C-allele)	3,62
	rs662799 (MA:G; 0.16)	Associated with HDL and intake of PUFAs (TT-genotype)	3,63
	rs3135506 (MA:C; 0.06)	Associated with high saturated fats and total fat consumption (GG-genotype)	3,63
APOE	rs429358 (MA:C; 0.15)	Associated with lipid metabolism disturbances	34,64
	rs7412 (MA:T; 0.08)	Associated with lipid metabolism disturbances	34,64
CLOCK	rs4580704 (MA:G; 0.28)	Associated with C-reactive protein levels and HDL/ApoA1 ratios (CC-genotype)	34,65
	rs1801260 (MA:G; 0.23)	Associated with body weight reduction (A-allele)	34,65
FTO	rs9930506 (MA:G; 0.29)	Associated with higher BMI and weight (G-allele)	3,66
	rs9939609 (MA:A; 0.34)	Associated with BMI, fat mass, weight, c-reactive protein, and leptin levels (A-allele)	3,63,67
	rs17817449 (MA:G; 0.31)	Associated with higher weight, BMI, waist-hip circumference, cholesterol, triglycerides, adiponectin and fasting glucose (GG-genotype)	3,68
INSIG2	rs12464355 (MA:G; 0.03)	Associated with LDL levels (G-allele)	3,69
	rs17047757 (MA:G; 0.12)	Associated with weight	3,69
	rs7566605 (MA:C; 0.29)	Associated with obesity (CC-genotype)	3,70
MC4R	rs2229616 (MA:T; 0.02)	Associated with features of metabolic syndrome and lower risk of obesity, and appetite control (I103 allele)	3,71,72
	rs17782313 (MA:C; 0.24)	Associated with obesity, and appetite control (C-allele)	34,71
MTHFR	rs1801133 (0.25)	Associated with obesity, high homocysteine and low folate	26,34,72
PPARA	rs1800206 (MA:G; 0.02)	Associated with lipid metabolism disturbances	34,71
PPARG	rs1801282 (MA:G; 0.07)	Associated with obesity and lipid parameters	34,71
TCF7L2	rs7903146 (MA:T; 0.23)	Associated with fat intake, and dietary components, nuclear and cytoplasm regulatory machinery for fat gain	34,71

Minor allele frequency was determined using the minor allele frequency from phase III populations: https://useast.ensembl.org/index.html.
Abbreviations: BMI, body mass index; HDL, high-density lipoproteins; LDL, low-density lipoproteins; PUFA, polyunsaturated fatty acids; SNP, single nucleotide polymorphism.

Table 2
Genes and Polymorphisms Related to T2DM

Gene	Prominent SNPs (Minor Allele Frequency)	Evidence Associations	References
ADIPOQ	rs1501299 (MA:T; 0.30)	Associated with higher fasting blood glucose and HbA1C, and insulin signaling (T-allele)	23,73
	rs2241766 (MA:G; 0.15)	Associated with decreased risk of T2DM, and insulin signaling (G-allele)	23,73
CAV2	rs2270188 (MA:G; 0.45)	Associated with higher risk of T2DM and insulin signaling (T-allele)	23,73
CLOCK	rs4580704 (MA:G; 0.28)	Associated with decreased risk of T2DM (G-allele)	23
	rs1801260 (MA:G; 0.23)	Associated with fasting insulin levels (C-allele)	73,74
CRY1	rs2287161 (MA:C; 0.46)	Associated with fasting insulin, an increase in HOMA-IR index, and a decrease in QUICK1 (C-allele)	23,73
FTO	rs9939609 (MA:A; 0.34)	Associated with lower risk of T2DM (A-allele)	23,73
	rs8050136 (MA:A; 0.32)	Associated with lower risk of T2DM (A-allele)	23
IRS1	rs7578326 (MA:G; 0.29)	Associated with decreased resistance to (plasma) insulin (G-allele)	23,63,71
	rs2943641 (MA: T; 0.25)	Associated with decreased resistance to (plasma) insulin, hyperinsulinemia, dyslipidemia and with HOMA-IR index (T-allele)	23,73,75,76
PLIN1	rs894160 (MA:T; 0.33)	Associated for HOMA-IR index in woman, and intake of fat and carbohydrates (A-allele)	23,77
	rs1052700 (MA:T; 0.28)	Associated with HOMA-IR and intake of fat and carbohydrates (A-allele)	23,73,77
PPARG	rs180282 (MA:C; 0.19)	Associated with higher risk of T2DM, and HOMA-IR index (G-allele)	23,73,75,76
SLC30A8	rs11558471 (MA:G; 0.26)	Associated with smaller levels of fasting plasma glucose (A-allele)	23,73,76
	rs13266634 (MA:T; 0.26)	Associated with T2DM risk (C-allele)	23,73,76
TCF7L2	rs7903146 (MA:T; 0.23)	Associated with T2DM risk (T-allele)	23,62,76
	rs12255372 (MA:G; 0.21)	Associated with T2DM risk (T-allele)	23,73,75,76
	rs12573128 (MA:G; 0.43)	Associated with HOMA-IR index and oral glucose tolerance (G-allele)	73,75,76
TRPM6	rs3750425 (MA:T; 0.18)	Associated for T2DM risk in woman (T-allele)	23
	rs2274924 (MA:C; 0.29)	Associated for T2DM risk in woman, and fasting glucose levels (T-allele)	23,73

Minor allele frequency was determined using the minor allele frequency from phase II populations: https://useast.ensembl.org/index.html.
Abbreviations: HbA1C, hemoglobin A1C; HOMA-IR, insulin resistance calculator; QUICK1, quantitative insulin sensitivity check index; SNP, single nucleotide polymorphism.

CVD encompasses numerous disorders such as heart disease, heart attack, stroke, congenital heart disease, and heart failure[3]. As of 2019 CVD had a prevalence of about 18.6 million people and was the leading global cause of death[24]. The American Heart Association has seven health factors to gauge the risk of CVD known as Life's Simple 7. Included in Life's Simple 7 are smoking, physical inactivity, nutrition, obesity, cholesterol, diabetes, and high blood pressure. Therefore, lifestyle, especially diet, impacts CVD risk both directly and indirectly[24,25]. As with obesity and T2DM, there is a large amount of interindividual variability with diet and CVD risk/mortality; thus, it is prudent to determine which genetic factors are linked with CVD and nutrition. **Table 3** is a representative example of genes linked to CVD that frequently appear in the literature.

As seen in the tables in this article, the same gene and polymorphism show up across diseases related to the metabolic syndrome. This connection is also seen in the disease states; obesity can lead to T2DM and CVD. For example, *FTO* is said to impact both obesity and T2DM. *FTO* is associated with higher body mass index and a higher body mass index can lead to T2DM. Additionally, *MTHFR* is associated with obesity and modest changes in homocysteine levels[3]. Of note, although common *MTHFR* variants were historically thought to be associated with mild hyperhomocysteinemia, leading to increased risk for thrombophilia, coronary heart disease, and recurrent miscarriage, currently, *MTHFR* genetic testing is thought to have limited clinical usefulness alone[26]. Interestingly, each of these genes may have a different impact depending on a person's diet. For example, the *APOE* gene harbors 3 different alleles that carry different probabilities of developing CVD and differing responses to environmental factors such as fat included in the diet[27].

Furthermore, many common cancers, such as breast cancer and colorectal cancer have been linked in part to metabolic syndromes[28]. The American Cancer Society notes that one in 3 individuals will be diagnosed with cancer within their lifetime[29]. Foods including processed meats are associated with several cancers and can alter gut microbiome forming a hospitable environment for tumorigenesis with 1 study showing 50 g of processed meat increasing colon cancer by 20%[30,31]. Similarly, high glycemic index foods present a risk for developing colon, breast, and endometrial cancers[32]. Previously discussed genes of *FTO*, *MTHFR*, *APOA*, and *APOE* have been implicated in cancer risk. Specifically, polymorphisms of *FTO* along with obesity increase cancer risk and thus play an active role in adipogenesis and tumorigenesis[33]. **Table 4** is a representative example of nutrigenomic genes linked to cancer that frequently appear in the literature.

Diet and the Gutome

The importance of nutrigenomics has been well-demonstrated through certain lineage diets. One such lineage diet, known as the Mediterranean diet, has been useful in enhancing the human gut microbiome. The Mediterranean diet consists of using olive oil as the principal source of fat for cooking, and choosing white meats, such as chicken or fish, over red meats[34]. Some studies have found red meat to be of increased risk of cancer owing to many being processed with nitrates and nitrites. These nitroso compounds can become beneficial S-nitroso compounds or carcinogenic, but it depends on dietary and environmental factors including food macronutrients such as fats and fiber, gastric acidity, and microbial flora[35]. Additionally, one reason that the Mediterranean diet is effective is that it alters the microbiome by increasing the levels of short-chain fatty acids and certain gut flora, including *Prevotella* and some fiber-degrading *Firmicutes*[36]. Meslier and colleagues[37] demonstrated that those adopting a Mediterranean diet for 2 months decreased their cholesterol,

Table 3
Genes and Polymorphisms Related to CVD

Gene	Prominent SNPs (Minor Allele Frequency)	Evidence Associations (Risk Allele)	References
APOA family	rs662799 (MA:G; 0.16)	Associated with elevated plasma triglycerides, increased risk of hypertriglyceridemia, VLDL and reduced HDL (C-allele)	3,78–80
	rs670 (MA:T; 0.19)	Associated with higher PUFA intake and higher HDL in woman (A-allele)	3,78–80
APOE	ε2/ε3/ε4	Associated with increased risk of CVD, CHD	3
CDKN2B	rs10757274 (MA: G; 0.40)	Associated with coronary heart disease, myocardial infarction, and atherosclerosis (C-allele)	81–83
	rs2383206 (MA:G; 0.49)	Associated with coronary heart disease, myocardial infarction, and atherosclerosis (G-allele)	81–83
	rs10757278 (MA: G; 0.41)	Associated with coronary heart disease, myocardial infarction, and atherosclerosis (C-allele	81,83,84
	rs1333049 (MA:C; 0.42)	Associated with coronary artery disease and myocardial infarction (C-allele)	81,83
MTHFR	rs1801133 (MA:A; 0.25)	Historically associated with modestly higher homocysteine levels and oxidative modification of LDL (C-allele); no longer believed to be a significant CVD factor alone.	3,78,80
PPARA	rs1800206 (MA:G; 0.02)	Associated with higher waist circumference, lipid oxidation, inflammation and telomere length	3,85

Minor allele frequency was determined using the minor allele frequency from phase III populations: https://useast.ensembl.org/index.html.
Abbreviations: CHD, congenital heart diseases; HDL, high-density lipoprotein; LDL, low-density lipoprotein; PUFA, polyunsaturated fatty acid; SNP, single nucleotide polymorphism; VLDL, very low-density lipoprotein.

Table 4
Genes and Polymorphisms Related to Cancer Risk

Gene	Prominent SNPs (Minor Allele Frequency)	Evidence associations (CRC/BC)	References
APOA family	rs1799837 (MA:T; <0.01)	(BC) Inhibit growth and invasion of tumor cells, variations lead to increased risk of BC (A-allele)	86
	rs5069 (MA:A; 0.12)	(BC) Inhibit growth and invasion of tumor cells, variations lead to increased risk of BC (T-allele)	86
	rs670 (MA:T; 0.19)	(BC) Poor surgery prognosis and increase risk of disease progression (A-allele)	87
	Nonspecified	(CRC) Increase elimination of bile acids leading to gut carcinogenesis	88
APOE	Nonspecified	(CRC) Increase elimination of bile acids leading to gut carcinogenesis; absence of e3 allele may increase risk with western diet in older individuals	88,89
	e4/e4	(BC) higher serum triglycerides leading to increased risk of BC depending on tumor staging	90,91
BRCA1	Nonspecified	(BC) Associated with familial cases of breast cancer. Lower risk with coffee consumption, genistein, folate and cobalamin intake, selenium supplementation, and fruit and veggie intake. Higher risk with iron consumption.	92,93
BRCA2	Nonspecified	(BC) Associated with familial cases of breast cancer. Lower risk with soy, genistein, fruits and vegetable intake	92,93
FTO	Nonspecified	(CRC) Dysregulated in CRC and may play a significant role in progression; regulates PD-L1 expression	94
	rs1558902 (MA:A; 0.23) rs8050136 (MA:A; 0.32) rs3751812 (MA:T; 0.22) rs9939609 (MA:A; 0.34)	(CRC) positive association with CRC (Minor Allele of each SNP associated with increased risk)	95
MTHFR	rs1801133 (MA:A; 0.25)	(CRC) decreased enzyme activity may lead to susceptibility especially with low folate intake and low vitamin B6. Additionally, increased risk of microsatellite-high tumors (T-allele)	88,92,96,97
	rs1801131 (MA:G; 0.25)	(BC) TT genotype may lead to increased risk of BC, along with intake of B-vitamins (T-allele)	
		(CRC) decreased enzyme activity may lead to susceptibility (CC-genotype)	88,98
PPARG	Nonspecified	(CRC) expression in tumors in associated with longer survival	99–101
		(BC) associated with disease free survival	

Minor allele frequency was determined using the minor allele frequency from phase III populations: https://useast.ensembl.org/index.html.

increased bile acid elimination, and improved insulin sensitivity; and there was enhanced diversity and increased amounts of microbiota species[32]. Additionally, the microbiome was enhanced to further house fiber-degrading *Faecalibacterium prausnitzii*, and there was also an increase of genes degrading microbial carbohydrates within the gut. Specifically, one gene upregulated to increase butyrate metabolism[37]. This is notable as butyrate is one of the most protective compounds known to reduce the risk of nonalcoholic steatohepatitis, atherosclerosis, IBD[38], and various cancers[39]. One study found the Mediterranean diet to be protective against the development of colon cancer through mediating DNA methylation of the CpG site cg-20674490-RUNX3 that prevents the onset of the disease[40].

Similarly, the Mediterranean diet also has clinical relevance for those with HER2+ breast cancers and carriers of *BRCA1/BRCA2* mutations owing to its ability to impact glucose regulation and insulin sensitivity, both of which are imperative in *BRCA1* and *BRCA2* mutation carriers[35,41,42]. Bruno and colleagues[43] found that in BRCA mutation carriers, the Mediterranean diet improved insulin sensitivity through insulin-like growth factor protein 1. Additionally, women observed a decrease in weight, a slimmer waistline and hips, and lowered cholesterol and triglycerides[43]. Thus, the nutrigenomics of some of the most concerning forms of breast cancer showed improved endocrine and immune balance through implementation of the Mediterranean diet.

In addition to the Mediterranean diet, certain religious diets including fasting have nutrigenomic effects on the microbiome. A small study conducted during the month of Ramadan by Özkul and colleagues[44] showed fasting improved the microbiome. Fasting increased bacteria known as *Akkermansia muciniphila* and *Bacteroides fragilis*. This finding is significant, because a deficiency in *A muciniphila* can be associated with chronic diseases including amyotrophic lateral sclerosis, Alzheimer's disease, and IBD, whereas the addition of *A muciniphila* to the gutome can slow the progression of amyotrophic lateral sclerosis[43–47]. A possible explanation for the benefits of fasting on the microbiome may be through by balancing nicotinamide, which is known to assist with the integrity of tissues, including skin and mucosal membranes, as well as enhancing detoxification processes through NADPH.

In contrast, an excess of *A muciniphila* has been associated with other diseases. In 1 study, a 4-fold increase of *A muciniphila* was found to be correlated with colon cancer[48,49]. As with colon cancer and other cancers, the -omics approaches may permit specific or targeted therapeutic options. These options include both diet and pharmacotherapy, including chemotherapy. Thus, therapeutic options should be based on the collaborative components of the gutome to be individualized. Nutrigenomics plays an interactive role in microbiome stability for some of the most serious diseases by way of supporting or thwarting specific species of microbes and expanding future therapy options.

DISCUSSION AND FUTURE PERSPECTIVES
Metabolic Syndromes and the Gutome

Understanding the role of nutrigenomics and the gutome provides windows of opportunity in shifting the nature of chronic disease. As noted elsewhere in this article, chronic disease is interactive, nonstatic, and can be altered if given the appropriate materials. This factor has significant consequences related to disease management, progression, therapeutics, and minimizing the burden on individuals and society. Nutrigenomics serves as an additional tool of prevention to enhance quality of life, alter chronic disease severity, and even diminish the severity of acute illness among those with existing chronic diseases including obesity, CVD, diabetes, and cancer.

One area of further interest related to nutrigenomics and the prevention of diabetes, metabolic disease, and CVD is to examine specific heterozygous and homozygous patterns related to the management of disease. As noted elsewhere in this article, lineage diets, including the Mediterranean diet, may serve as an additional tool in therapeutic options and management. One such study compared the Mediterranean and Central European diets, where individual carriers of *FTO* and *PPARG* were assessed in relationship to blood pressure, obesity, cholesterol, and body habitus. The study assessed postmenopausal women with central obesity[50]. Both diets over 16 weeks showed metabolic improvements in some form. Yet the study further explored *FTO* (rs9939609) and *PPARG* (rs1801282) heterozygous and homozygous status in relation to these 2 ancestral diets. Among those on the Central European Diet, *PPARG* rs1801282 G carriers had a greater reduction in weight and high-density lipoproteins than those homozygous for the C allele. Additionally, *FTO* rs9939609 T allele homozygotes showed superior outcomes in diastolic blood pressure when compared with G allele carriers. Stratifying by those on the Mediterranean diet, greater fat reduction was observed in *PPARG* rs1801282 G allele carriers[50]. Similarly, the Mediterranean Diet was also assessed in relationship to MTHFR C677 T and potential positive metabolic changes[51]. Over 12 weeks of dietary changes, both individuals who did and did not carry the T allele showed a reduction of overall weight and body fat. However, 71.4% of individuals with a C/C genotype were able to lose weight and total body fat as compared with only 28.6% of T allele carriers. Additionally, T allele carriers were more likely to lose lean body mass when compared with C/C individuals[51]. Thus, specific polymorphisms may guide diet selection as an additional therapeutic tool in the prevention and reversal of metabolic syndromes.

Another notable and timely example is seen with acute disease in those who contracted coronavirus disease 2019 (COVID-19). As observed globally, not all people share equal risk of severity or mortality. In fact, those with CVD, diabetes, and obesity had a higher risk of hospitalizations and mortality. Numerous studies found that the gut microbiome may serve as a contributor to increased COVID hospitalizations and mortality among these individuals[52]. In fact, gut dysbiosis was found in hospitalized patients with COVID-19 with a lower diversity of flora, specifically *Lactobacillus and Bifidobacterium*. These same individuals with chronic disease maintained a higher level of pathogenic bacteria of *Actinomyces*, *Rothia*, and *Streptococcus*[53]. Once again, CVD, diabetes, and obesity are not isolated diseases, but their foundation of the gut biome plays a role in morbidity and mortality even in cases of acute disease.

As noted elsewhere in this article, apolipoprotein E is correlated with obesity and CVD and more recently the apolipoprotein E e4e4 genotype is associated with a 4-fold increase in mortality from COVID-19[54]. The ability to prevent severe acute infection for those with metabolic disease and CVD may not be random, but instead housed within the biome where epigenetics not only play a role in progression of chronic disease, but alter the immune response during times of acute disease. Therefore, nutrigenomics may be beneficial in the prevention of acute disease among those with CVD and obesity in addition to well-established hygienic practices and vaccination. It is this understanding that serves as a window of opportunity to further identify those at greatest risk and to minimize further morbidity or mortality.

The Gutome and Cancer

As noted elsewhere in this article, a more balanced microbiome yields advantageous effects on health including protection against certain diseases. One such example includes estrogen receptor-positive breast cancer[55]. The gut microbiome has a unique ability to regulate and metabolize estrogens using the same phase II detoxification reactions that metabolize medications, including glucuronidation, methylation, gluta-thione conjugation, and sulfation. With an unbalanced or dysbiotic biome, unmetabo-lized and unbound estrogens increase. Estrogen regulation of the gut may alter total body estrogen and impact the breast tissue, increasing the risk of estrogen recep-tor-positive breast cancer[56]. This process is so significant that it serves as its own ecosystem, known as the estrobolome, referring to the intestinal bacterial microbiome that metabolizes and regulates circulating estrogens[55]. Beta-glucuronidase serves as an important enzyme in carbohydrate degradation, but, in excess, can cleave key bonds of the intestinal lining leading to leaky gut. It also serves as a competitor to glu-curonidation, thus impairing estrogen degradation. Certain microbes alter beta-glucuronidase, including bacteriodes, bifidobacterium, and lactobacillus[55]. Thus, in balance and under the best of circumstances the human microbiome can serve as a protector against cancer. Nutrients also impact estrogen receptor-positive and HER2-positive breast cancer, where fat-soluble vitamins including A, D, and E alter the flora and are correlated to more positive outcomes[57-59]. Fish oil, cod liver oil, and foods that contain essential fatty acids also show specific promise in improving the flora. Additionally, vitamins A, D, and E have shown to enhance the benefits of certain chemotherapy and aromatase inhibitors and even reduce drug resistance[60,61].

SUMMARY

Nutrigenomics is ever evolving. Owing to extensive recent research, the role of the microbiome, both in terms of impact on chronic disease and how it influences the ef-ficacy of specialized diets and pharmacotherapies, is beginning to be better under-stood. Our approach to chronic disease should continue to advance in therapeutic options based on the individual. In recent years, pharmacogenomics has been increasingly incorporated into clinical practice. Perhaps in the future, the micro-biome's role in drug metabolism could be used to further refine medication selection. Nutrigenetic advances may be used in the future to guide selection of specialized diets that could be used as an adjunct to pharmacotherapy, as well as to influence the composition of the microbiome. Finally, further interventions to alter the microbiome (eg, probiotics, fecal transplantation, or alteration through nutrient intake) may be used as additional approaches to improve health and treat disease. Using genetics and epigenetics in each of these contexts, a patient's therapeutic response can be maximized. These improved outcomes serve to reduce morbidity and mortality and enhance quality of life.

DISCLOSURE

The authors have nothing to disclose related to this article.

REFERENCES

1. Dimitrov DV. The human gutome: nutrigenomics of the host–microbiome interac-tions. Omi A J Integr Biol 2011;15(7–8):419–30.

2. Ferguson JF, Allayee H, Gerszten RE, et al. Nutrigenomics, the microbiome, and gene-environment interactions: new directions in cardiovascular disease research, prevention, and treatment. Circ Cardiovasc Genet 2016;9(3): 291–313. Available at: https://www.ahajournals.org/doi/10.1161/HCG. 0000000000000030.

3. Peña-Romero AC, Navas-Carrillo D, Marín F, et al. The future of nutrition: nutrigenomics and nutrigenetics in obesity and cardiovascular diseases. Crit Rev Food Sci Nutr 2018;58(17):3030–41.

4. Cresci GAM, Izzo K. Gut microbiome. In: Adult short bowel syndrome. Elsevier; 2019. p. 45–54. https://doi.org/10.1016/B978-0-12-814330-8.00004-4.

5. Ratsika A, Codagnone MC, O'Mahony S, et al. Priming for life: early life nutrition and the microbiota-gut-brain axis. Nutrients 2021;13(2). https://doi.org/10.3390/nu13020423.

6. Petra AI, Panagiotidou S, Hatziagelaki E, et al. Gut-microbiota-brain axis and its effect on neuropsychiatric disorders with suspected immune dysregulation. Clin Ther 2015;37(5):984–95.

7. Yamamoto EA, Jørgensen TN. Relationships between vitamin D, gut microbiome, and systemic autoimmunity. Front Immunol 2019;10:3141.

8. Yang Q, Liang Q, Balakrishnan B, et al. Role of dietary nutrients in the modulation of gut microbiota: a narrative review. Nutrients 2020;12(2).

9. Bäumler AJ, Sperandio V. Interactions between the microbiota and pathogenic bacteria in the gut. Nature 2016;535(7610):85–93.

10. Knoop KA, Holtz LR, Newberry RD. Inherited nongenetic influences on the gut microbiome and immune system. Birth Defects Res 2018;110(20):1494–503.

11. Prince AL, Chu DM, Seferovic MD, et al. The perinatal microbiome and pregnancy: moving beyond the vaginal microbiome. Cold Spring Harb Perspect Med 2015;5(6). https://doi.org/10.1101/cshperspect.a023051.

12. Dunlop AL, Mulle JG, Ferranti EP, et al. Maternal microbiome and pregnancy outcomes that impact infant health: a review. Adv Neonatal Care 2015;15(6): 377–85.

13. Yao Y, Cai X, Fei W, et al. Regulating gut microbiome: therapeutic strategy for rheumatoid arthritis during pregnancy and lactation. Front Pharmacol 2020; 11:594042.

14. Gominak SC. Vitamin D deficiency changes the intestinal microbiome reducing B vitamin production in the gut. The resulting lack of pantothenic acid adversely affects the immune system, producing a "pro-inflammatory" state associated with atherosclerosis and autoimmunity. Med Hypotheses 2016;94:103–7.

15. Marchesi JR, Adams DH, Fava F, et al. The gut microbiota and host health: a new clinical frontier. Gut 2016;65(2):330–9.

16. Khan I, Ullah N, Zha L, et al. Alteration of gut microbiota in inflammatory bowel disease (IBD): cause or consequence? IBD treatment targeting the gut microbiome. Pathog (Basel, Switzerland) 2019;8(3). https://doi.org/10.3390/pathogens8030126.

17. Salem F, Kindt N, Marchesi JR, et al. Gut microbiome in chronic rheumatic and inflammatory bowel diseases: Similarities and differences. United Eur Gastroenterol J 2019;7(8):1008–32.

18. Wilson ID, Nicholson JK. Gut microbiome interactions with drug metabolism, efficacy, and toxicity. Transl Res 2017;179:204–22.

19. Tuteja S, Ferguson JF. Gut microbiome and response to cardiovascular drugs. Circ Genomic Precis Med 2019;12(9). https://doi.org/10.1161/CIRCGEN.119.002314.

20. Prevention C for DC and. Adult obesity facts. Overweight and obesity. Available at: https://www.cdc.gov/obesity/data/adult.html. Accessed March 30, 2021.

21. Saltiel AR, Olefsky JM. Inflammatory mechanisms linking obesity and metabolic disease. J Clin Invest 2017;127(1):1–4.

22. Organization WH. Diabetes. Health topics. 2021. Available at: https://www.who.int/health-topics/diabetes#tab=tab_1. Accessed March 30, 2021.

23. Ortega Á, Berná G, Rojas A, et al. Gene-diet interactions in type 2 diabetes: the chicken and egg debate. Int J Mol Sci 2017;18(6). https://doi.org/10.3390/ijms18061188.

24. Virani SS, Alonso A, Aparicio HJ, et al. Heart disease and stroke statistics—2021 update. Circulation 2021;143(8). https://doi.org/10.1161/CIR.0000000000000950.

25. Barrea L, Annunziata G, Bordoni L, et al. Nutrigenetics—personalized nutrition in obesity and cardiovascular diseases. Int J Obes Suppl 2020;10(1):1–13.

26. Hickey SE, Curry CJ, Toriello HV. ACMG practice guideline: lack of evidence for MTHFR polymorphism testing. Genet Med 2013;15(2):153–6.

27. Nutrigenomics MM. The genome – food interface. Environ Health Perspect 2007;115(12):A582–9.

28. Esposito K, Chiodini P, Colao A, et al. Metabolic syndrome and risk of cancer: a systematic review and meta-analysis. Diabetes Care 2012;35(11):2402–11.

29. ACS. American Cancer Society. Available at: https://www.cancer.org/. Accessed March 30, 2021.

30. Publishing HH. Cancer and diet: what's the connection? Harvard Men's Health Watch. Available at: https://www.health.harvard.edu/cancer/cancer-and-diet-whats-the-connection. Accessed March 30, 2021.

31. Anderson JJ, Darwis NDM, Mackay DF, et al. Red and processed meat consumption and breast cancer: UK Biobank cohort study and meta-analysis. Eur J Cancer 2018;90:73–82.

32. Sieri S, Krogh V. Dietary glycemic index, glycemic load and cancer: an overview of the literature. Nutr Metab Cardiovasc Dis 2017;27(1):18–31.

33. Deng X, Su R, Stanford S, et al. Critical enzymatic functions of FTO in obesity and cancer. Front Endocrinol (Lausanne) 2018;9. https://doi.org/10.3389/fendo.2018.00396.

34. de Toro-Martín J, Arsenault BJ, Després JP, et al. Precision nutrition: a review of personalized nutritional approaches for the prevention and management of metabolic syndrome. Nutrients 2017;9(8):1–28.

35. Kobayashi J. Effect of diet and gut environment on the gastrointestinal formation of N-nitroso compounds: a review. Nitric Oxide Biol Chem 2018;73:66–73.

36. Bruno E, Manoukian S, Venturelli E, et al. Adherence to Mediterranean diet and metabolic syndrome in BRCA mutation carriers. Integr Cancer Ther 2018;17(1):153–60.

37. Meslier V, Laiola M, Roager HM, et al. Mediterranean diet intervention in overweight and obese subjects lowers plasma cholesterol and causes changes in the gut microbiome and metabolome independently of energy intake. Gut 2020;69(7):1258–68.

38. Liu H, Wang J, He T, et al. Butyrate: a double-edged sword for health? Adv Nutr 2018;9(1):21–9.

39. McNabney SM, Henagan TM. Short chain fatty acids in the colon and peripheral tissues: a focus on butyrate, colon cancer, obesity and insulin resistance. Nutrients 2017;9(12). https://doi.org/10.3390/nu9121348.

40. Fasanelli F, Giraudo MT, Vineis P, et al. DNA methylation, colon cancer and Mediterranean diet: results from the EPIC-Italy cohort. Epigenetics 2019;14(10):977–88.

41. Castelló A, Pollán M, Buijsse B, et al. Spanish Mediterranean diet and other dietary patterns and breast cancer risk: case–control EpiGEICAM study. Br J Cancer 2014;111(7):1454–62.

42. Kiechle M, Dukatz R, Yahiaoui-Doktor M, et al. Feasibility of structured endurance training and Mediterranean diet in BRCA1 and BRCA2 mutation carriers - an interventional randomized controlled multicenter trial (LIBRE-1). BMC Cancer 2017;17(1):752.

43. Bruno E, Oliverio A, Paradiso AV, et al. A Mediterranean dietary intervention in female carriers of BRCA mutations: results from an Italian prospective randomized controlled trial. Cancers (Basel) 2020;12(12). https://doi.org/10.3390/cancers12123732.

44. Özkul C, Yalınay M, Karakan T. Islamic fasting leads to an increased abundance of Akkermansia muciniphila and Bacteroides fragilis group: a preliminary study on intermittent fasting. Turk J Gastroenterol 2019;30(12):1030–5.

45. Ou Z, Deng L, Lu Z, et al. Protective effects of Akkermansia muciniphila on cognitive deficits and amyloid pathology in a mouse model of Alzheimer's disease. Nutr Diabetes 2020;10(1):12.

46. Haran JP, Bhattarai SK, Foley SE, et al. Alzheimer's disease microbiome is associated with dysregulation of the anti-inflammatory P-glycoprotein pathway. MBio 2019;10(3). https://doi.org/10.1128/mBio.00632-19.

47. Inacio P. Gut microbiome may help slow ALS progression, study indicates. ALS News Today. 2019. Available at: https://alsnewstoday.com/news-posts/2019/07/25/gut-microbiome-slow-als-progression-study/. Accessed December 3, 2021.

48. Bian X, Wu W, Yang L, et al. Administration of Akkermansia muciniphila ameliorates dextran sulfate sodium-induced ulcerative colitis in mice. Front Microbiol 2019;10:2259.

49. Weir TL, Manter DK, Sheflin AM, et al. Stool microbiome and metabolome differences between colorectal cancer patients and healthy adults. PLoS One 2013;8(8):e70803.

50. Chmurzynska A, Muzsik A, Krzyżanowska-Jankowska P, et al. PPARG and FTO polymorphism can modulate the outcomes of a central European diet and a Mediterranean diet in centrally obese postmenopausal women. Nutr Res 2019;69:94–100.

51. Di Renzo L, Rizzo M, Iacopino L, et al. Body composition phenotype: Italian Mediterranean diet and C677T MTHFR gene polymorphism interaction. Eur Rev Med Pharmacol Sci 2013;17(19):2555–65. Available at: http://www.ncbi.nlm.nih.gov/pubmed/24142599.

52. Viana SD, Nunes S, Reis F. ACE2 imbalance as a key player for the poor outcomes in COVID-19 patients with age-related comorbidities - role of gut microbiota dysbiosis. Ageing Res Rev 2020;62:101123.

53. Xu K, Cai H, Shen Y, et al. [Management of corona virus disease-19 (COVID-19): the Zhejiang experience]. Zhejiang Da Xue Xue Bao Yi Xue Ban 2020;49(1):147–57.

54. Kuo C-L, Pilling LC, Atkins JL, et al. ApoE e4e4 genotype and mortality with COVID-19 in UK Biobank. J Gerontol A Biol Sci Med Sci 2020;75(9):1801–3.

55. Kwa M, Plottel CS, Blaser MJ, et al. The intestinal microbiome and estrogen receptor-positive female breast cancer. J Natl Cancer Inst 2016;108(8). https://doi.org/10.1093/jnci/djw029.

56. Baker JM, Al-Nakkash L, Herbst-Kralovetz MM. Estrogen–gut microbiome axis: physiological and clinical implications. Maturitas 2017;103:45–53.

57. Miro Estruch I, de Haan LHJ, Melchers D, et al. The effects of all-trans retinoic acid on estrogen receptor signaling in the estrogen-sensitive MCF/BUS subline. J Recept Signal Transduct Res 2018;38(2):112–21.

58. Bak MJ, Das Gupta S, Wahler J, et al. Inhibitory effects of γ- and δ-tocopherols on estrogen-stimulated breast cancer in vitro and in vivo. Cancer Prev Res (Phila) 2017;10(3):188–97.

59. Tam K-W, Ho C-T, Lee W-J, et al. Alteration of α-tocopherol-associated protein (TAP) expression in human breast epithelial cells during breast cancer development. Food Chem 2013;138(2–3):1015–21.

60. Koay DC, Zerillo C, Narayan M, et al. Anti-tumor effects of retinoids combined with trastuzumab or tamoxifen in breast cancer cells: induction of apoptosis by retinoid/trastuzumab combinations. Breast Cancer Res 2010;12(4):R62.

61. Tiwary R, Yu W, Sanders BG, et al. α-TEA cooperates with chemotherapeutic agents to induce apoptosis of p53 mutant, triple-negative human breast cancer cells via activating p73. Breast Cancer Res 2011;13(1):R1.

62. Corella D, Peloso G, Arnett DK, et al. APOA2, dietary fat, and body mass index: replication of a gene-diet interaction in 3 independent populations. Arch Intern Med 2009;169(20):1897–906.

63. Domínguez-Reyes T, Astudillo-López CC, Salgado-Goytia L, et al. Interaction of dietary fat intake with APOA2, APOA5 and LEPR polymorphisms and its relationship with obesity and dyslipidemia in young subjects. Lipids Health Dis 2015; 14:106.

64. Koopal C, Van Der Graaf Y, Asselbergs FW, et al. Influence of APOE-2 genotype on the relation between adiposity and plasma lipid levels in patients with vascular disease. Int J Obes 2015;39(2):265–9.

65. Garaulet M, Corbalán MD, Madrid JA, et al. CLOCK gene is implicated in weight reduction in obese patients participating in a dietary programme based on the Mediterranean diet. Int J Obes (Lond) 2010;34(3):516–23.

66. Scuteri A, Sanna S, Chen W-M, et al. Genome-wide association scan shows genetic variants in the FTO gene are associated with obesity-related traits. Plos Genet 2007;3(7):e115.

67. Qi Q, Kilpeläinen TO, Downer MK, et al. FTO genetic variants, dietary intake and body mass index: insights from 177,330 individuals. Hum Mol Genet 2014; 23(25):6961–72.

68. Duicu C, Mărginean CO, Voidăzan S, et al. FTO rs 9939609 SNP is associated with adiponectin and leptin levels and the risk of obesity in a cohort of Romanian children population. Medicine (Baltimore) 2016;95(20):e3709.

69. Kaulfers A-M, Deka R, Dolan L, et al. Association of INSIG2 polymorphism with overweight and LDL in children. PLoS One 2015;10(1):e0116340.

70. Heid IM, Huth C, Loos RJF, et al. Meta-analysis of the INSIG2 association with obesity including 74,345 individuals: does heterogeneity of estimates relate to study design? Plos Genet 2009;5(10):e1000694.

71. Martínez JA. Perspectives on personalized nutrition for obesity. J Nutrigenet Nutrigenomics 2014;7(1):6–8.

72. Di Renzo L, Gualtieri P, Romano L, et al. Role of personalized nutrition in chronic-degenerative diseases. Nutrients 2019;11(8):1–24.

73. Berná G, Oliveras-López MJ, Jurado-Ruíz E, et al. Nutrigenetics and nutrigenomics insights into diabetes etiopathogenesis. Nutrients 2014;6(11):5338–69.

74. Corella D, Asensio EM, Coltell O, et al. CLOCK gene variation is associated with incidence of type-2 diabetes and cardiovascular diseases in type-2 diabetic

subjects: dietary modulation in the PREDIMED randomized trial. Cardiovasc Diabetol 2016;15:4.

75. Dedoussis GVZ, Kaliora AC, Panagiotakos DB. Genes, diet and type 2 diabetes mellitus: a review. Rev Diabet Stud 2007;4(1):13–24.

76. Ali O. Genetics of type 2 diabetes. World J Diabetes 2013;4(4):114–23.

77. Corella D, Qi L, Sorlí JV, et al. Obese subjects carrying the 11482G>A polymorphism at the perilipin locus are resistant to weight loss after dietary energy restriction. J Clin Endocrinol Metab 2005;90(9):5121–6.

78. Engler MB. Nutrigenomics in cardiovascular disease: implications for the future. Prog Cardiovasc Nurs 2009;24(4):190–5.

79. Iacoviello L, Santimone I, Latella MC, et al. Nutrigenomics: a case for the common soil between cardiovascular disease and cancer. Genes Nutr 2008;3(1):19–24.

80. Ordovas JM, Kaput J, Corella D. Nutrition in the genomics era: cardiovascular disease risk and the Mediterranean diet. Mol Nutr Food Res 2007;51(10):1293–9.

81. Do R, Xie C, Zhang X, et al. The effect of chromosome 9p21 variants on cardiovascular disease may be modified by dietary intake: evidence from a case/control and a prospective study. Plos Med 2011;8(10). https://doi.org/10.1371/journal.pmed.1001106.

82. Aleyasin SA, Navidi T, Davoudi S. Association between rs10757274 and rs2383206 SNPs as genetic risk factors in Iranian patients with coronary artery disease. J Tehran Heart Cent 2017;12(3):114–8. Available at: http://www.ncbi.nlm.nih.gov/pubmed/29062378.

83. Hannou SA, Wouters K, Paumelle R, et al. Functional genomics of the CDKN2A/B locus in cardiovascular and metabolic disease: what have we learned from GWASs? Trends Endocrinol Metab 2015;26(4):176–84.

84. Niemiec P, Gorczynska-Kosiorz S, Iwanicki T, et al. The rs10757278 polymorphism of the 9p21.3 locus is associated with premature coronary artery disease in Polish patients. Genet Test Mol Biomarkers 2012;16(9):1080–5.

85. Aberle J, Hopfer I, Beil FU, et al. Association of peroxisome proliferator-activated receptor delta +294T/C with body mass index and interaction with peroxisome proliferator-activated receptor alpha L162V. Int J Obes (Lond) 2006;30(12):1709–13.

86. Zhou Y, Luo G. Apolipoproteins, as the carrier proteins for lipids, are involved in the development of breast cancer. Clin Transl Oncol 2020;22(11):1952–62.

87. Pirro M, Ricciuti B, Rader DJ, et al. High density lipoprotein cholesterol and cancer: marker or causative? Prog Lipid Res 2018;71:54–69.

88. Caramujo-Balseiro S, Faro C, Carvalho L. Metabolic pathways in sporadic colorectal carcinogenesis: a new proposal. Med Hypotheses 2021;148:110512.

89. Slattery ML, Sweeney C, Murtaugh M, et al. Associations between apoE genotype and colon and rectal cancer. Carcinogenesis 2005;26(8):1422–9.

90. Moysich KB, Freudenheim JL, Baker JA, et al. Apolipoprotein E genetic polymorphism, serum lipoproteins, and breast cancer risk. Mol Carcinog 2000;27(1):2–9.

91. Porrata-Doria T, Matta JL, Acevedo SF. Apolipoprotein E allelic frequency altered in women with early-onset breast cancer. Breast Cancer (Auckl) 2010;4:43–8. Available at: http://www.ncbi.nlm.nih.gov/pubmed/20697532.

92. Riscuta G, Dumitrescu RG. Nutrigenomics: implications for breast and colon cancer prevention. Methods Mol Biol 2012;343–58. https://doi.org/10.1007/978-1-61779-612-8_22.

93. Sellami M, Bragazzi NL. Nutrigenomics and breast cancer: state-of-art, future perspectives and insights for prevention. Nutrients 2020;12(2):512.
94. Liu X, Liu L, Dong Z, et al. Expression patterns and prognostic value of m6A-related genes in colorectal cancer. Am J Transl Res 2019;11(7):3972–91. Available at: http://www.ncbi.nlm.nih.gov/pubmed/31396313.
95. Yamaji T, Iwasaki M, Sawada N, et al. Fat mass and obesity-associated gene polymorphisms, pre-diagnostic plasma adipokine levels and the risk of colorectal cancer: the Japan Public Health Center-based Prospective Study. PLoS One 2020;15(2):e0229005.
96. Davis CD. Nutrigenomics and the prevention of colon cancer. Pharmacogenomics 2007;8(2):121–4.
97. Levine AJ, Figueiredo JC, Lee W, et al. Genetic variability in the MTHFR gene and colorectal cancer risk using the Colorectal Cancer Family Registry. Cancer Epidemiol Biomarkers Prev 2010;19(1):89–100.
98. Cecchin E, Perrone G, Nobili S, et al. MTHFR-1298 A>C (rs1801131) is a predictor of survival in two cohorts of stage II/III colorectal cancer patients treated with adjuvant fluoropyrimidine chemotherapy with or without oxaliplatin. Pharmacogenomics J 2015;15(3):219–25.
99. Ogino S, Shima K, Baba Y, et al. Colorectal cancer expression of peroxisome proliferator-activated receptor γ (PPARG, PPARgamma) is associated with good prognosis. Gastroenterology 2009;136(4):1242–50.
100. Girnun G. PPARG: a new independent marker for colorectal cancer survival. Gastroenterology 2009;136(4):1157–60.
101. Papadaki I, Mylona E, Giannopoulou I, et al. PPARgamma expression in breast cancer: clinical value and correlation with ERbeta. Histopathology 2005;46(1):37–42.

Blood Group Genotyping

Jensyn K. Cone Sullivan, MD[a,b], Nicholas Gleadall, PhD[c],
William J. Lane, MD, PhD[d,e,*]

KEYWORDS

- Next generation sequencing • Red blood cells • Erythrocyte antigens
- Blood groups • Blood group antigens • Array • Genomics

KEY POINTS

- Erythrocyte antigens-surface structures capable of eliciting specific, humoral immune responses-were historically characterized by antibody-based methodologies, occasionally precluding accurate phenotyping and compatible blood transfusion.
- Single-nucleotide variants (SNVs) code for most blood group antigens, although there are also many well-characterized indels, structural variants, copy number variants, or regulatory region variants.
- Next Generation Sequencing (NGS) accurately calls SNV erythrocyte phenotypes. Adding long-, paired-end, and split reads and copy number analysis accurately calls more challenging blood group systems.
- NGS aids analysis of challenging serologic cases, phenotypes without requiring blood samples, identifies rare blood donors and prevents alloimmunization via improved blood product matching.
- Similarly, array technology advances allow rapid, inexpensive, and nearly exhaustive identification of known (and predicted) variants.

Red blood cell (RBC) antigens are inherited, intrinsic or adsorbed surface structures provoking specific humoral immune response. Historically, serologic—antibody-based and relatively unchanged since the early 20th century—assays imperfectly defined these antigens, at times hindering accurate phenotyping and compatible RBC transfusion and solid organ transplantation. Single-nucleotide variants (SNV),

This article originally appeared in *Advances in Molecular Pathology*, Volume 4, Issue 1, November 2021.

[a] Department of Pathology, The Neely Cell Therapy Center, Tufts Medical Center, 800 Washington Street, #826, Boston, MA 02111, USA; [b] Tufts University School of Medicine, Boston, MA, USA; [c] Department of Haematology, University of Cambridge, University of Cambridge Biomedical Campus, Long Road, Cambridge, CB2 0PT, UK; [d] Department of Pathology, Brigham and Women's Hospital, Hale Building for Transformative Medicine, Room 8002L, 60 Fenwood Road, Boston, MA 02115, USA; [e] Harvard Medical School, Boston, MA, USA
* Corresponding author. Department of Pathology, Brigham and Women's Hospital, Hale Building for Transformative Medicine, Room 8002L, 60 Fenwood Road, Boston, MA 02115.
E-mail address: wlane@bwh.harvard.edu
Twitter: @bloodantigens (W.J.L.)

and less frequently structural variants, copy number variants or regulatory region variants encode RBC antigens. Whole genome, whole exome, and targeted next-generation sequencing (NGS) characterize these antigens more reliably and specifically than serology. Furthermore, long-reads, paired-end reads, split reads, and copy number analysis allow accurate prediction of challenging blood group systems including ABO, Rh, and MNS. NGS enriches analysis of challenging serologic cases by producing accurate phenotype data when blood samples are unobtainable, by screening the existing donor pool for rare blood identifying compatible blood for recipients via more rigorous standards and by preventing alloimmunization and hemolytic transfusion reactions. Similarly, recent array technology rapidly, accurately, inexpensively, and nearly exhaustively identifies known (and predicted) variants. Owing to significant time, cost, and clinical and research benefits, utilization of molecular RBC typing is expanding rapidly.

INTRODUCTION
Red Blood Cell Antigen Phenotypes and Blood Groups

Red blood cell antigens
Red blood cell (RBC) antigens are inherited, polymorphic, intrinsic or adsorbed cell-surface protein or carbohydrate structures capable of eliciting a specific, humoral immune response (**Fig. 1**A). RBC phenotyping, performed serologically with a spectrum of monoclonal reagents, deems antigens present on the RBC surfaces "positive" and those absent "negative". Antigen variants include weak, el, mod, and partial antigens. Weak antigens are present lower in number than expected, while mod and el are present in such low numbers that sensitive serologic methods (ie, absorption-elution) must be used to identify them. Partial variants lack portions of the antigen structure and may produce alloantibodies targeting the absent portions.

Blood groups
Blood groups consist of one or multiple related antigens coded by a single gene or by closely linked genes (**Table 1**; **Fig. 1**B). The International Society for Blood Transfusion (ISBT) recognizes 43 blood group systems[1].

Blood group systems must
- Possess an erythrocyte surface structure
- Have known genetic basis
- Be targeted by a specific antibody

Functionally, the gene products that define RBC antigen expression fill many cellular roles, acting as
- Enzymes (ABO, *ABO*, glycosyltransferases)
- Surface receptors (Duffy, *DARC*, chemokine receptors)
- Cell adhesion molecules (Lutheran, *BCAM*, B-cell adhesion molecule)
- Channels (Colton, *AQP1*, aquaporin)
- Bacterial and parasite receptors (MNS, *GYPA/GYPB*, glycophorins)
- Complement defense (Cromer, *CD55*, decay-inhibiting factor).

Historical blood group testing (serology) and transfusion
RBC transfusion, a form of an allotransplantation, exposes recipients to nonself donor antigens and leads to development of specific antibodies targeting nonself antigens. Chronically transfused patients of African ancestry form alloantibodies more frequently than transfusion recipients broadly (>50% vs approximately 3%, respectively)[2]. Sensitization increases the risk of hemolytic transfusion reaction, hemolytic disease of the fetus and newborn (HDFN)[3], further alloimmunization[4], and the difficulty

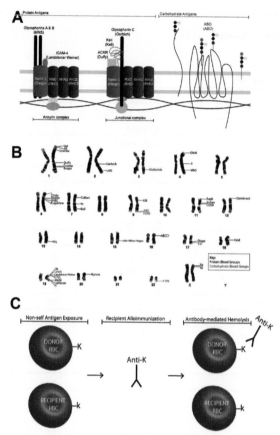

Fig. 1. (*A*) Schematic of selected protein and carbohydrate RBC antigens, including protein antigens housed within structural complexes and carbohydrate antigens located on surface glycoproteins. Structures names are listed, with corresponding blood group in parentheses. Black or white typeface denotes protein antigens and associated structures. Red typeface denotes carbohydrate antigens. (*B*) Blood group antigen coding genes by chromosomal location. Black typeface denotes blood groups with protein antigens. Red typeface denotes blood groups with carbohydrate antigens. (*C*) Schematic representation of the process of alloimmunization: A recipient encounters a nonself antigen and produces a specific alloantibody targeting the nonself antigen. The alloantibody is capable of producing hemolysis.

of finding compatible donor blood. Compatible units must contain RBCs that are negative for antigens targeted by the recipient's alloantibodies to prevent acute hemolysis (**Fig. 1**C). Posttransfusion complications in sensitized patients range from minor hemolysis to death and follow 3% to 30%[5] of transfusions.

Pretransfusion testing includes serologic ABO and Rh donor and recipient typing and recipient alloantibody identification. Notwithstanding the gold standard status, serologic studies are labor- and time-intensive and may be erroneous, particularly in the case of variant Rh antigens which are more common in individuals of African ancestry.

Serologic studies
- Require fresh recipient RBCs (potentially challenging or dangerous to obtain from fetuses, neonates, children, and severely anemic patients)

Table 1
Blood Group Antigen Systems

System Number	System Name	Gene(s)	Number of Antigens	Chromosomal Location
1	ABO	ABO	4	9q34.2
2	MNS	GYPA, GYPB, GYPE	50	4q31.21
3	P1PK	A4GALT	3	22q13.2
4	Rh	RHD, RHCE	55	1p36.11
5	Lutheran	BCAM	27	19q13.2
6	Kell	KEL	36	7q33
7	Lewis	FUT3	6	19p13.3
8	Duffy	ACKR1	5	1q21-q22
9	Kidd	SLC14A1	3	18q11-q12
10	Diego	SCL4A1	22	17q21.31
11	Yt	ACHE	5	7q22
12	Xg	XG, MIC2	2	Xp22.32
13	Scianna	ERMAP	9	1p34.2
14	Dombrock	ART4	10	12p13-p12
15	Colton	AQP1	4	7p14
16	Landsteiner-Wiener	ICAM4	3	19p13.2
17	Chido/Rogers	C4A, C4B	9	6p21.3
18	H	FUT1	1	19q13.33
19	Kx	XK	1	Xp21.1
20	Gerbich	GYPC	13	2q14-q21
21	Cromer	CD55	20	1q32
22	Knops	CR1	12	1q32.2
23	Indian	CD44	6	11p13
24	Ok	BSG	3	19p13.3
25	Raph	CD151	1	11p15.5
26	John Milton Hagan	SEMA7A	8	15q22.3-q23
27	I	GCNT2	1	6p24.2
28	Globoside	B3GALNT1	2	3q25
29	Gill	AQP3	1	9p13
30	Rh-associated glycoprotein	RHAG	4	6p12.3
31	FORS	GBGT1	1	9q34.13-q34.3
32	JR	ABCG2	1	4q22.1
33	LAN	ABCB6	1	2q36
34	Vel	SMIM1	1	1p36.32
35	CD59	CD59	1	11p13
36	Augustine	SLC29A1	4	6p21.1
37	Kanno	PRNP	1	20p13
38	SID	BGALNT2	1	17q21.32
39	CTL2	SCL44A2	2	19p13.2
40	PEL	ABCC4	1	13q32.1

(continued on next page)

System Number	System Name	Gene(s)	Number of Antigens	Chromosomal Location
41	MAM	EMP3	1	19q13.33
42	EMM	PIGG	1	4p16.3
43	ABCC1	ABCC1	1	16p13.11

Table 1
(*continued*)

Adapted from Table of Blood Group Systems. International Society of Blood Transfusion (ISBT) Working Party on Red Cell Immunogenetics and Blood Group Terminology; 2021. https://www.isbtweb.org/fileadmin/user_upload/Table_of_blood_group_systems_v._9.0_03-FEB-2021.pdf; with permission.

- Cannot identify rare antigens (ie, no Dombrock antisera widely exist[6])
- Inconsistently type variants
- Require separate testing for identification of each RBC antigen[7].

In contrast, genotyping rapidly and increasingly inexpensively analyzes DNA from any cell source (and some acellular sources), accurately characterizes rare antigens, and exhaustively types both blood and platelet antigens[8].

Call out 1: Blood group terms

Blood Group Genetic Changes

Terminology
Alleles—alternate nucleotide sequences inhabiting specific genomic locations (loci) within coding sequences (CDS)—produce alternate gene products. The Genome Reference Consortium maintains a widely used, composite, idealized human reference genome (HRG), hg38[9]. Comparing next-generation sequencing (NGS) sequences against hg38 allows variant allele calling. Genomic coordinates denote specific loci, such as genes, by chromosome number (chr7) and positional base number along the chromosome for locus start and end (eg, chr9:133233278-133276024 denotes the *ABO* gene in the GRCh38 reference genome).

Variant databases
Various resources compile blood group antigens, their variants, and their alleles (**Table 2**). Blood Group Antigen FactsBook[14], initially published in 1997, provides a clinically relevant summary. BGMUT[10,11] and dbRBC[12] databases, merged in 1999 and closed in 2017, listed common antigens and rare variants. RheususBase[13] and Erythrogene[13,15] (both 2014-present) contain similar information. The ISBT updates and curates portable document format (PDF) allele tables for each blood group system[17], describing broadly, not exhaustively, antigen variants' genetic bases. No centralized resource unites all known data, although a *recent compilation* united the aforementioned resources, providing one of the most exhaustive known databases at the time of publication[5]. Algorithms seeking to accurately identify antigens via genetic sequence must use such pools of variant data.

Variant types
Multiple variant types affect antigen expression on RBCs. One or multiple single-nucleotide variants (SNVs) (and single-nucleotide polymorphisms [SNPs], SNVs present in less than 1% of a given population) account for well-documented structures and the cell-surface density of most antigens.

Table 2
Databases of Variant Alleles Coding for Blood Group Antigens

BGMUT[10,11]	(From" Blood Group antigen gene MUTation") Human blood group antigen variant allele database with concurrent serologic phenotypes, created through the Human Genome Variation Society (HGVS). Active from 1999 until transferred under the National Center for Biotechnology Information (NCBI) and National Institute of Health (NIH)'s dbRBC (database Red Blood Cells).
dbRBC[12]	NCBI and NIH's human blood group antigen variant allele database. Included common through extremely rare single-instance variants. BGMUT merged in 1999. Supported through 2017. Foundational to current databases.
RheususBase[13]	At publication (2014), the largest database of variant alleles coding for Rh group antigens.
Blood Group Antigens FactsBook[14]	Published in 1997, updated in 2003 and 2012, this succinct desktop reference outlines 33 blood group systems' antigens, phenotypes and molecular bases.
Erythrogene[13,15]	Database of variant alleles coding for blood group antigens extracted from a diverse cohort of samples (1000 Genomes Project[16], n = 2504 samples from 26 population groups).
bloodantigens.com[5]	Curated database of all known blood group and HPA variants. Publicly available website. Forms the basis for bloodTyper interpretations.

SNVs alter antigen expression through
- Nonsense mutations
- Missense mutations
- Regulatory region alterations[18]
- Structural alterations.

Structural variants (SVs)—gene conversions, large insertions, deletions, copy number variants, and translocations—also alter antigen expression. Glycosyltransferases (ABO, *ABO;* Lewis, *FUT2, FUT3*) transfer immunodominant sugars A, B, and H onto the RBC surface, creating carbohydrate antigens. SNV and SV in *ABO* and *FUT* genes alter enzyme action, decreasing or obliterating sugar installation. Homologous genes (Rh's *RHD* and *RHCE,* or MNS' *GYPA, GYPB,* and *GYPE*) undergo gene conversion: recombination of homologous regions, producing hybrid genes and altered gene products. Additionally, RBC structural changes such as South Asian ovalocytosis (variant *SLC4A1* coding variant band 3 protein) depress numerous antigens' surface expression[19]. Algorithms inferring antigens from genetic sequence must recognize all variant types.

Weak

Weak variants decrease surface antigen expression, although residual expression prevents alloantibody formation. For example,
- A_{weak}: variants encode weak enzymatic forms of ABO glycosyltransferases including single or multiple SNVs[20,21], minisatellite repeats[22], deletions[23], and splice-site-mutation-produced hybrid genes[24].

- Fy(b + w): Variants encode for forms of the ACKR1 protein with weaker serologic reactivity of the Fy^b antigen often due to missense variants[6].
- Del: Significantly decreases surface antigen expression of D antigen; due to many types of variants—splice site mutations, intronic SNVs[25], or exon 8 deletions[26].
- K_{mod}: Variants encode for forms of the Kel protein with altered and weaker serologic reactivity of the K antigen often due to missense variants[6].

Null. Null allele-coding variants obliterate antigen expression, potentially resulting in alloantibodies targeting the missing structure.

Common ABO null variants:
- NM_020469.2:c.261delG truncates the glycosyltransferase, preventing group A's immunodominant sugar from being transferred to RBCs.

Common RHD Null Variants
- Complete *RHD* deletion with fusion of upstream and downstream Rhesus boxes (most common in all ethnicities)
- Pseudogene $RHD^*\Psi$[27], an intron 3-exon 4 duplication producing a premature stop codon (common among Africans)

Combined RhD and RhCE null variants (Rh_{null})
- Amorph
- Regulator

Other null mutations decrease expression of all Rh gene products in both *RHD* and *RHCE* (Rh_{null}). The "amorph"-type Rh_{null} variant is caused by mutations (*RHCE* frameshift, deletion frameshift, or intronic splice site[6]) producing truncated or misfolded structures either unstable after membrane insertion or never inserted into the membrane. "Regulator"-type variants follow mutations (SNVs, SNV leading to partial exon skipping, frameshift or intronic splice site[6]) preventing surface expression of the Rh-stabilizing integral surface protein RhAG. U-(null) RBCs commonly follow complete deletions of *GYPB*[28].

Partial. Partial allele-coding variants lack epitopes, portions of the antigen structure. Partial variants may test serologically antigen positive, but similar to null variants, they may provoke alloantibodies which target lacking epitopes. Partial Rh variants DIIIa, DAR, and DIV and DVI result from multiple SNVs.

Other. Hybrid alleles alter antigen expression by changing enzyme activity (A hybrid B-O gene produced a product with group A transferase activity[29]), altering antigen expression (Hybrid RHD-CE-Ds have only partial C expression.) or by creating new antigens (low-frequency antigens HIL, MINY, Dantu follow *GYPA-GYPB* hybrid recombination). Conversely, variants in one blood group system may alter expression of a dependent blood group system: Gerbich-negative variants may decrease Kell expression, Kpa-antigen trans (on the opposite chromosome to) K antigen decreases K expression, and variation in the Xk protein destabilizes Kell, significantly decreasing expression, producing the McLeod phenotype[6].

Call out 2: Allele terminology
Call out 3: Blood group governance

SIGNIFICANCE
Next-Generation Sequencing

Many advances undergird NGS utilization for blood group prediction. The discovery of ABO group antigens in 1901[30] and the creation of Sanger sequencing in 1977[31] made discovery of the genetic basis ABO possible in 1990[32]; after this, the completion of the Human Genome Project in 2001[33,34] and the rise of NGS in the early 21st century led to the first instance of NGS utilization for ABO typing in 2011[35], followed by the proof of concept work demonstrating NGS exhaustive blood group antigen prediction[8].

Method overview

High-throughput massively parallel sequencing begins with DNA extraction and degradation. Then, library preparation adds oligonucleotide adaptors to dsDNA's 3′ and 5′ fragment ends. Barcoding and/or indexing-specific libraries allow simultaneous sequencing of multiple libraries (multiplexing). After this, the library may be clonally amplified. Sequencing proceeds via the chosen methodology. Then, mapping aligns sequenced reads with concurrent reference genome areas.

Sequence interpretation

History. Many recent approaches to genotyping include SNP-based assays or SNP-focused genomic analysis. Although a leap forward compared with serology, such assays cannot identify novel and rare SNPs not targeted by the assay. *An early algorithm*[36] based on Hidden Markov Modeling (HMM) and the BGMUT database called 94.2% samples (n = 67/71) correctly. Nonetheless, HMM is difficult to iteratively improve, and the allele tables used are not regularly updated. Other algorithms were based on 1000 Genomes[15,37]. Unfortunately, the underlying input coverage included only 15x mean coverage, insufficient to fully resolve heterozygous SNVs and SVs. The bioinformatic basis for NGS RBC genotyping is evolving.

Current algorithms. Specific algorithms facilitate variant calling (**Fig. 2** and **Table 3**). *One algorithm*[5,8] aligned 30x mean coverage whole genome sequencing (WGS) data to the RefSeq transcript database, making variant calls for RBC and platelet antigens where nucleotides differed from the HRG. Aligning HRG and cDNA RefSeq

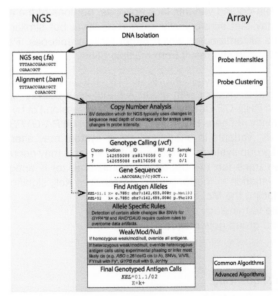

Fig. 2. Flowchart illustrating common and advanced algorithm processes for predicting blood group antigens from NGS sequencing data.

allowed genomic coordinate conversion from variant calling into conventional CDS, allowing comparison with variant allele tables and comprehensive prediction of blood and platelet antigens. Subsequent updates automated and iteratively improved the process via samples' serologic typing and built a collective variant database[5] and permitted whole exome sequencing (WES)[38] input, allowing high-accuracy antigen calling (**Table 3**).

Interpretation of specific variants

Single nucleotide variants and indels. Simplest among variants to call, exonic SNVs account for the majority of RBC antigen variants. As noted previously, resources list variants in cDNA format, requiring conversion to CDS. Accurate and complete calling of SNVs requires a RefSeq transcript (otherwise variants may be overlooked) and also requires a database containing a thorough compilation of known variants[5,8,15].

Structural variants. Early NGS data analysis for blood group genotyping primarily focused on targeted sequencing able to identify well-defined SNV alterations encoding protein antigens. Now, we and other researchers have used WGS to predict SVs[5,39,40].

Final predicted phenotype depends on accurate SV analysis, but homologous blood group systems with hybrid alleles (eg, Rh and MNS) are seen which are challenging to call with traditional genotyping methods. Much progress, especially in the Rh system, has been made to call these complex SV from NGS data using several different analysis methods including copy number depth analysis (ie, Read Depth Analysis) and split read analysis (SRA)[28,41,42].

An ancestral RHD exon 2 conversion event produced the *RHCE*C* sequence. Thus, this sequence commonly misaligns to *RHD* exon 2 in NGS analysis. Assessment of copy number through sequence depth of coverage can identify this misalignment and correctly call the C/c antigens in both WGS[5,41] and WES[38,43]. Similarly, M antigen sequences align to RefSeq with low efficiency, likely due to RefSeqs encoding only the N, not M, antigen or due to misalignment of M antigen's *GYPA* sequence to a homologous region on *GYPE*. This can be addressed by looking in *GYPE* for misaligned sequence reads with one M-specific and one *GYPA*-specific SNP[38].

Transcription factors. Multiple blood group systems depend on transcription factor function[44]. The *A4GALT*-encoded galactosyl transferase attaches galactose on an RBC glycolipid, producing P1 antigen. A RUNX-1 transcription factor (TF) binding site SNP rs5751348 (NM_017436:c.-188 + 3010G > T) alters the expression of A4GALT, with the G nucleotide associated with P1-positive and T nucleotide with P1-negative phenotypes[45]. Xg^a antigen expression, produced by the X-linked gene XG, requires GATA-1 TF binding activity[46]. A GATA-1 TF binding site SNP rs311103 (NC_000023.11:g.2748343 G > C) alters expression of Xg^a, with the G nucleotide producing Xg^a-positive and C producing Xg^a-negative phenotypes. Lane and colleagues screened WGS data to find the same TF changes and integrated them into their *algorithm's variant database*[44]. However, it is only possible to genotype for the Xg^a-associated SNVs in males because the X and Y chromosomes share virtually identical copies of a region called PAR1 that includes the Xg^a TF binding location. Thus, females can have off-target genotyping[44,46].

WGS versus WES versus targeted sequencing. Multiple approaches to sequencing exist (**Fig. 3**). Whole genome sequencing allows analysis of ~three billion base pairs[34]. Benefits include identification of rare or not previously observed variants and analysis of intronic mutations affecting gene expression. Drawbacks include

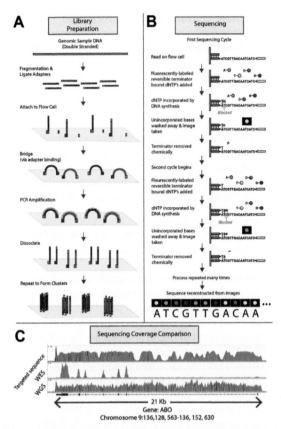

Fig. 3. Description of next-generation sequencing, including library preparation (A) and sequencing (B). (C) Comparison of NGS versus other molecular methods' coverage when sequencing the ABO blood group system's genes.

time and cost of sequencing and analysis and data storage space required (150 GB/genome without backup[47]). Whole exome sequencing generally sequences only exons and immediately adjacent introns, sequencing only ~thirty million base pairs[34], reducing cost, time to sequence, and storage space required, but precluding analysis of some deep intronic variants and requiring pipeline adjustments for accurate calls[38]. Additionally, enrichment may create capture bias, skewing copy number calculations used to call antigens in the Rh and MNS blood group systems. Targeted sequencing, requiring analysis of only 150,000 base pairs (<0.5% of the exome), further compresses time, money, and analytical and storage requirements. Targeted sequencing is least likely of the three methods to sufficiently sequence intronic regions and identify variants therein. An excellent review documents previous studies and approaches undertaken in each[48].

Short read versus long read. Commonly used short-read sequencing produces ~50 to 400 base pair read lengths. Many platforms use short reads for rapid, parallel, accurate sequencing (>99%). Nonetheless, mapping short reads to homologous genes in the HRG is challenging. Similarly, short reads cannot always resolve cis/trans ambiguities. Compared with short-read sequencing, long-read sequencing is generally more expensive, and some methods are less accurate, but long reads allow for essentially unambiguous cis/trans phasing and virtually eliminate ambiguities. Several groups have used long reads in ABO genotyping to phase SNVs[49,50]. Long read have also been used to resolve compound heterozygous SV underlying the U-antigen phenotype[28].

Call out 4: NGS terminology

DNA Microarrays

Introduction

DNA microarrays are a high-throughput and cost-effective tool for ascertaining individual genotypes pertaining to a predetermined set of genetic variants, selected during array design. They were adopted and popularized by early population scale genotyping studies such as The International HapMap project which used several different DNA microarrays to genotype 1397 individuals from several ethnic backgrounds[51]. The aim of the study was to identify loci in the genome for assessing risk of common diseases and variants which control quantitative traits of biomedical interest such as height, weight, and blood cell metrics. In 2006, the Wellcome Trust Case Control Consortium (WTCCC) conducted the first genome-wide association study (GWAS) in which donor samples were used. In this study, DNA samples from 14,000 English National Health Service patients with seven common diseases and 3000 healthy controls (1500 of which were UK blood donors) were genotyped on the Affymetrix GeneChip Mapping Array which contained probes for typing 500,000 DNA variants and captured about 60% of the then known common sequence variation in the genome. The WTCCC study discovered 24 genetically independent loci associated with disease risk, thus validating that DNA microarray-based GWAS could be used as a hypothesis-free method to identify risk loci for human diseases[52].

Today, DNA microarrays are widely used for a wide variety of purposes, and many different array designs exist. The genome-wide typing arrays in recent large-scale studies such as UK BioBank, which used the ThermoFisher Axiom UK BioBank array, now type over 800,000 genetic variants which have been specifically selected to allow for statistical inference of genotypes for untyped variants via imputation and GWAS[53]. There are also large numbers of highly specialized arrays which type a limited number of genetic variants such as the BioArray HEA BeadChip (Immucor, Norcross, GA) for typing select red cell antigens or the CytoScan 750k (Affymetrix, Santa Clara, CA) for genomic copy number characterization of patients with diseases such as hematological cancers[54,55].

How DNA microarrays work

Many different DNA microarray technologies exist, and it would be infeasible to discuss them all within a single book chapter. The authors have therefore selected the ThermoFisher Axiom genotyping platform as an exemplar of how these platforms generally work.

The Thermo Fisher Scientific Axiom ligation-based microarray genotyping platform uses 30-mer DNA oligonucleotide "probe sets", synthesized in situ on "array slides" to genotype-specific genetic variants. Numerous 3-μm squares—"features"—populate glass array slide surfaces. Each feature contains millions of unique 30 base pair oligonucleotide probes complementary to the genomic sequence flanking the variant of interest (forward or reverse). Replicating features numerous times on each array improves specific SNP resolution and protects against failure by adding redundancy. Two fluorescent color channels and each probe's recorded array slide spatial position detect genotypes. A<>T and C<>G variation must also be represented by two spatially separated features as only two dyes are used, one for bases A and T, and another for bases C and G.

In a standard genotyping experiment sample, DNA, amplified by PCR, fragmented, hybridizes to the probe/array complex. A solution of detection probes, many DNA probes representing every possible combination of 9 DNA bases labeled with a base-specific "hapten", wash over the array and covalently bond to the array-probe/genomic-DNA complex. A stringent wash cycle removes unbound solution probes and genomic DNA. After fluorescently labeled antibody staining, laser excitation produces a signal, and fluorescent intensity measurements denote genotype.

An overview of the Axiom genotyping process is given in **Fig. 4**.

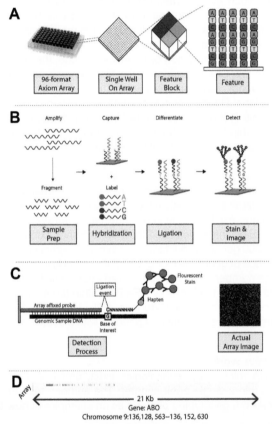

Fig. 4. Overview of Axiom array genotyping. (*A*) A zoomed diagram showing the construction of an Axiom array. (*B*) Axiom genotyping workflow. From left to right, Genomic DNA is amplified then fragmented, fragments are captured and labeled via hybridization to array probes and detection probes, ligation then covalently bonds the genomic DNA to the array/detection probe complex, finally fluorescent staining is performed followed by excitation and imaging. (*C*) Cartoon representation of the genomic DNA and array/detection probe complex. An actual image of array fluorescence during genotyping is included for reference. (*D*) Example array probe coverage for the *ABO* locus, red marks indicate the positions in the locus where probesets for measuring specific DNA changes have been incorporated into the array design.

Variant calling

Further statistical analysis of all samples' fluorescence intensity data calculates and extracts genotype information for each typed variant—"genotype clustering"[56]. In simple terms, each probe set on the array consists of two components, an A or B probe. During clustering, the A and B probe fluorescence for each measured variant are used to group samples with similar fluorescence patterns. If all fluorescence is accounted for by probe A, then the individual is of genotype homozygous *AA*, and similarly, if all fluorescence is accounted for by probe B, then the individual is of genotype homozygous *BB*. If fluorescence signal is detected for both probes A and B, then the individual is of genotype AB, or a heterozygote.

Fig. 5 shows a "genotype call plot" and illustrates the separation of samples via A and B probe fluorescence intensity.

For SNPs and indels where the genetic variation being measured is an A|T <> C|G change for which two different colored fluorescent dyes are used, the intensity of each color for each sample is compared and genotype inferred. In the case if A<>T or C<>G changes, for which the same color dye is used, the probes are physically separated on the surface of the array slide. Importantly, indel identification queries only a particular set of variants consistent with indel presence or absence. No direct, complete indel sequencing occurs.

DNA microarrays may measure larger scale genomic structural variation using "copy number probes." These probes target nonpolymorphic sites spread throughout the genome. The average total fluorescence intensity produced by the copy number probes determines a "baseline" assumed to represent copy number 2. Comparing the average fluorescence intensity of probes in a region of interest to this baseline intensity allows copy number assessment.

DNA microarrays for typing blood group antigens

Owing to being low cost and high throughput, DNA microarrays provide an excellent platform for genotyping large numbers of blood donors for the variants that underpin antigen expression. The main commercial assays on the market today are the HEA BeadChip and the BloodChip assay. The HEA BeadChip is based on a short extension reaction of oligonucleotide probes bound to color-encoded beads using a PCR product as template. The test can type for a few antigens in the RHCE, KEL, FY, DO, LW, CO, SC, LU, DI, JK, and MNS blood group systems but lacks the ability to type for many clinically important antigens[57].

The BloodChip assay is based on allele- and spatial-specific hybridization of PCR products to complementary oligonucleotides affixed to glass arrays and can be used for clinical typing of 13 RBC antigens (JK, FY, KEL, RH, MNS, and DO)[58]. Studies using DNA microarrays in combination with antibody-based typing have shown that the typing data produced can dramatically increase the availability of antigen-negative blood, with *one group reporting* that they were able to provide blood for 99.8% of complex blood requests using just 43,066 donors genotyped for a limited number of antigens[13].

Although the benefits of the previously described assays are clear, they have not been widely applied to all donors by the global blood supply organizations. This is because the currently commercially available RBC antigen genotyping assays can only detect a limited number of antigens, and in comparison to traditional serologic methods, they are expensive for the number of antigens they type. In 2020, an international group of researchers sought to overcome these limitations and redesigned the UK BioBank Axiom genotyping array, a cheap population genetics screening test capable of assaying approximately 800,000 DNA variants, with blood donor

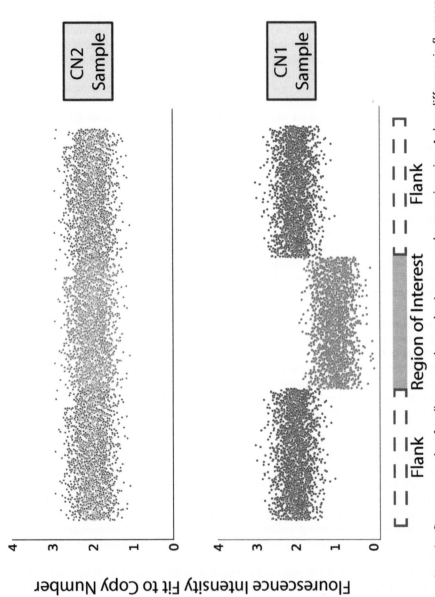

Fig. 5. Fluorescence intensity, fit to copy number, for all copy number probes in an example genomic region. A clear difference in fluorescence intensity over the region of interest can be observed between the copy number one and two samples.

genotyping in mind. In the study, 7984 English and Dutch donors were genotyped, and blood types were inferred from the resulting data using the bloodTyper algorithm. In 89,371 comparisons between genotype and serologically determined antigen types, 99.9% concordance was observed, and the total number of antigen typing results was raised from 110,980 to over 1.2 million for the typed donors. The researchers were also able to infer platelet (HPA) and leukocyte (HLA) antigen types from the same data, observing 99.97% and 99.03% concordance in 3016 and 9289 comparisons for HPA and HLA, respectively. Once these tests have achieved regulatory approval and their results can be used for labeling blood products, it is likely that they will be applied to vast numbers of donors worldwide ushering in an era of genomics-based precision transfusion medicine.

PRESENT RELEVANCE AND FUTURE AVENUES TO CONSIDER OR TO INVESTIGATE
Clinical Indications for Genotyping

Applications of NGS genotyping for RBC antigen prediction range wide—from selecting healthy donors to provide rare products, diagnosing potentially pathogenic alternate antigens between mother and fetus, and to providing well-matched product for chronically transfused populations (**Table 3**).

- Patients requiring chronic transfusion: The challenge of providing blood to chronically transfused populations (often patients with sickle cell anemia or thalassemia) is compounded by population-based genetic diversity. Antigen variants (specifically those providing malarial resistance) occur at higher frequency in Black populations, while United States blood donors are predominantly White and predisposed to be poorly matched. Matching transfusions to patients with sickle cell disease for additional antigens (C, E, and K) decreases alloimmunization. Genotyping presents the alluring ability to identify and match donors and patients not only for serologic, low-resolution types, or even for the variants included on current commercial array-based technology, but for many, or all, potentially clinically significant (alloimmunization inducing) antigens.
- Challenging serologic workups
  - *Diagnosis of unusual alloantibodies* against low- or high-frequency antigens requires rare or unavailable reagents. NGS identifies antigens a patient lacks against which they may become alloimmunized, informing alloantibody identification.
  - *Warm or cold autoantibodies* bind self erythrocytes, obscuring serologic identification of some antigens and alloantibodies and increasing risk of further alloimmunization and hemolysis. Serologic techniques remove autoantibodies from plasma but require time and remove other potentially hemolytic alloantibodies. NGS can accurately, exhaustively predict phenotype, expediting compatible product delivery and preventing alloimmunization.
  - *Therapeutic monoclonals* anti-CD38 and anti-CD47 monoclonal antibodies bind patient red cells and populate patient plasma causing false positive serologic phenotyping results and "reverse" ABO typing, respectively. As mentioned previously, NGS can accurately, exhaustively predict phenotype, expediting compatible product delivery and preventing alloimmunization.
- Challenging samples: Recently transfused patients' typing reflects both donor and recipient antigens. NGS typing, collected from recipient nonblood or leukocyte sources, accurately identifies recipient-only type.
- Insufficient sample: HDFN occurs when a pregnant woman forms an alloantibody targeting a fetal RBC antigen. These antibodies may cross into fetal circulation,

Table 3 Genotyping Software	
BOOGIE[36]	First WGS predictive algorithm for a subset of blood group systems. First machine learning-guided software for predicted typing. Called 94.2% samples (n = 67/71) correctly. Difficult to iteratively improve. Not updated with new allele tables.
bloodTyper[5,8,38,44]	Comprehensive genotyping of all known blood group and HPA variants. A curated, regularly updated allele database (bloodantigens.com). Analyzed NGS data producing exhaustive RBC and HPA antigen genotyping from WGS, WES, targeted NGS, and high-density DNA arrays with >99% accuracy. Includes expansive SV support for Rh and MNS hybrids.
RHtyper[42]	Comprehensive, high-throughput RH-typing algorithm utilizing RHD zygosity, allele zygosity and hybrid alleles via coverage profiling, and allele pair prediction via haplotype associations. Open access[59].
Omixon[60]	Monotype ABO amplifies ABO exons 2–7 for NGS sequencing, designed for solid organ transplant compatibility analysis[61].
Erythrogene[15,62]	Imported 1000 Genomes variant data and population information. Compared inputs with a composite antigen table curated from ISBT, Blood Group Antigen Factsbook, and dbRBC. Available as a searchable, online database. 15x input coverage limits SVs identification.
Schoeman et.al. Software[63–66]	Utilizes targeted exome data to interpret 35 blood group systems.
Montemayor-Garcia Software[37]	Evaluated 1000 Genomes data for single SNV and short indels of 42 blood group genes (excluding ABO, Rh and MNS). Extracted coordinates and superpopulation frequencies.

destroying fetal RBCs (anti-D) or blood-producing cells (anti-K). Neonatal alloimmune thrombocytopenia (NAIT) similarly destroys platelets. Early RBC and platelet typing confirms HDFN and/or NAIT allowing treatment. Fetal blood sampling is impossible early in pregnancy and, later, poses significant fetal risk. Cell-free fetal DNA circulates in maternal plasma. This DNA can predict Rh typing[67], Kell typing[68], and recently Rh, Kell, Duffy, Kidd, MNS, and 5 HPA antigens (implicated in NAIT)[69]. Similarly, sufficient blood for serologic workup can be challenging to obtain from neonates, pediatric patients, and anemic adults. NGS can sequence DNA from nonblood sources, facilitating testing when blood is not available.

- Blood donor screening: Blood donor samples are laboriously serologically typed, antigen by antigen. Additionally, serologic typing cannot reliably recognize variants. NGS typing all donors would undoubtedly reveal numerous rare (or heretofore unrecognized) blood types. Such units could be directed to needy, compatible recipients, and donors' information could be collected and stored for future use.
- Transplant screening: ABO compatibility affects time to engraftment of allogeneic hematopoietic stem cell transplants. Stem cell donor HLAs of recipients are commonly gathered via genotyping pretransplant, and ABO is gathered

serologically. Extending genotyping to include *ABO* could allow for screening of stem cell transplant donors from buccal swabs before the collection of a blood sample. Many deceased donors undergo massive transfusion with type O emergency release blood. *ABO* genotyping of deceased donors could help identify deceased donors who have converted their serologic ABO and aid in the resolution of discordant ABO due to these transfusions.

Many challenges to widespread adoption of NGS for blood typing remain[70]:

- Cost and accessibility: Despite decreasing costs, NGS's current cost may still be prohibitive for many. Similarly, storage requirements for the large volumes of information generated by NGS are significant, and ensuring balanced data security and accessibility (ideally for all clinicians caring for a given patient) remain problematic.

- Databases and pipelines: No single, exhaustive source documents all known antigen variants. An exceedingly large number of interacting mutations' effects on antigen expression must be considered. Pipelines continue to reckon with these challenges.

- Clinical significance? NGS frequently identifies novel variations and polymorphisms of unknown significance. Current modeling techniques often cannot accurately predict their effects on antigen structure.

- Alignment: Alignment of sequenced reads—mapping—allows variant calling, but blood group systems coded by multiple homologous chromosomes (Rh, MNS) are particularly challenging, often mapping to either homologue irrespective of origin, preventing variant calls[35,63,71]. Depth of coverage analysis identifies inaccurate mapping. Paired end reads and SRA further inform correct algorithmic placement.

- Rare null alleles: Although NGS can evaluate entire gene regions, it can miss novel null alleles, especially those produced by the introduction of stop codons or exonic indels. It can be especially difficult to predict the effect of novel changes in promoter or intronic regions which can, in theory, affect expression and lead to null states. Miscalling nulls could result in incompatible transfusion, alloimmunization, and hemolysis. Maintaining current, thorough, widely curated variant databases would decrease, but not prevent this, especially in cases of previously undescribed alleles. Encouragingly, recently produced microarrays encompass not only known but also predicted (ie, not yet observed) variants.

Future directions

Historically, serologic antigen or antigen variant discovery precipitated a search for the underlying CDS. As observed in many fields in medicine, NGS analysis commonly inverts this process, identifying variants of unknown clinical significance. As such, by sequencing larger collections of samples and then correlating concurrent serologically typed samples will allow a more complete understanding of the serologic effect of variants. Similarly, historically, blood group discovery proceeded from interesting serologic findings ("Ah! This antibody is confounding my serologic work-up! Huh. It does not target any common known antigens. I should try to identify it!") to erythrocyte surface structure identification and to underlying genetic basis determination. This process undergirds the identification of ABO, Rh, and other blood groups throughout the 20th and early 21st century. Only recently has new blood group identification begun with genetic observations, followed by confirmatory serologic discovery.

Mismatches between blood donor and blood recipient phenotypes theoretically increase the risk for alloimmunization. Such mismatches occur commonly when transfusing patients with sickle cell disease in the United States, where the donor population consists primarily of people who are white. Analysis of other geographic regions of broad-scale blood donor and recipient mismatch would highlight areas where increased alloimmunization surveillance is beneficial. Finally, RBC antigens function in a variety of cellular processes, and varying antigens and/or antigen variants may produce susceptibility or confer resistance to diseases from severe acute respiratory syndrome coronavirus 2 (SARS-CoV-2)[72] to malaria[73]. Gene-wide association studies focused on blood group antigens will likely deepen insight into such connections.

SUMMARY

Historical antibody-based RBC antigen typing accurately calls common antigens but poorly calls many variant antigens. Inaccurately phenotyped blood samples increase the risk of incompatible blood transfusion, potentially resulting in hemolysis and death. SNVs code most blood group antigens, but indels, SVs, and copy number variants or regulatory region variants code others, including variants which are often particularly challenging to phenotype. Enriching standard short-read NGS analysis with copy number, paired end read, and SRA allows accurate prediction of challenging blood group systems such as Rh. Recent advances in array technology provide nearly comparable clinical information. Such NGS and array technology allows challenging serologic case analysis, provides phenotype information when sample blood cannot be obtained, identifies rare blood donors from the donor population, and allows product matching for patients at risk of alloimmunization.

DEFINITIONS
Call Out 1: Blood Group Terms

- Antigen: RBC-surface protein or sugar structure capable of provoking a specific humoral response. Include RBC antigens, human platelet antigens, and "human leukocyte antigens," although RBC antigens are the main focus of the chapter.
- Blood group: Antigen or antigens encoded by a single (or multiple homologous) gene(s).
- Phenotyping: Determining antigen identity, commonly through serologic (antibody) reagents.
- Weak: Lower antigen expression than expected.
- Modified (mod): Significantly lower antigen expression than expected.
- El (from "eluate"): Significantly lower antigen expression than expected, requiring sensitive serologic techniques (absorbtion-elution) to identify.
- Partial: Lack some surface structure portion (some epitope or epitopes) characteristic of the antigen.

Call Out 2: Allele Terminology

- Locus: Gene's fixed chromosomal location.
- Allele: Alternate gene iterations.
- CDS (from "coding sequence"): Sum of an organism's protein-coding sequences.
- Genome Reference Consortium: Multi-institutional collaborative maintaining human reference genomes.
- Contig: Overlain DNA sequences forming a consensus sequence.
- Human reference genome: A representative genome. Not one human's DNA sequence, rather an idealized "normal" human genome composite. Built of contigs.

- hg38[9]: Human genome reference build, released December 2013, widely used in NGS to make variant calls.
- Genomic coordinates: Denote gene location in relation to the reference genome. Include chromosome number and gene start and end positions.
- Format: File formats relaying NGS data. Include FASTA (reference sequence; eg, RefSeq), FASTQ (unaligned NGS reads with quality scores), SAM (aligned NGS reads), BAM (binary format sequence of SAM files), and VCF (variant call format).
- Single nucleotide variant (SNV): At one genomic position, interchanging one nucleotide with another.
- Single nucleotide polymorphism: SNV occurring in greater than 1% of a population.
- Structural variant: Large changes in chromosome structural (generally >1kb). Include insertions, deletions, translocations, duplications, and *copy number variants*.
- Indels: Nucleotide sequences inserted or deleted, typically less than 100 nucleotides.
- Gene conversion: Interchanging one sequence with a homologue, producing a hybrid gene.
- Hybrid gene: Product of gene conversion.
- Deletion: Nucleotide sequence loss, via removal or nonreplication.
- Insertion: Nucleotide sequence addition.
- Multiallelic site: Genomic position where greater than 2 alternative alleles (or variants) have been detected.

Call Out 3: Blood Group Governance

The ISBT defines blood group antigens under the governance of the Red Cell Immunogenetics and Blood Group Terminology working party, a collaborative of blood group antigen serology and genetics world experts. ISBT recognizes greater than 330 blood group antigen phenotypes across 43 blood group systems, defined by greater than 1700 alleles[74].

Call Out 4: Next Generation Sequencing Terminology

- Read: Nucleotide sequence copied from reference DNA.
- Sequence read: Number of separate sequence reads copying a locus[75].
- Paired read: Two reads separated by a known distance, flanking the sequenced area. Read distance variation from expected implies structural variation. Algorithms use read distance to improve mapping in repetitive portions of the genome.
- Split read: Presumed contiguous read mapping to two separate areas in the reference genome. Indicates structural variation.
- Phased sequencing, "Phasing": Delineating mapped allele maternal versus paternal origin. Allows[76],
  - Compound heterozygote analysis
  - Allele-specific expression measurement
  - Variant linkage identification.

Call Out 5: Array Terminology

- Probe: Oligonucleotide hybridizing with a specific nucleotide target sequence.
- Feature: Geographic array constituent; a "spot" of probes designed to hybridize with one specific target sequence.

- Probeset: Multiple probes targeting one transcript. Separate probes hybridizing with varying transcript sequence lengths.
- Array: Collection of spots identifying selected transcripts.
- Copy number probe: Oligonucleotides hybridizing with transcripts of a specific copy number.
- Probe intensity: Fluorescent antibodies bind probe-transcript hybrids. High fluorescence implies successful hybridization. Genotype (delineated by known feature position) is inferred by degree of fluorescence.
- Cluster plot: Specific genotypes produce repeatable array fluorescence patterns. Statistical analysis of fluorescence intensity data allows variant calling.
- Contrast: Ratio between fluorescence signal from probe A and probe B in array genotyping determines separability of different genotype clusters. Equals log2 (A signal intensity/B signal intensity).
- Strength: The average strength of the fluorescence signal from probe A and probe B in array genotyping. Usefully highlights signal strength differences between genotype clusters. Equals (log2(A signal)+log2(B signal))/2.

CLINIC CARE POINTS

- Conventional serologic testing and PCR based genotyping cannot be used to routinely identify all known clinically significant blood group antigens, potentially leading to incompatible transfusions.
- Conversely, next generation sequencing (NGS) and high-density DNA array genotyping can identify nearly all known blood group antigens, promoting more compatible transfusions and prevent alloantibody formation.
- Therefore, NGS and high-density DNA array-based genotyping are valuable testing modalities to supplement serologic testing in multiply transfused patients, patients for whom blood samples are not available and patients with complicated serologic workups.

DISCLOSURE

W.J. Lane reports receiving personal consulting fees from CareDx, Inc, and his institution is a founding member of the Blood transfusion Genomics Consortium (BGC) that has received fees from Thermo Fisher Scientific Inc. to help codevelop a high-density DNA genotyping array. J.K. Cone Sullivan has nothing to disclose. N. Gleadall's institution is a founding member of the Blood transfusion Genomics Consortium (BGC) that has received fees from Thermo Fisher Scientific Inc. to help codevelop a high-density DNA genotyping array.

REFERENCES

1. Table of blood group systems. ISBT. 2021. Available at: https://www.isbtweb.org/fileadmin/user_upload/Table_of_blood_group_systems_v._9.0_03-FEB-2021.pdf. Accessed March 16, 2021.
2. Hendrickson JE, Tormey CA, Shaz BH. Red blood cell alloimmunization mitigation strategies. Transfus Med Rev 2014;28(3):137–44.
3. Tormey CA, Stack G. The persistence and evanescence of blood group alloantibodies in men. Transfusion 2009;49(3):505–12.
4. Schonewille H, van de Watering LMG, Brand A. Additional red blood cell alloantibodies after blood transfusions in a nonhematologic alloimmunized patient

cohort: is it time to take precautionary measures? Transfusion 2006;46(4): 630–5.

5. Lane WJ, Westhoff CM, Gleadall NS, et al. Automated typing of red blood cell and platelet antigens: a whole-genome sequencing study. Lancet Haematol 2018; 5(6):e241–51.

6. Daniels G. Human blood groups. Hoboken, NJ: John Wiley & Sons; 2008.

7. Westhoff CM. Blood group genotyping. Blood 2019;133(17):1814–20.

8. Lane WJ, Westhoff CM, Uy JM, et al. Comprehensive red blood cell and platelet antigen prediction from whole genome sequencing: proof of principle. Transfusion 2016;56(3):743–54.

9. Genome browser FAQ. Available at: https://genome.ucsc.edu/FAQ/FAQreleases. html#release1. Accessed March 18, 2021.

10. Patnaik SK, Helmberg W, Blumenfeld OO. BGMUT database of allelic variants of genes encoding human blood group antigens. Transfus Med Hemother 2014; 41(5):346–51.

11. Patnaik SK, Helmberg W, Blumenfeld OO. BGMUT: NCBI dbRBC database of allelic variations of genes encoding antigens of blood group systems. Nucleic Acids Res 2012;40(Database issue):D1023–9.

12. Index of/pub/mhc/rbc/Final archive. Available at: https://ftp.ncbi.nlm.nih.gov/ pub/mhc/rbc/Final%20Archive/. Accessed March 21, 2021.

13. Wagner FF, Flegel WA. The rhesus site. Transfus Med Hemother 2014;41(5): 357–63.

14. Reid ME, Lomas-Francis C, Olsson ML. The blood group antigen factsBook. Hoboken, NJ: Academic Press; 2012.

15. Möller M, Jöud M, Storry JR, et al. Erythrogene: a database for in-depth analysis of the extensive variation in 36 blood group systems in the 1000 Genomes Project. Blood Adv 2016;1(3):240–9.

16. 1000 Genomes Project Consortium, Auton A, Brooks LD, et al. A global reference for human genetic variation. Nature 2015;526(7571):68–74.

17. [No title]. Available at: http://www.isbtweb.org/fileadmin/user_upload/Working_ parties/WP_on_Red_Cell_Immunogenetics_and/004_RHCE_alleles_v4.0_ 180208.pdf. Accessed March 18, 2021.

18. Tournamille C, Colin Y, Cartron JP, et al. Disruption of a GATA motif in the Duffy gene promoter abolishes erythroid gene expression in Duffy–negative individuals. Nat Genet 1995;10(2):224–8.

19. Booth PB, Serjeantson S, Woodfield DG, et al. Selective depression of blood group antigens associated with hereditary ovalocytosis among melanesians. Vox Sang 1977;32(2):99–110.

20. Ogasawara K, Yabe R, Uchikawa M, et al. Molecular genetic analysis of variant phenotypes of the ABO blood group system. Blood 1996;88(7):2732–7.

21. Olsson ML, Irshaid NM, Hosseini-Maaf B, et al. Genomic analysis of clinical samples with serologic ABO blood grouping discrepancies: identification of 15 novel A and B subgroup alleles. Blood 2001;98(5):1585–93.

22. Seltsam A, Wagner FF, Grüger D, et al. Weak blood group B phenotypes may be caused by variations in the CCAAT-binding factor/NF-Y enhancer region of the ABO gene. Transfusion 2007;47(12):2330–5.

23. Yamamoto F-I, McNeill PD, Hakomori S-I. Human histo-blood group A2 transferase coded by A2 allele, one of the A subtypes, is characterized by a single base deletion in the coding sequence, which results in an additional domain at the carboxyl terminal. Biochem Biophys Res Commun 1992;187(1):366–74.

24. Hosseini-Maaf B, Smart E, Chester MA, et al. The Abantu phenotype in the ABO blood group system is due to a splice-site mutation in a hybrid between a new O1-like allelic lineage and the A2 allele. Vox Sanguinis 2005;88(4):256–64.

25. Wagner FF, Frohmajer A, Flegel WA. RHD positive haplotypes in D negative Europeans. BMC Genet 2001;2:10.

26. Richard M, Perreault J, Constanzo-Yanez J, et al. A newDELvariant caused by exon 8 deletion. Transfusion 2007;47(5):852–7.

27. Olsson ML, Chester MA. A rapid and simple ABO genotype screening method using a novel B/O2 versus A/O2 discriminating nucleotide substitution at the ABO locus. Vox Sang 1995;69(3):242–7.

28. Lane WJ, Gleadall NS, Aeschlimann J, et al. Multiple GYPB gene deletions associated with the U- phenotype in those of African ancestry. Transfusion 2020;60(6): 1294–307.

29. Suzuki K, Iwata M, Tsuji H, et al. A de novo recombination in the ABO blood group gene and evidence for the occurrence of recombination products. Hum Genet 1997;99.

30. Landsteiner K. On agglutination of normal human blood. Transfusion 1961;1:5–8.

31. Sanger F, Nicklen S, Coulson AR. DNA sequencing with chain-terminating inhibitors. Proc Natl Acad Sci U S A 1977;74(12):5463–7.

32. Yamamoto F, Clausen H, White T, et al. Molecular genetic basis of the histo-blood group ABO system. Nature 1990;345(6272):229–33.

33. Lander ES, Linton LM, Birren B, et al. Initial sequencing and analysis of the human genome. Nature 2001;409(6822):860–921.

34. Venter JC, Adams MD, Myers EW, et al. The sequence of the human genome. Science 2001;291(5507):1304–51.

35. Stabentheiner S, Danzer M, Niklas N, et al. Overcoming methodical limits of standard RHD genotyping by next-generation sequencing. Vox Sang 2011;100(4): 381–8.

36. Giollo M, Minervini G, Scalzotto M, et al. BOOGIE: predicting blood groups from high throughput sequencing data. PLoS One 2015;10(4):e0124579.

37. Montemayor-Garcia C, Karagianni P, Stiles DA, et al. Genomic coordinates and continental distribution of 120 blood group variants reported by the 1000 Genomes Project. Transfusion 2018;58(11):2693–704.

38. Lane WJ, Vege S, Mah HH, et al. Automated typing of red blood cell and platelet antigens from whole exome sequences. Transfusion 2019. https://doi.org/10. 1111/trf.15473.

39. Pirooznia M, Goes FS, Zandi PP. Whole-genome CNV analysis: advances in computational approaches. Front Genet 2015;6:138.

40. Baronas J, Westhoff CM, Vege S, et al. RHD zygosity determination from whole genome sequencing data. J Blood Disord Transfus 2016;7(5). https://doi.org/ 10.4172/2155-9864.1000365.

41. Wheeler MM, Lannert KW, Huston H, et al. Genomic characterization of the RH locus detects complex and novel structural variation in multi-ethnic cohorts. Genet Med 2019;21(2):477–86.

42. Chang T-C, Haupfear KM, Yu J, et al. A novel algorithm comprehensively characterizes human RH genes using whole-genome sequencing data. Blood Adv 2020;4(18):4347–57.

43. Chou ST, Flanagan JM, Vege S, et al. Whole-exome sequencing for RH genotyping and alloimmunization risk in children with sickle cell anemia. Blood Adv 2017; 1(18):1414–22.

44. Lane WJ, Aguad M, Smeland-Wagman R, et al. A whole genome approach for discovering the genetic basis of blood group antigens: independent confirmation for P1 and Xga. Transfusion 2019;59(3):908–15.
45. Westman JS, Stenfelt L, Vidovic K, et al. Allele-selective RUNX1 binding regulates P1 blood group status by transcriptional control of A4GALT. Blood 2018;131(14): 1611–6.
46. Möller M, Lee YQ, Vidovic K, et al. Disruption of a GATA1-binding motif upstream of XG/PBDX abolishes Xga expression and resolves the Xg blood group system. Blood 2018;132(3):334–8.
47. Storage and computation requirements. Available at: https://www.strand-ngs.com/support/ngs-data-storage-requirements. Accessed March 29, 2021.
48. Orzinska A, Guz K, Brojer E. Potential of next-generation sequencing to match blood group antigens for transfusion. IJCTM 2019;7:11–22.
49. Lang K, Wagner I, Schöne B, et al. ABO allele-level frequency estimation based on population-scale genotyping by next generation sequencing. BMC Genomics 2016;17:374.
50. Wu PC, Lin Y-H, Tsai LF, et al. ABO genotyping with next-generation sequencing to resolve heterogeneity in donors with serology discrepancies. Transfusion 2018; 58(9):2232–42.
51. International HapMap Consortium. The international HapMap project. Nature 2003;426(6968):789–96.
52. Wellcome Trust Case Control Consortium. Genome-wide association study of 14,000 cases of seven common diseases and 3,000 shared controls. Nature 2007;447(7145):661–78.
53. Bycroft C, Freeman C, Petkova D, et al. The UK Biobank resource with deep phenotyping and genomic data. Nature 2018;562(7726):203–9.
54. Veldhuisen B, van der Schoot CE, de Haas M. Blood group genotyping: from patient to high-throughput donor screening. Vox Sang 2009;97(3):198–206.
55. Berry NK, Scott RJ, Rowlings P, et al. Clinical use of SNP-microarrays for the detection of genome-wide changes in haematological malignancies. Crit Rev Oncol Hematol 2019;142:58–67.
56. Rabbee N, Speed TP. A genotype calling algorithm for affymetrix SNP arrays. Bioinformatics 2006;22(1):7–12.
57. Hashmi G, Shariff T, Seul M, et al. A flexible array format for large-scale, rapid blood group DNA typing. Transfusion 2005;45(5):680–8.
58. Beiboer SHW, Wieringa-Jelsma T, Maaskant-Van Wijk PA, et al. Rapid genotyping of blood group antigens by multiplex polymerase chain reaction and DNA microarray hybridization. Transfusion 2005;45(5):667–79.
59. Company Profiles: DNAnexus Inc. Available at: https://platform.dnanexus.com/app/RHtyper. Accessed August 13, 2021.
60. HLA Typing. Available at: https://www.omixon.com/. Accessed March 17, 2021.
61. Monotype ABOTM. Available at: https://www.omixon.com/products/monotype-abo/. Accessed March 17, 2021.
62. Möller M, Hellberg Å, Olsson ML. Thorough analysis of unorthodox ABO deletions called by the 1000 Genomes project. Vox Sang 2018;113(2):185–97.
63. Schoeman EM, Roulis EV, Liew Y-W, et al. Targeted exome sequencing defines novel and rare variants in complex blood group serology cases for a red blood cell reference laboratory setting. Transfusion 2018;58(2):284–93.
64. Sano R, Nakajima T, Takahashi K, et al. Expression of ABO blood-group genes is dependent upon an erythroid cell-specific regulatory element that is deleted in persons with the B(m) phenotype. Blood 2012;119(22):5301–10.

65. Schoeman EM, Lopez GH, McGowan EC, et al. Evaluation of targeted exome sequencing for 28 protein-based blood group systems, including the homologous gene systems, for blood group genotyping: SEQUENCING FOR BLOOD GROUP GENOTYPING. Transfusion 2017;57(4):1078–88.

66. RBC-FluoGeneNX ABO plus. Published May 12, 2020.Available at: https://www.inno-train.de/en/news/produkte/details/detail/rbc-fluogenenx-abo-plus/. Accessed March 17, 2021.

67. Lo YM, Hjelm NM, Fidler C, et al. Prenatal diagnosis of fetal RhD status by molecular analysis of maternal plasma. N Engl J Med 1998;339(24):1734–8.

68. Rieneck K, Bak M, Jønson L, et al. Next-generation sequencing: proof of concept for antenatal prediction of the fetal Kell blood group phenotype from cell-free fetal DNA in maternal plasma. Transfusion 2013. https://doi.org/10.1111/trf.12172.

69. Orzińska A, Guz K, Mikula M, et al. Prediction of fetal blood group and platelet antigens from maternal plasma using next-generation sequencing. Transfusion 2019;59(3):1102–7.

70. Montemayor-Garcia C, Westhoff CM. The "next generation" reference laboratory? Transfusion 2018;58(2):277–9.

71. Fichou Y, Le Maréchal C, Bryckaert L, et al. Variant screening of the RHD gene in a large cohort of subjects with D phenotype ambiguity: report of 17 novel rare alleles. Transfusion 2012;52(4):759–64.

72. Wu S-C, Arthur CM, Wang J, et al. The SARS-CoV-2 receptor-binding domain preferentially recognizes blood group A. Blood Adv 2021;5(5):1305–9.

73. Rowe JA, Opi DH, Williams TN. Blood groups and malaria: fresh insights into pathogenesis and identification of targets for intervention. Curr Opin Hematol 2009;16(6):480–7.

74. E T. Red Cell Immunogenetics and Blood Group Terminology. Available at: https://www.isbtweb.org/working-parties/red-cell-immunogenetics-and-blood-group-terminology. Accessed March 18, 2021.

75. Sims D, Sudbery I, Ilott NE, et al. Sequencing depth and coverage: key considerations in genomic analyses. Nat Rev Genet 2014;15(2):121–32.

76. Phased sequencing. Available at: https://www.illumina.com/techniques/sequencing/dna-sequencing/whole-genome-sequencing/phased-sequencing.html. Accessed March 21, 2021.

Cell-free Nucleic Acids in Cancer

Current Approaches, Challenges, and Future Directions

Liron Barnea Slonim, MD, Kathy A. Mangold, PhD,
Mir B. Alikhan, MD, Nora Joseph, MD, Kalpana S. Reddy, MD,
Linda M. Sabatini, PhD, Karen L. Kaul, MD, PhD*

KEYWORDS

- Cell-free DNA • ctDNA • Companion diagnostics • PCR • Early detection
- Liquid biopsy

KEY POINTS

- Tumors shed fragmented DNA and nucleic acids into the blood, generally during apoptosis.
- Technical advances now allow highly sensitive detection of tumor genomic alterations in a background of normal DNA.
- Cell-free DNA is a potential new tool for the clinical assessment of human tumors resistance.

Histologic and cytologic evaluation of tissue and cells remains the mainstay of cancer diagnosis and assessment, though pathologists have long worked to develop novel and improved approaches. Indeed, many biopsy and tissue sampling protocols, new immunostains, and other molecular assays have been implemented over the years to improve cancer detection and management. Recent technologic advances have allowed the evaluation of genomic change in tumor-derived nucleic acids found in blood samples, opening the door to a potentially extremely impactful and minimally invasive method for the detection and characterization of cancer.

Cell-free DNA (cfDNA) has been used for clinical purposes for a decade or more; noninvasive prenatal testing (NIPT) has become routine for screening at 10 to 12 weeks

This article previously appeared in *Advances in Molecular Pathology*, Volume 4, Issue 1, November 2021.
Department of Pathology and Laboratory Medicine, NorthShore University HealthSystem, 2650 Ridge Avenue, Evanston, IL 60201
* Corresponding author.
E-mail address: kkaul@northshore.org

gestation[1,2]. cfDNA enters the blood following apoptosis—of normal cells, inflammatory cells, cells from the placenta, or tumor cells. Initial applications of NIPT focused on the detection of numeric chromosomal abnormalities such as trisomy 21, but more sensitive methods such as next-generation sequencing allow detection of other genetic abnormalities as well. The proportion of fetal DNA in maternal blood during pregnancy is at least tenfold greater than circulating tumor DNA (ctDNA) when present; however, NIPT has in many respects paved the way for current efforts in the detection and characterization of cell-free tumor DNA.

Although tumor-derived DNA can enter the bloodstream following cellular necrosis or by active secretion, the majority appears to arise from apoptosis, based on the size correspondence to nucleosomes[3,4]. The typical fragment size approximates 166 bp, though smaller and larger fragments can also be recovered. Newer analytical approaches are ideal for these smaller fragments.

Different tumor types show variable release of cfDNA fragments, which has a great impact on the clinical sensitivity of these tests. Bladder, colorectal, gastroesophageal, and ovarian cancers show the highest amount of plasma cfDNA, whereas little is detectable from glioma and thyroid tumors[5]. Furthermore, detection of cfDNA rises with the stage tumor[5]. The impact of other factors such as timing, treatment, and various histologic features remains unknown.

PREANALYTICAL REQUIREMENTS

Successful liquid biopsy analysis starts in the preanalytical phase. This includes use of the appropriate specimen, proper collection and processing, and storage[3,6,7] to provide sufficient cfDNA or RNA for analysis. Many biofluids (sputum, CSF, and more) can be used as liquid biopsy specimens[8,9], but blood is the most common source. Early studies used serum samples instead of plasma because of a greater yield of total cfDNA, but the fraction of ctDNA is actually less because of DNA release from leukocytes during blood clotting; most studies therefore favor plasma[10,11]. Cellular lysis should be avoided during blood collection using proper phlebotomy technique[7,12]. Frozen whole blood is not acceptable because of hemolysis.

The biofluid should be processed quickly[12]; standard EDTA tubes can be used for plasma if processing will occur within 6 hours (optimally 1–3 hr); longer delays result in hemolysis and lymphocyte lysis as well as reduced plasma volume[7]. Specialized tubes containing stabilizers can extend the preprocessing time up to 14 days (3 days optimum)[11–15]. Within these time limits, several studies showed equivalent ctDNA yield and variant allele frequency (VAF) when either EDTA or specialized tubes were used[7,11,14,16]. Although some analyses have reported success with very low plasma volume, 1 mL of plasma on average yields only 3000 whole genomic equivalents[17]. If a typical 10 mL blood draw yields 4 mL of plasma, a theoretic assay sensitivity of ∼0.01% would detect only one ctDNA copy among 12,000 wild-type copies, corresponding to an ∼1 cm^3 tumor, assuming that early-stage tumor is actively shedding ctDNA into the bloodstream. To increase the amount of ctDNA available for variant analysis, increasing the plasma input volume and minimizing the extraction volume optimizes the downstream ctDNA analysis without altering the VAF[15,17–19].

Processing blood samples begins with 2 centrifugation steps for at least 10 minutes each[7]. The first low g force centrifugation separates the plasma from cells without damaging the latter (200–2500 × g). The second centrifugation (1600–18,400 × g) reduces cellular genomic DNA in the final sample. No statistically significant changes between the varied g forces have been found for either cfDNA yield or VAF[16]. If necessary, a second high-speed centrifugation can be performed if single-spun samples were stored frozen to obtain useable cfDNA[20–22]. The spun plasma should be stored at −80°C with minimal freeze-thaws[12].

The final preanalytical step is cfDNA extraction. Although greater than 40 cfDNA extraction kits are available, the most used remains QIAamp Circulating Nucleic Acid Kit (Qiagen, Germantown, MD, USA)[7]. Note that cfDNA sizes obtained may differ between kits, and the significance of this is unknown[3,7,23,24]. Some extraction kits recover all DNA in the sample, including high molecular weight DNA from cellular lysis, protected DNA in tri-, di-, and mono-nucleosomes, or even less than 100 bp fragmented DNA, as well as smaller circulating mitochondrial DNA not protected by histones[25]. Most analyses rely on the ~166 bp fragments corresponding to protected DNA in mononucleosomes[4] with minimal extraction volumes to increase ctDNA concentrations[7]. The flexibility shown above in preanalytical steps will permit successful transfer to the clinical testing environment, but standardization will enhance downstream analyses[12].

TECHNICAL APPROACHES

Detection of ctDNA is challenging because of the presence of normal cfDNA and the need to discriminate normal from tumor, the low levels of ctDNA, and the need to quantify the mutant fragments in a sample[26]. Many strategies have been used and include both limited and broad candidate gene panels, and less commonly whole exome and whole genome approaches. Single or limited gene panels require less DNA and can detect mutations with good sensitivity[27]. Although sensitivity is an advantage, these methods may be limited in their ability to detect novel genomic changes. Broader ctDNA analysis includes large gene panels and exome- and genome-wide analysis of mutations[28], require more ctDNA and have lower sensitivity and therefore would be less useful for early stage and MRD situations. Select commercially available methods are described in **Table 1**.

Limited Target Analysis

Many limited target assays exist and are often PCR-based platforms concentrating on one or few targets, such as specific hotspot mutational variants in a small panel of genes in the context of a specific type of cancer (eg, *EGFR* in non-small cell lung cancer [NSCLC]; **Table 1**).

Digital PCR is an ultrasensitive, quantitative method to detect point mutations in ctDNA at low allele fractions. Digital PCR includes ddPCR and BEAMing; in both, the sample is split into nanoliter droplets, which partition parallel fluorescence-emitting PCR reactions each amplifying a single DNA molecule from the sample. Fluorescence is measured by flow cytometry[28,29].

Broader Genomic Analysis

NGS-based broad gene panel testing is widely performed using LDPs, kits from the main NGS platform providers Illumina (TruSight Oncology 500 ctDNA) and Ion-Torrent (Oncomine cfDNA) and by some commercial labs (eg, Guardant, Foundation One (see **Table 1**). Some NGS-based methods have incorporated further modifications to increase the sensitivity of ctDNA detection, as described below.

Cancer personalized profiling by deep sequencing (CAPP-seq) is a targeted NGS-based method in which patient-specific genomic alterations are first identified then sought in cfDNA. This method optimizes library preparation for low DNA input, allows tracking of multiple mutations per patient, and achieves low levels of detection[30]. The CAPP-Seq method has been used to assess plasma ctDNA in NSCLC for both

Table 1
Examples of commercially available ctDNA detection assays

Test name	Category	Targets	Purpose	Test specifications/ Technology
cobas® EGFR Mutation Test v2[a]	Multiplex real-time PCR	EGFR mutations: exon 19 deletions; L858R in exon 21; T790M in exon 20; G719X in exon 18; S768I in exon 20; exon 20 insertion mutations; L861Q in exon 21	Qualitative detection of defined mutations of EGFR in cfDNA from plasma in NSCLC patients and formalin-fixed, paraffin-embedded (FFPE)	Allele-specific PCR amplification and fluorescent detection.
therascreen PIK3CA RGQ PCR test[b]	Multiplex real-time PCR	PIK3CA gene mutations: Exon 7: C420R; Exon 9: E542K, E545A, E545D [1635G>T only], E545G, E545K, Q546E, Q546R; and Exon 20: H1047L, H1047R, H1047Y.	Qualitative PCR test for the detection of PIK3CA gene mutations ctDNA from plasma (or tumor FFPE) of patients with breast cancer	Fluorescent detection using mutation-specific PCR primers.
FoundationOne® Liquid CDx[c]	NGS (hybridization-based capture)	Substitutions, insertions, and deletions (indels) in 311 genes, rearrangements in 3 genes (ALK, BRCA1, BRCA2), and copy number variations in 3 genes (BRCA1, BRCA2, ERBB2).	FDA approved for detection of BRCA1/ BRCA2 alterations in metastatic castration-resistant prostate cancer and patients with epithelial ovarian cancer; EGFR activating mutations (Exon 19 deletions and L858R) in patients with advanced and metastatic NSCLC; ALK rearrangements in NSCLC; PIK3CA mutations	A whole-genome indexed library is amplified from plasma cfDNA Hybridization-based capture of all coding exons of 309 genes with select intronic regions of 3 genes. Deep sequencing performed using the NovaSeq6000 platform. A subset of targeted regions in 75 genes is baited for added sensitivity.

		patients with breast cancer		
Guardant360® CDx[d]	NGS (hybridization-based capture)	FDA approved for identification of *EGFR* exon 19 deletions, *EGFR* L858R, and *EGFR* T790M in NSCLC patients	Single nucleotide variants, insertions and deletions in 55 genes, copy number amplifications in 2 genes (*ERBB2, MET*), and fusions in 4 genes (*ALK, NTRK1, RET, ROS1*)	Barcoded library construction/ amplification from cfDNA, with NGS on the Illumina NextSeq 550. Alterations in 55 genes are reported.
Ion Torrent Oncomine™ [e]	NGS (amplicon-based method)	Focused disease specific (lung, breast, or colon cancer) or comprehensive pan-cancer genomic profiling	Five different tumor type-specific assays (10–12 genes) or a 52-gene pan-cancer assay, are available. The latter covers >900 hotspots and insertion deletions, 96 fusions 12 copy number variants and MET exon 14 skipping	For the pan-cancer assay, a single library is constructed from plasma cfDNA and RNA following multiplex PCR. 272 amplicons are used, and sequencing is performed on the Ion GeneStudio S5. A quick 2-d turnaround time is enabled by this approach. Variants present at an allele frequency as low as 0.1% can be detected with a 20 ng DNA input.
Illumina TruSight™ Oncology 500 ctDNA[f]	NGS (hybridization-based capture)	Pan-cancer comprehensive genomic profiling	Analysis of the full coding sequence of 523 genes for single nucleotide variants, insertions and deletions, copy number variants and fusions. Microsatellite instability	This method combines UMIs for library construction. Sequencing is performed on the NovaSeq 6000. Error correction software (and UMI use) enable error rate reduction even at

(continued on next page)

Table 1 (continued)				
Test name	Category	Targets	Purpose	Test specifications/ Technology
		and tumor mutational burden are also assessed		low VAFs. 30 ng of cfDNA are required. With 30 ng, the analytical sensitivity at 0.2% VAF is 82.59% at 15,000× raw coverage depth.
BIO-RAD ddPCR™ Mutation Detection Assays[9]	digital droplet PCR	Primers can be designed for over >400 mutations from the COSMIC database, >200 validated targets for detection of KRAS G12/G13, KRAS Q61, NRAS G12, NRAS G12/G13, NRAS Q61, BRAF V600 mutations and EGFR exon 19 deletions, with other designs available. Copy number variant detection for >700 variants and 60 targets available	Detection/quantification of genomic alterations including mutations and copy number variations. This test has multiple other applications (such as gene expression profiling, or DNA quantification before NGS)	Emulsion droplet amplification of cfDNA fragments fluorescence detection to quantify the amount of target DNA 5 ng of plasma cfDNA is required to detect a mutation present at 0.2%.
OncoBEAM[h]	BEAM (beads, emulsion, amplification, magnetics), a form of digital PCR	Available formats: (tumor-specific) Acute myeloid leukemia glioma breast cancer colorectal cancer lung cancer, melanoma, pancreatic cancer, prostatic cancer Single gene tests: AKT1, ALK,	Detection and quantification of mutations	cfDNA from plasma is multiplex amplified using primers of specific regions of interest. Amplicons are bead captured and further amplified using emulsion PCR. Fluorescent flow

AR, BRAF, EGFR, ESR1, IDH1 IDH2, KRAS, NRAS, PIK3CA, and ROS1. Multigene tests: AKT1, ESR1, PIK3CA; ALK-ROS; BRAF-EGFR-KRAS; BRAF-KRAS-NRAS; BRAF-NRAS; IDH1-IDH2.	cytometric assessment of the proportions of WT/ mutant DNA. Reported sensitivity ranges from 0.1% to 0.02% depending on the specific assay and sample.

Abbreviation: UMIs, unique molecular identifiers.

[a] Administration UFaD. cobas EGFR Mutation Test v2. https://www.accessdata.fda.gov/cdrh_docs/pdf15/P150047A.pdf. Published 2016. Accessed April 28, 2021.

[b] Administration UFaD. therascreen PIK3CA RGQ PCR kit. https://www.accessdata.fda.gov/cdrh_docs/pdf19/P190004A.pdf. Published 2019. Accessed April 28, 2021.

[c] Administration UFaD. FoundationOne Liquid CDx (F1 Liquid CDx). https://www.accessdata.fda.gov/cdrh_docs/pdf20/P200016A.pdf. Published 2020. Accessed April 28, 2021.

[d] Administration UFaD. Guardant360CDx. https://www.accessdata.fda.gov/cdrh_docs/pdf20/P200010A.pdf. Published 2020. Accessed April 28, 2021, 2021.

[e] Thermo Fisher Scientific Inc. Ion Torrent Oncomine. https://www.thermofisher.com/order/catalog/product/A37664?SID=srch-srp-A37664#/A37664?SID=srch-srp-A37664. Accessed April 28, 2021, 2021.

[f] Illumina Inc. TruSight Oncology 500. https://www.illumina.com/products/by-type/clinical-research-products/trusight-oncology-500.html. Accessed April 28, 2021, 2021.

[g] Bio-Rad Laboratories Inc. ddPCR mutation detection assays, Validated. https://www.bio-rad.com/webroot/web/pdf/lsr/literature/10033487.pdf. Published 2015. Accessed April 28, 2021, 2021.

[h] Sysmex Inostics I. OncoBEAM: Benchmark-Setting Liquid Biopsy Technology. https://www.sysmex-inostics.com/sysmex-oncobeam-technology-overview. Accessed April 28, 2021, 2021.

disease monitoring and minimal residual disease detection with ctDNA detection rates[31]. The sensitivity can be further increased when combined with integrated digital error suppression, a computational error correction method that uses molecular barcoding and removes nonbiological background errors introduced during library preparation and sequencing for the efficient recovery of cfDNA molecules[32].

Targeted error correction sequencing (TEC-Seq) allows ultrasensitive evaluation of sequence changes in cfDNA using massively parallel sequencing directed at a panel of 58 cancer-related genes. This method has proven sensitive for early-stage colorectal, breast, lung, and ovarian cancer, in which somatic mutations were detected in 71%, 59%, 59%, and 68%, respectively, in the plasma of patients with stage I or II disease[33].

Safe-Seq is an NGS approach that incorporates unique molecular identifiers (UMIs or UIDs) to each DNA molecule in the sample to identify duplicate reads of that molecule. The use of UMIs allows for error correction and enables the detection and quantification of rare mutations, and this approach is now commonly used in cfDNA NGS platforms[34].

TAm-Seq (Tagged-amplicon deep sequencing)[35] is used for deep sequencing of genomic regions spanning thousands of bases from as little as a single copy of fragmented DNA. This technique uses a combination of short amplicons, two-step amplification, sample barcodes, and high-throughput PCR. Because the first-round amplicons are short, this method effectively amplifies even small amounts of fragmented DNA. The two-step amplification includes a limited-cycle preamplification step where all primer sets are used to capture the starting molecules present in the sample, followed by individual amplification specific for intended targets. This permits primer multiplexing which enables amplification and sequencing of relatively large genomic regions by tiling short amplicons without loss of fidelity. Duplicate sequencing of each sample is performed to avoid incorporation of PCR errors. Allele frequencies as low as 0.2% can be detected with this method with reported sensitivity and specificity of greater than 97%[35].

In addition to the aforementioned methods, enrichment steps used before NGS can be used to greatly improve ctDNA analysis yield. Multiplex PCR (mPCR) provides an alternative to capture hybridization for targeted NGS. This enrichment technique is used in the CancerSEEK platform and the Tracking Cancer Evolution Through Therapy (TRACERx) platform (Signatera)[36]. In this mPCR approach, each template molecule is uniquely labeled with a DNA barcode, minimizing errors and enabling the use of small amounts of cfDNA. The reaction is divided into multiple aliquots and the assay is performed independently on each replicate, thus increasing sensitivity and the signal-to-noise ratio[36].

Other Markers Found in Plasma

DNA methylation changes are implicated in carcinogenesis and tumor progression, and can be used as a biomarker detectable in ctDNA[37,38]. Most methods use bisulfite to convert nonmethylated cytosine residues to uracil. The target can then be sequenced and methylation can be assessed and compared to a standard[39]. This can be performed on a whole genome level (methylome), or for specific biologically relevant CpG islands[38,40]. Differential methylation patterns are also used for the enrichment of ctDNA to enhance sensitivity and specificity, such as the platform designed by GRAIL technologies[41].

MicroRNA (miRNA) expression profiles serve as biomarkers for prognosis or even classification of certain cancers[42–44]. Circulating free or exosomal miRNA or can be isolated from plasma and converted to complementary DNA (cDNA), followed by quantitative real-time PCR (qRT-PCR), allowing relative quantitation of miRNA expression. Although qRT-PCR is a common method for the detection of miRNA, other options include in situ hybridization, enzymatic luminescence miRNA assay and northern blotting, microarrays, NGS, and nanopore technology[45].

CLINICAL APPLICATIONS

The current investigation of ctDNA for clinically significant alterations is primarily focused on patients with late-stage malignancies for targeted treatment selection and monitoring of response to systemic therapy. However, other applications, such as detection of early recurrence and emerging treatment resistance before imaging-detectable relapse, have great potential. Even more promising and challenging is the identification of ctDNA within an asymptomatic population for screening and initial detection of early-stage cancers[3,46,47]. These applications are summarized in **Table 2**.

Screening and Early Detection of Cancer

A major goal in cancer management is early identification, and cfDNA offers great potential as a screening tool[48,49]. Numerous studies have demonstrated detectable cfDNA in early-stage disease, before the presence of symptoms, and up to 2 years before cancer diagnosis[3]. However, high sensitivity and specificity is reported only in patients with a known diagnosis of cancer; testing an asymptomatic patient population with no known cancer history has proven to be more challenging because of the limited amount of cfDNA in the circulation. Ideally, ctDNA screening will be effective in detecting occult cancer, and incorporated into routine clinical care without unnecessary and invasive follow-up testing.

The CancerSeek assay profiles mutations in ctDNA from 16 genes and 9 protein biomarkers in a novel assay that has shown promise in stage I-III cancers for which traditional screening tests are not available, including ovary, liver, stomach, pancreas, esophagus, colorectal, and lung. CancerSEEK detected the majority of cancers along with tissue of origin, with sensitivities ranging from 69% to 98% and specificity greater than 99%[36]. This assay has been used in large screening study[36] of women with no history of cancer (DETECT-A); patients with positive results were referred for PET-CT[50]. A follow-up clinical trial (ASCEND) is underway to address issues of sensitivity and specificity, as well as tissue of origin identification[46].

Similarly, GRAIL Technologies has applied their methylation-based techniques to interrogate plasma ctDNA from solid and hematologic malignancies. The Circulating Cell-free Genome Atlas Consortium (CCGA)[41] recently published promising results on the detection and localization of multiple early- and late-stage cancers. Currently, there are several ongoing large-scale clinical trials using GRAILs multiplexed methylation-based assays to identify early cancers as part of general population-based screening programs[51].

Other ctDNA approaches to screen asymptomatic patients include the DNA evaluation of fragments for early interception (DELFI) platform[52], Epi proColon, an FDA-approved colorectal cancer screening test detecting methylation status of *SEPT9* promoter in blood[53], the LUNG Cancer Likelihood in Plasma (Lung-CLiP) assay[54] and CAncer Personalized Profiling by deep Sequencing (CAPP-Seq) to name a few[31].

Guiding Treatment

Currently, the most established clinical use for liquid biopsies is guiding first-line or subsequent systemic therapy in patients with metastatic tumors. ctDNA analysis is becoming the standard of care for patients with certain tumors, particularly NSCLC.

Table 2
Clinical Applications of Cell-free Nucleic Acid

Applications	Use/Impact	Advantages	Disadvantages
Screening/Early Detection	Routine screen for cf-NA in healthy individuals	• Earlier intervention • Help identify tissue of origin • May select patients for imaging	• Need low false positives • Risk of false negatives • Possible tumor localization • Cost
Diagnostics & Staging	Clarify diagnosis in suspect cases (eg, Lung nodule) Potential adjunct to traditional staging	• Can aid diagnosis in cases with limited tissue or access	• Tissue-based testing remains the gold standard
Prognostic & Predictive Markers	May aid therapy choice and planning	• Can aid diagnosis in cases with limited tissue or access	• Tissue-based testing is the gold standard
Monitoring for: • Therapeutic response • MRD • Recurrence	Longitudinal testing for therapy response, resistance, early relapse	• Earlier detection of disease • May reduce imaging • Tracking clonal evolution • Detection of emerging resistance • Improved outcome?	• Need more definitive data to show improved outcomes

Current NCCN recommendations for NSCLC directly address cfDNA testing, and support the use of cfDNA when a tissue biopsy is medically unsafe or if there is insufficient tissue for molecular testing and a follow-up tissue-based assay will be performed if no significant variants are identified (NCCN NSCLC v4.2021)[55]. However, the guidelines also state that cfDNA should not be used for the diagnosis of NSCLC.

Both FDA-approved and lab-developed assays are used to guide first or second-line systemic therapy for solid tumors. The Cobas EGFR mutation test v2 was the first liquid biopsy assay approved by the FDA as a companion diagnostic test to identify EGFR mutations in patients with advanced-stage NSCLC being considered for erlotinib (EGFR TKI therapy)[56]. The Guardant360 CDx assay has been approved for treatment decisions for any solid malignancy after positive results from the NILE study[57,58]. Based on results from the SOLAR-1 trial, PIK3CA RGQ PCR (Therascreen) assay is FDA approved for patients with HR+/HER2- advanced/metastatic breast cancer who progress after prior aromatase inhibitor therapy[59]. Foundation One Liquid CDx interrogates 324 genes and has been approved to identify druggable targets for advanced stage/metastatic disease in patients with solid tumors. Lastly, Resolution HRD is a cfDNA assay being developed to detect homologous recombination deficiency (HRD) in patients with metastatic castration-resistant prostate cancer who could benefit from PARP inhibitor therapy[60]. Although ctDNA analysis has been incorporated into routine clinical practice, it is important to note that a significant proportion of patients may have insufficient ctDNA, even with late-stage cancers, or alterations outside the scope of these assays[5].

Monitoring disease progression, early identification of relapse and drug resistance
Serial ctDNA sampling may be useful in monitoring disease, early detection of relapse, and determining when adjuvant in treatment is necessary. For example, ctDNA has been used to monitor patients with breast cancer after surgery, and positive results were highly correlated with metastatic relapse months later[61]. In further studies, surveillance of early-stage treated breast cancer patients for patient-specific mutations in ctDNA detected molecular relapse nearly a year before clinical signs[62]. Similarly, Signatera, a custom test for treatment monitoring and MRD assessment, generates a patient-specific "tumor signature" from whole exome sequencing of the primary tumor and matched normal control, which is then used to monitor plasma ctDNA[63]. A positive test predicted relapse with a positive predictive value (PPV) of over 98% across multiple solid tumors[64,65]. This technology can also be used to select patients for immune checkpoint blockade[66].

In addition, the development of resistance and emergence of subclones can be identified using cfDNA[67]. However, ctDNA alone is not yet used for routine monitoring of treatment response; while ctDNA can detect progression earlier than imagining, improved clinical outcomes have not yet been demonstrated following treatment decisions based on changes in ctDNA. In several tumor types, evaluation of ctDNA is currently used for patients who show clinical signs of relapse and progression when a tissue biopsy is either insufficient or cannot be tolerated[47].

Challenges in the Implementation of Cell-free Nucleic Acid Testing

Challenges in interpretation
ctDNA testing is complex, and interpretation of the results poses additional challenges. The results, if not understood correctly, can lead to considerable confusion among pathologists, clinicians, and patients. This necessitates that the report is clear with respect to the limitations of the analysis and what unexpected results may indicate.

Implications of a negative test result must be clearly understood; the negative predictive value can be as low as 60% depending on the tumor type, the clinical context, and timing of the test[68]. Conversely, a positive result seen during screening of healthy patients may be a harbinger of future malignancy, though these may occur more than 10 years later[18].

Another cause of misleading positive results stems from the detection of pathogenic mutations arising in myeloid cells, detected in cfDNA analysis. The most common would be clonal hematopoiesis of indeterminate potential (CHIP)[69], and related changes such as age-related clonal hematopoiesis[70]. These often involve mutations in *DNMT3A*, *TET2*, *ASXL1*, and even *TP53*, which would indicate an increased risk of development of myeloid neoplasms such as myelodysplastic syndrome. Patients with such mutations are also at increased risk of developing cardiovascular disease[71]. The allele frequencies in which these mutations are present, as well as the total number of mutations, factors into the risk of developing disease[72].

CHIP-like mutations may be detected in emerging therapy-related myeloid neoplasms (t-MNs). These are aggressive diseases in patients treated with radiation and/or chemotherapy and may develop months or years after completion of treatment. This is an important consideration when monitoring patients for residual solid tumor following therapy. Mutations in what are thought of as myeloid-related genes can be present in solid tumors, such as DNMT3A[73]. In addition, mutations in TP53 are also common in myeloid neoplasms, particularly t-MNs. These factors must be taken into account when interpreting positive results from ctDNA testing that involves these gene targets.

Challenges in standardization

Lastly, as molecular oncology evolves at break-neck speed, it is challenging to rapidly establish guidelines to standardize the performance and interpretation of cfDNA molecular analysis. Owing to multiple strategies used for cfDNA analysis, there is lack of standardization across workflows, and sometimes a lack of concordance between assays[74,75]. Concordance studies have also been flawed by the timing of sample collection and other issues. Lack of concordance is most problematic at low allele fractions.

Multiple groups have convened to outline best practices and set guidelines (**Table 3**) for clinical implementation of cfDNA analysis[76–80]. There are also numerous publications on individual laboratory validation efforts[81,82]. Standardization should also address the intended use. Qualitative assays would have different validation protocols than quantitative panels. Further technologic advances (molecular barcoding, digital PCR strategies) may improve quantification efforts in the future[83,84].

Table 3
Current Efforts to Develop Guidelines in cfDNA Testing

Project	Group	Reference
American Society Clinical Oncology and the College of American Pathologists, Joint Review	ASCO-CAP	78
Blood profiling atlas consortium, analytical variables working group	BloodPAC	76
Innovative Medicines Initiative Consortium	CANCER-ID	79
International Liquid Biopsy Standardization Alliance	ILSA	80
Multi-stakeholder invitational workshop		77

Efforts are underway to help develop cancer-specific guidelines[80] to aid clinicians and pathologists in the use of these tests, though keeping such guidelines up to date will be challenging[78]. If there is near universal adaptation of guidelines, cfDNA testing can become more uniform and reliable for patient care.

Challenges in reimbursement

Cost of testing and reimbursement are necessary considerations as well. As with any test, the laboratory must weigh the practical benefits of bringing ctDNA testing in-house against the cost of sending the test to a reference laboratory. The technical challenges and bioinformatics requisite for such complex testing can be a substantial effort and expense.

Regardless of where the test is performed, reimbursement for ctDNA testing has increased from 2015 for both private payer and Medicare coverage[85]. Data from both coverage determinations favor cancer-specific approvals, such as coverage for NSCLC testing. However, the overall trend is toward coverage of pan-cancer panels, allowing testing for a significant subset of patients with cancer. In addition, there are draft and future local coverage determinations that would cover non–FDA-approved cfDNA testing[85].

Part of the challenge of cfDNA use is assessing the overall cost-benefit of the testing. One study focusing on screening for early cancer determined that as the cost of testing reaches $200, there is an overall benefit[85]. Others have shown that monitoring post-treatment may not be cost-effective[86]. As cost declines and the potential clinical impact of the test becomes more certain, payers will increasingly provide coverage, all promising for the widespread use of cfDNA testing over a range of tumor types.

SUMMARY

Since the first observation of cfDNA in blood samples in 1948[87], great strides have been made in the biology, detection and clinical applications of this analyte. The tremendous improvements in our technical capabilities leading to greater analytical sensitivity, coupled with a growing understanding of the source and biology of ctDNA, will pave the way for the further advances needed. A clear understanding of factors affecting the release of ctDNA will help us understand how to best use this biomarker in various tumors and different clinical scenarios. In time, the use of ctDNA will be a valuable tool, used across the full range of clinical applications in patients with cancer.

CLINICS CARE POINTS

- Many technical approaches now exist to interrogate cell-free DNA from tumors in plasma.
- Cell-free DNA approaches are becoming standard for the assessment of drug resistance.
- Ongoing studies are needed to establish the role of cfDNA in early detection and monitoring of cancer.

DISCLOSURE

The authors have nothing to disclose.

REFERENCES

1. American College of Obstetrics and Gynecologists' Committee on Practices: Bulletins-Obstetrics, American College of Obstetrics and Gynecologists' Committee on Genetics, Society of Maternal-fetal Medicine. Screening for Fetal Chromosomal Abnormalities: ACOG Practice Bulletin, Number 226. Obstet Gynecol 2020;136(4):e48–69.

2. Lo YM, Corbetta N, Chamberlain PF, et al. Presence of fetal DNA in maternal plasma and serum. Lancet 1997;350(9076):485–7.

3. Bronkhorst AJ, Ungerer V, Holdenrieder S. The emerging role of cell-free DNA as a molecular marker for cancer management. Biomol Detect Quantif 2019;17: 100087.

4. Snyder MW, Kircher M, Hill AJ, et al. Cell-free DNA Comprises an In Vivo Nucleosome Footprint that Informs Its Tissues-Of-Origin. Cell 2016;164(1–2):57–68.

5. Bettegowda C, Sausen M, Leary RJ, et al. Detection of circulating tumor DNA in early- and late-stage human malignancies. Sci Transl Med 2014;6(224):224ra224.

6. Bronkhorst AJ, Ungerer V, Holdenrieder S. Comparison of methods for the isolation of cell-free DNA from cell culture supernatant. Tumour Biol 2020;42(4). 1010428320916314.

7. Ungerer V, Bronkhorst AJ, Holdenrieder S. Preanalytical variables that affect the outcome of cell-free DNA measurements. Crit Rev Clin Lab Sci 2020;57(7): 484–507.

8. Fettke H, Kwan EM, Azad AA. Cell-free DNA in cancer: current insights. Cell Oncol 2019;42(1):13–28.

9. Peng M, Chen C, Hulbert A, et al. Non-blood circulating tumor DNA detection in cancer. Oncotarget 2017;8(40):69162–73.

10. Lampignano R, Kloten V, Krahn T, et al. Integrating circulating miRNA analysis in the clinical management of lung cancer: Present or future? Mol Aspects Med 2020;72:100844.

11. Schneegans S, Luck L, Besler K, et al. Pre-analytical factors affecting the establishment of a single tube assay for multiparameter liquid biopsy detection in melanoma patients. Mol Oncol 2020;14(5):1001–15.

12. Greytak SR, Engel KB, Parpart-Li S, et al. Harmonizing Cell-Free DNA Collection and Processing Practices through Evidence-Based Guidance. Clin Cancer Res 2020;26(13):3104–9.

13. Sorber L, Zwaenepoel K, Jacobs J, et al. Specialized Blood Collection Tubes for Liquid Biopsy: Improving the Pre-analytical Conditions. Mol Diagn Ther 2020; 24(1):113–24.

14. van Dessel LF, Beije N, Helmijr JC, et al. Application of circulating tumor DNA in prospective clinical oncology trials - standardization of preanalytical conditions. Mol Oncol 2017;11(3):295–304.

15. van Dessel LF, Martens JWM, Lolkema MP. Fundamentals of liquid biopsies in metastatic prostate cancer: from characterization to stratification. Curr Opin Oncol 2020;32(5):527–34.

16. Risberg B, Tsui DWY, Biggs H, et al. Effects of Collection and Processing Procedures on Plasma Circulating Cell-Free DNA from Cancer Patients. J Mol Diagn 2018;20(6):883–92.

17. Bronkhorst AJ, Ungerer V, Holdenrieder S. Early detection of cancer using circulating tumor DNA: biological, physiological and analytical considerations. Crit Rev Clin Lab Sci 2019;1–17.

18. Alborelli I, Generali D, Jermann P, et al. Cell-free DNA analysis in healthy individuals by next-generation sequencing: a proof of concept and technical validation study. Cell Death Dis 2019;10(7):534.

19. de Kock R, Deiman B, Kraaijvanger R, et al. Optimized (Pre) Analytical Conditions and Workflow for Droplet Digital PCR Analysis of Cell-Free DNA from Patients with Suspected Lung Carcinoma. J Mol Diagn 2019;21(5):895–902.

20. Barrett AN, Thadani HA, Laureano-Asibal C, et al. Stability of cell-free DNA from maternal plasma isolated following a single centrifugation step. Prenat Diagn 2014;34(13):1283–8.

21. Cavallone L, Aldamry M, Lafleur J, et al. A Study of Pre-Analytical Variables and Optimization of Extraction Method for Circulating Tumor DNA Measurements by Digital Droplet PCR. Cancer Epidemiol Biomarkers Prev 2019;28(5):909–16.

22. Swinkels DW, Wiegerinck E, Steegers EA, et al. Effects of blood-processing protocols on cell-free DNA quantification in plasma. Clin Chem 2003;49(3):525–6.

23. Beije N, Martens JWM, Sleijfer S. Incorporating liquid biopsies into treatment decision-making: obstacles and possibilities. Drug Discov Today 2019;24(9):1715–9.

24. van Dessel LF, Vitale SR, Helmijr JCA, et al. High-throughput isolation of circulating tumor DNA: a comparison of automated platforms. Mol Oncol 2019;13(2):392–402.

25. Diefenbach RJ, Lee JH, Kefford RF, et al. Evaluation of commercial kits for purification of circulating free DNA. Cancer Genet 2018;228-229:21–7.

26. Diaz LA Jr, Bardelli A. Liquid biopsies: genotyping circulating tumor DNA. J Clin Oncol 2014;32(6):579–86.

27. Heitzer E, Haque IS, Roberts CES, et al. Current and future perspectives of liquid biopsies in genomics-driven oncology. Nat Rev Genet 2019;20(2):71–88.

28. Elazezy M, Joosse SA. Techniques of using circulating tumor DNA as a liquid biopsy component in cancer management. Comput Struct Biotechnol J 2018;16:370–8.

29. Hindson BJ, Ness KD, Masquelier DA, et al. High-throughput droplet digital PCR system for absolute quantitation of DNA copy number. Anal Chem 2011;83(22):8604–10.

30. Chaudhuri AA, Chabon JJ, Lovejoy AF, et al. Early Detection of Molecular Residual Disease in Localized Lung Cancer by Circulating Tumor DNA Profiling. Cancer Discov 2017;7(12):1394–403.

31. Newman AM, Bratman SV, To J, et al. An ultrasensitive method for quantitating circulating tumor DNA with broad patient coverage. Nat Med 2014;20(5):548–54.

32. Newman AM, Lovejoy AF, Klass DM, et al. Integrated digital error suppression for improved detection of circulating tumor DNA. Nat Biotechnol 2016;34(5):547–55.

33. Phallen J, Sausen M, Adleff V, et al. Direct detection of early-stage cancers using circulating tumor DNA. Sci Transl Med 2017;9(403):eaan2415.

34. Abbosh C, Birkbak NJ, Swanton C. Early stage NSCLC - challenges to implementing ctDNA-based screening and MRD detection. Nat Rev Clin Oncol 2018;15(9):577–86.

35. Forshew T, Murtaza M, Parkinson C, et al. Noninvasive identification and monitoring of cancer mutations by targeted deep sequencing of plasma DNA. Sci Transl Med 2012;4(136):136ra168.

36. Cohen JD, Li L, Wang Y, et al. Detection and localization of surgically resectable cancers with a multi-analyte blood test. Science 2018;359(6378):926–30.

37. Guo S, Diep D, Plongthongkum N, et al. Identification of methylation haplotype blocks aids in deconvolution of heterogeneous tissue samples and tumor tissue-of-origin mapping from plasma DNA. Nat Genet 2017;49(4):635–42.

38. Zeng H, He B, Yi C, et al. Liquid biopsies: DNA methylation analyses in circulating cell-free DNA. J Genet Genomics 2018;45(4):185–92.

39. Legendre C, Gooden GC, Johnson K, et al. Whole-genome bisulfite sequencing of cell-free DNA identifies signature associated with metastatic breast cancer. Clin Epigenet 2015;7:100.

40. Wen L, Li J, Guo H, et al. Genome-scale detection of hypermethylated CpG islands in circulating cell-free DNA of hepatocellular carcinoma patients. Cell Res 2015;25(11):1250–64.

41. Liu MC, Oxnard GR, Klein EA, et al. Sensitive and specific multi-cancer detection and localization using methylation signatures in cell-free DNA. Ann Oncol 2020; 31(6):745–59.

42. He FC, Meng WW, Qu YH, et al. Expression of circulating microRNA-20a and let-7a in esophageal squamous cell carcinoma. World J Gastroenterol 2015;21(15): 4660–5.

43. Lan H, Lu H, Wang X, et al. MicroRNAs as potential biomarkers in cancer: opportunities and challenges. Biomed Res Int 2015;2015:125094.

44. Markou A, Liang Y, Lianidou E. Prognostic, therapeutic and diagnostic potential of microRNAs in non-small cell lung cancer. Clin Chem Lab Med 2011;49(10): 1591–603.

45. de Planell-Saguer M, Rodicio MC. Detection methods for microRNAs in clinic practice. Clin Biochem 2013;46(10–11):869–78.

46. Detecting Cancers Earlier Through Elective Plasma-based CancerSEEK Testing (ASCEND). 2021. Available at: https://clinicaltrials.gov/ct2/show/NCT04213326. [Accessed 28 April 2021].

47. Ignatiadis M, Sledge GW, Jeffrey SS. Liquid biopsy enters the clinic - implementation issues and future challenges. Nat Rev Clin Oncol 2021;18(5):297–312.

48. Kalinich M, Haber DA. Cancer detection: Seeking signals in blood. Science 2018; 359(6378):866–7.

49. Liu MC. Transforming the landscape of early cancer detection using blood tests-Commentary on current methodologies and future prospects. Br J Cancer 2021; 124(9):1475–7.

50. Lennon AM, Buchanan AH, Kinde I, et al. Feasibility of blood testing combined with PET-CT to screen for cancer and guide intervention. Science 2020;(6499):369.

51. GRAIL Clinical Research Program. 2020. Available at: https://grail.com/clinical-studies/. [Accessed 28 April 2001].

52. Cristiano S, Leal A, Phallen J, et al. Genome-wide cell-free DNA fragmentation in patients with cancer. Nature 2019;570(7761):385–9.

53. Potter NT, Hurban P, White MN, et al. Validation of a real-time PCR-based qualitative assay for the detection of methylated SEPT9 DNA in human plasma. Clin Chem 2014;60(9):1183–91.

54. Chabon JJ, Hamilton EG, Kurtz DM, et al. Integrating genomic features for noninvasive early lung cancer detection. Nature 2020;580(7802):245–51.

55. Network NCC. NCCN Guidelines Non-Small Cell Lung Cancer v4.2021. 2021. Available at: https://www.nccn.org/professionals/physician_gls/pdf/nscl.pdf. [Accessed 28 April 2021].

56. Malapelle U, Sirera R, Jantus-Lewintre E, et al. Profile of the Roche cobas(R) EGFR mutation test v2 for non-small cell lung cancer. Expert Rev Mol Diagn 2017;17(3):209–15.
57. Aggarwal C, Rolfo CD, Oxnard GR, et al. Strategies for the successful implementation of plasma-based NSCLC genotyping in clinical practice. Nat Rev Clin Oncol 2021;18(1):56–62.
58. Leighl NB, Page RD, Raymond VM, et al. Clinical Utility of Comprehensive Cell-free DNA Analysis to Identify Genomic Biomarkers in Patients with Newly Diagnosed Metastatic Non-small Cell Lung Cancer. Clin Cancer Res 2019;25(15):4691–700.
59. Andre F, Ciruelos E, Rubovszky G, et al. Alpelisib for PIK3CA-Mutated, Hormone Receptor-Positive Advanced Breast Cancer. N Engl J Med 2019;380(20):1929–40.
60. Teyssonneau D, Margot H, Cabart M, et al. Prostate cancer and PARP inhibitors: progress and challenges. J Hematol Oncol 2021;14(1):51.
61. Garcia-Murillas I, Schiavon G, Weigelt B, et al. Mutation tracking in circulating tumor DNA predicts relapse in early breast cancer. Sci Transl Med 2015;7(302):302ra133.
62. Garcia-Murillas I, Chopra N, Comino-Mendez I, et al. Assessment of Molecular Relapse Detection in Early-Stage Breast Cancer. JAMA Oncol 2019;5(10):1473–8.
63. Abbosh C, Birkbak NJ, Wilson GA, et al. Phylogenetic ctDNA analysis depicts early-stage lung cancer evolution. Nature 2017;545(7655):446–51.
64. Christensen E, Birkenkamp-Demtroder K, Sethi H, et al. Early Detection of Metastatic Relapse and Monitoring of Therapeutic Efficacy by Ultra-Deep Sequencing of Plasma Cell-Free DNA in Patients With Urothelial Bladder Carcinoma. J Clin Oncol 2019;37(18):1547–57.
65. Coombes RC, Page K, Salari R, et al. Personalized Detection of Circulating Tumor DNA Antedates Breast Cancer Metastatic Recurrence. Clin Cancer Res 2019;25(14):4255–63.
66. Bratman SV, Yang SYC, Iafolla MAJ, et al. Personalized circulating tumor DNA analysis as a predictive biomarker in solid tumor patients treated with pembrolizumab. Nat Cancer 2020;1(9):873–81.
67. Parikh AR, Leshchiner I, Elagina L, et al. Liquid versus tissue biopsy for detecting acquired resistance and tumor heterogeneity in gastrointestinal cancers. Nat Med 2019;25(9):1415–21.
68. Cavallone L, Aguilar-Mahecha A, Lafleur J, et al. Prognostic and predictive value of circulating tumor DNA during neoadjuvant chemotherapy for triple negative breast cancer. Sci Rep 2020;10(1):14704.
69. Steensma DP, Bejar R, Jaiswal S, et al. Clonal hematopoiesis of indeterminate potential and its distinction from myelodysplastic syndromes. Blood 2015;126(1):9–16.
70. Jaiswal S, Fontanillas P, Flannick J, et al. Age-related clonal hematopoiesis associated with adverse outcomes. N Engl J Med 2014;371(26):2488–98.
71. Jaiswal S, Natarajan P, Silver AJ, et al. Clonal Hematopoiesis and Risk of Atherosclerotic Cardiovascular Disease. N Engl J Med 2017;377(2):111–21.
72. Gondek LP, DeZern AE. Assessing clonal haematopoiesis: clinical burdens and benefits of diagnosing myelodysplastic syndrome precursor states. Lancet Haematol 2020;7(1):e73–81.
73. Zhang W, Xu J. DNA methyltransferases and their roles in tumorigenesis. Biol Res 2017;5:1.

74. Kuderer NM, Burton KA, Blau S, et al. Comparison of 2 Commercially Available Next-Generation Sequencing Platforms in Oncology. JAMA Oncol 2017;3(7): 996–8.

75. Stetson D, Ahmed A, Xu X, et al. Orthogonal Comparison of Four Plasma NGS Tests With Tumor Suggests Technical Factors are a Major Source of Assay Discordance. JCO Precision Oncol 2019;(3):1–9.

76. Godsey JH, Silvestro A, Barrett JC, et al. Generic Protocols for the Analytical Validation of Next-Generation Sequencing-Based ctDNA Assays: A Joint Consensus Recommendation of the BloodPAC's Analytical Variables Working Group. Clin Chem 2020;66(9):1156–66.

77. IJzerman MJ, de Boer J, Azad A, et al. Towards Routine Implementation of Liquid Biopsies in Cancer Management: It Is Always Too Early, until Suddenly It Is Too Late. Diagnostics 2021;11(1):103.

78. Merker JD, Oxnard GR, Compton C, et al. Circulating Tumor DNA Analysis in Patients With Cancer: American Society of Clinical Oncology and College of American Pathologists Joint Review. J Clin Oncol 2018;36(16):1631–41.

79. Weber S, Spiegl B, Perakis SO, et al. Technical Evaluation of Commercial Mutation Analysis Platforms and Reference Materials for Liquid Biopsy Profiling. Cancers (Basel) 2020;12(6).

80. Connors D, Allen J, Alvarez JD, et al. International liquid biopsy standardization alliance white paper. Crit Rev Oncol Hematol 2020;156:103112.

81. Verma S, Moore MW, Ringler R, et al. Analytical performance evaluation of a commercial next generation sequencing liquid biopsy platform using plasma ctDNA, reference standards, and synthetic serial dilution samples derived from normal plasma. BMC Cancer 2020;20(1):945.

82. Fettke H, Steen JA, Kwan EM, et al. Analytical validation of an error-corrected ultra-sensitive ctDNA next-generation sequencing assay. BioTechniques 2020; 69(2):133–40.

83. Johansson G, Andersson D, Filges S, et al. Considerations and quality controls when analyzing cell-free tumor DNA. Biomol Detect Quantif 2019;17:100078.

84. Yu Q, Huang F, Zhang M, et al. Multiplex picoliter-droplet digital PCR for quantitative assessment of EGFR mutations in circulating cell-free DNA derived from advanced non-small cell lung cancer patients. Mol Med Rep 2017;16(2): 1157–66.

85. Douglas MP, Gray SW, Phillips KA. Private Payer and Medicare Coverage for Circulating Tumor DNA Testing: A Historical Analysis of Coverage Policies From 2015 to 2019. J Natl Compr Canc Netw 2020;18(7):866–72.

86. Sanchez-Calderon D, Pedraza A, Mancera Urrego C, et al. Analysis of the Cost-Effectiveness of Liquid Biopsy to Determine Treatment Change in Patients with Her2-Positive Advanced Breast Cancer in Colombia. Clin Outcomes Res 2020; 12:115–22.

87. Mandel P, Metais P. Nuclear Acids In Human Blood Plasma. C R Seances Soc Biol Fil 1948;142(3–4):241–3.

Review of SARS-CoV-2 Antigen and Antibody Testing in Diagnosis and Community Surveillance

Robert D. Nerenz, PhD[1], Jacqueline A. Hubbard, PhD*,[1], Mark A. Cervinski, PhD

KEYWORDS

- COVID-19 • SARS-CoV-2 • Antigen • Antibody • Serology • Vaccine • Pfizer
- Moderna

KEY POINTS

- SARS-CoV-2 antigen tests offer short turnaround time and high specificity but the lower sensitivity relative to nucleic acid testing increases the risk of further transmission by patients with false-negative antigen test results.
- Although numerous SARS-CoV-2 antibody detection methods exist, the lack of harmonization and correlation with neutralizing antibodies limits their clinical usefulness.
- SARS-CoV-2 antibody titers are higher after vaccination than after a natural infection, but antibody longevity and the frequency at which vaccine re-immunization will be needed remain unknown.

INTRODUCTION

The severe acute respiratory syndrome coronavirus 2 (SARS-CoV-2), identified as the cause of the coronavirus disease 2019 (COVID-19) global pandemic, is a single-stranded RNA virus belonging to the coronavirus family. It consists of structural spike proteins that interact with angiotensin-converting enzyme 2 receptors to infect host cells, nucleocapsid protein that encapsulates the RNA, and envelope protein that surrounds the nucleocapsid[1]. Commercially available antibody assays have predominantly been developed to target antibodies to either the spike or nucleocapsid

This article originally appeared in *Advances in Molecular Pathology*, Volume 4, Issue 1, November 2021.

Department of Pathology and Laboratory Medicine, Dartmouth-Hitchcock Medical Center, 1 Medical Center Drive, Lebanon, NH 03756, USA

[1] Authors contributed equally to this article.

* Corresponding author.

E-mail address: Jacqueline.a.hubbard@hitchcock.org

proteins. Although the nucleocapsid protein is highly conserved and less susceptible to genetic variation, the spike protein is the target of neutralizing antibodies, which are hypothesized to correlate with immunity[2–5].

Despite public health efforts to encourage masking, social distancing, and surveillance testing, the SARS-CoV-2 virus continued to spread at an alarming rate. As a result, significant effort was dedicated to the development of vaccines against SARS-CoV-2. After rapid development and deployment, several manufacturers began clinical trials on their vaccine within just months of the sequencing of the SARS-CoV-2 virus[6]. All vaccines available at the time of this publication target the spike protein, and immunocompetent individuals who receive the vaccine develop only antispike antibodies. In contrast, after a natural infection, both antispike and antinucleocapsid antibodies are detectable. Additional longitudinal studies are required to determine the longevity of antibodies after a natural infection or vaccination.

The gold standard for diagnosing a SARS-CoV-2 infection is nucleic acid amplification testing with throat or nasopharyngeal swabs[6]. However, difficulty of sample collection, slow turnaround time owing to batch mode testing and limited instrument availability, and supply chain shortages for reagents and consumables limited the ability to produce quick diagnostic results in many laboratories. As a result, several manufacturers developed rapid antigen-based assays for the diagnosis of SARS-CoV-2. Although these tests offer several logistical advantages, including rapid identification of infected individuals and ease of implementation in a nonlaboratory setting, antigen testing is considered less sensitive than molecular diagnostic techniques. Furthermore, the performance may vary considerably depending on whether it is used to diagnose symptomatic individuals, or to screen for asymptomatic individuals[7].

The essential role of rapid and accurate clinical laboratory testing has been highlighted during the SARS-CoV-2 global pandemic. In this review, we discuss the design and performance characteristics of commercially available antibody platforms. We then review antibody response after natural infection and after vaccination, with an emphasis on development of the 3 vaccines currently authorized for use in the United States (Pfizer-BioNtech, Moderna, and Janssen Biotech, Inc). Finally, we consider the use of antigen testing as an alternative diagnostic tool to nucleic acid testing. Taken together, we emphasize the essential contributions of laboratory medicine professionals in the global effort to detect, contain, and eradicate SARS-CoV-2.

ANTIBODY TESTING

The appearance of and subsequent spread of SARS-CoV-2 has challenged health care systems on a global scale. The accurate and rapid detection of the SARS-CoV-2 virus has propelled the laboratory community, particularly molecular pathology and microbiology laboratories, into the spotlight. As the pandemic has grown and evolved, new assay modalities focusing on the human host's adaptive immune response to SARS-CoV-2 have become available.

By April of 2020 the US Food and Drug Administration (FDA) began to grant emergency use authorization (EUA) for a limited number of immunoassays designed to detect the presence of antibodies specific to the SARS-CoV-2 virus[8]. Importantly these serology tests are not designed to detect current infection with the SARS-CoV-2 virus, because the immunoglobulins specific to viral proteins may not have developed in the time between infection and symptom onset. Consequently, a diagnosis of active SARS-CoV-2 infection is best achieved using nucleic acid techniques, or via specific detection of SARS-CoV-2 viral proteins.

Despite these limitations, numerous in vitro diagnostic companies and clinical laboratories devoted considerable resources to develop serologic methods to detect SARS-CoV-2 specific IgM and IgG antibodies with the expectation that these assays may fill an unmet laboratory testing need.

Assay Format

At the time of this report, 52 assays have attained EUA from the FDA, with the exclusion of point-of-care lateral flow immunoassays and laboratory developed tests. These EUA SARS-CoV-2 serology assays fall into 2 general methodologic categories, antibody isotype specific, and nonspecific or total immunoglobulin assays (**Fig. 1, Table 1**). Within the isotype-nonspecific and -specific categories, there are also methodologic differences in the antigen immobilization scheme used, with assays using microparticle or paramagnetic/magnetic particles predominating over the more traditional microwell- or plate-based formats.

Given the close homology of SARS-CoV-2 proteins with those of other coronaviruses, including the SARS-CoV-1 virus that caused the more limited SARS outbreak between 2002 and 2004, there was concern that serology assays would be subject to frequent false-positive results owing to prior exposure to related human coronaviruses (HCoV). The spike proteins of the related betacorona viruses infecting humans display varying degrees of sequence homology (SARS-CoV-1 = 76%, Middle Eastern respiratory syndrome [MERS]-CoV = 42%, HCoV-OC43 = 30%, and HCoV-HKU1 = 29%). Although HCoV-OC43 and HCoV-HKU1 are endemic and seroprevalence is high, the sequence differences in spike proteins between them and SARS-CoV-2 are sufficient to prevent measurable or significant cross-reactivity[9]. Although there is predicted to be intermediate cross-reactivity between spike antibodies to SARS-CoV-1 and MERS-CoV for SARS-CoV-2 spike serology assays, the low seroprevalence for these 2 coronaviruses cause them to be less of a concern[10].

The low cross-reactivity for spike proteins from human betacoronaviruses was a welcomed discovery, and this feature also extends to assays targeting the SARS-CoV-2 nucleocapsid protein. Although the nucleocapsid protein of the closely related SARS-CoV-1 virus and MERS-CoV display homology with SARS-CoV-2, the amino acid sequence differences between SARS-CoV-2 nucleocapsid and the other endemic coronaviruses[11–13] are sufficient to limit predicted cross-reactivity.

Data from subsequent publications examining available serologic assays from in vitro diagnostic manufacturers has confirmed these predictions. These publications demonstrated very low false-positive rates across multiple test manufacturers and platforms by testing sera from either well-characterized SARS-CoV-2 polymerase chain reaction (PCR)-negative patients, or samples collected before December 2019, the generally accepted date associated with SARS-CoV-2 spread[14–17].

These articles also characterized the persistence of antibody up to 200 days after a positive SARS-CoV-2 PCR test result[15]. When the data of these publications are normalized to the number of days after a positive SARS-CoV-2 PCR test, the in vitro diagnostic platforms examined (**Table 2**) display sensitivities ranging from 75% to 99%[14–17].

Further, these articles also provide indirect evidence as to the clear lack of usefulness in diagnosing active SARS-CoV-2 infection. The sensitivity for detecting a specific antibody response at approximately 7 days after a positive SARS-CoV-2 PCR result ranged from 58% to 96%. This wide range in sensitivity is surprising, particularly in that the same platform in one publication displayed a sensitivity of 59% between 3 and 7 days post positive PCR result, whereas in another the sensitivity was reported as 96% for samples collected less than 7 days after a positive PCR test[15,17]. One

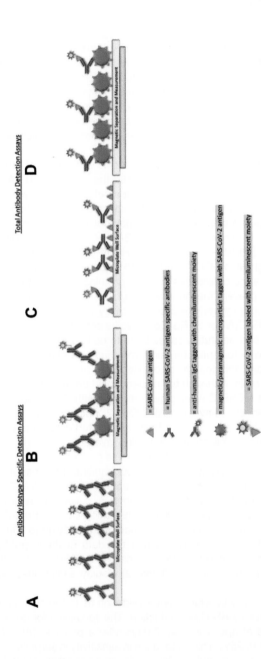

Fig. 1. SARS-CoV-2 serology assays fall into 2 distinct groups, those that are antibody isotype specific (*A, B*), and those that are total antibody assays that cannot distinguish between IgA, IgG, and IgM antibody isotype (*C, D*). The assays also differ in regards to separation technology with SARS-CoV-2 antigen immobilized on a microwell or microtiter plate (A, C), or a paramagnetic or magnetic microparticle (**B, D**).

Table 1
SARS-CoV-2 Serology Assays

Test Name	Antibody Target	Antibody Isotype(s)	Assay Format[d]	Qualitative (Q) or Semiquantitative (SQ)
Abbott AdviseDX SARS-CoV-2 IgG II	RBD	IgG	B	SQ
Abbott AdviseDX SARS-CoV-2 IgM	Spike	IgM	B	Q
Abbott SARS-CoV-2 IgG[a]	Nucleocapsid	IgG	B	Q
Beckman Coulter Access SARS-CoV-2 IgG	RBD	IgG	B	Q
Beckman Coulter Access SARS-CoV-2 IgG II	RBD	IgG	B	SQ
Beckman Coulter Access SARS-CoV-2 IgM II	RBD	IgM	B	Q
bioMerieux VIDAS SARS-CoV-2 IgG	RBD	IgG	A	Q
bioMerieux VIDAS SARS-CoV-2 IgG	RBD	IgM	A	Q
Bio-Rad Platelia SARS-CoV-2 Total Ab	Nucleocapsid	IgA, IgG, IgM	C	Q
DiaSorin Liaison SARS-CoV-2 IgM	RBD	IgM	B	Q
DiaSorin Liaison SARS-CoV-2 S1/S2 IgG	S1 and S2	IgG	B	Q
Diazyme DZ-Lite SARS-CoV-2 IgG	Nucleocapsid and spike	IgG	B	Q
Diazyme DZ-Lite SARS-CoV-2 IgM	Nucleocapsid and spike	IgM	B	Q
Euroimmun Anti-SARS-CoV-2	S1	IgG	A	Q
IDS SARS-CoV-2 IgG	Nucleocapsid and spike	IgG	B	Q
Inova Diagnostics, QUANTA Flash SARS-CoV-2 IgG	Nucleocapsid and spike	IgG	B	SQ
Luminex xMAP SARS-CoV-2 Multi-Antigen IgG Assay	S1, RBD, nucleocapsid	IgG	B	Q
Ortho-Clinical Diagnostics VITROS Anti-SARS-CoV-2 IgG	Spike	IgG	A	Q
Ortho-Clinical Diagnostics VITROS Anti-SARS-CoV-2 Total	Spike	IgA, IgG, IgM	C	Q
Phadia AB ELIA SARS-CoV-2-Sp1 IgG	Spike	IgG	A	SQ
Roche Elecsys Anti-SARS-CoV-2	Nucleocapsid	IgA, IgG, IgM	D	Q
Roche Elecsys Anti-SARS-CoV-2 s	Spike	IgA, IgG, IgM	D	SQ

(continued on next page)

Table 1
(continued)

Test Name	Antibody Target	Antibody Isotype(s)	Assay Format[d]	Qualitative (Q) or Semiquantitative (SQ)
Siemens Healthcare Diagnostics SARS-COV-2 IgG[b]	RBD	IgG	B	SQ
Siemens Healthcare Diagnostics SARS-CoV-2 Total[b]	RBD	IgA, IgG, IgM	D	SQ
Siemens Healthcare Diagnostics Dimension/Dimension EXL SARS-CoV-2 IgG[c]	RBD	IgG	Other	SQ
Siemens Healthcare Diagnostics Dimension/Dimension EXL SARS-CoV-2 Total[c]	RBD	IgA, IgG, IgM	Other	Q
Thermo Fisher OmniPATH COVID-19	Spike	IgA, IgG, IgM	C	Q
Zeus Scientific ELISA SARS-CoV-2 IgG	Spike and nucleocapsid	IgG	A	Q
Zeus Scientific ELISA SARS-CoV-2 Total	Spike and nucleocapsid	IgA, IgG, IgM	C	Q

Abbreviations: RBD, receptor binding domain; S1, S1 domain of SARS-CoV-2 spike protein; S2, S2 domain of SARS-CoV-2 spike protein.

[a] Abbott Alinity i SARS-CoV-2 and Abbott ARCHITECT SARS-CoV-2 use the same assay format and are shown here in one row.

[b] Siemens ADIVA Centaur and Atellica assays utilize the same assay format and are show here in one row per assay format (IgG vs Total Immunoglobulin).use

[c] Siemens Dimension and Dimension EXL SARS-CoV-2 assays use the LOCI (luminescent oxygen channeling assay) technology not depicted in **Fig. 1**.

[d] Assay format described in Figure 1.

Table 2		
In Vitro Diagnostic Platform Performance Characteristics		
Assay Manufacturer	**Sensitivity (%)**	**References**
Abbott SARS-CoV-2 IgG	81[a]–99	(Poore et al,[15] 2021; Tang et al, 2020)
Beckman Coulter Access SARS-CoV-2 IgG	78	(Poore et al,[15] 2021)
Diazyme DZ-Lite SARS-CoV-2 IgG	96	(Suhandynata et al,[16] 2020)
Euroimmun Anti-SARS-CoV-2	75[a]	(Tang et al,[17] 2020)
Roche Elecsys Anti-SARS-CoV-2	87–96	(Poore et al,[15] 2021; Suhandynata et al., 2020)

[a] Sensitivity defined as positive serology result at either *≥14 d or ≥15 d after a positive SARS-CoV-2 PCR result.

possible explanation for the discrepancy in sensitivity is a difference in time between symptom onset and performance of the PCR test.

Serology Correlation with Neutralizing Antibody Titer

Of the numerous hurdles limiting the clinical usefulness of SARS-CoV-2 serology testing are the lack of assay harmonization or international standardization, as well as the currently sparse data correlating serology antibody result with neutralizing antibody titer. In 2 recent publications, this question of correlation of serology result to neutralizing titer was examined[18,19]. Both publications demonstrated that a positive correlation exists between automated serology assay signal and neutralizing antibody titer. The limitation of these studies is that neither article contains data from quantitative or semiquantitative serology assays, but rather rely on the ratio of assay signal to a positive calibrator or cut-off signal.

In the publication by Tang and colleagues[19], the authors demonstrate that at a neutralizing titer of 1:64, the positive percent agreement (PPA) for the Abbott, Roche, and Euroimmun assays are 96%, 100%, and 92%, respectively, when using the manufacturers' specified positive ratio thresholds. At the manufacturer specified positive thresholds the negative predictive agreement of the 3 were 50%, 70%, and 47%, respectively. The authors also calculated assay-specific ideal ratios for the 3 assays which slightly decreased the PPA, but increased the negative predictive agreement for each assay.

In an article by Suhandynata and colleagues[20], the authors examined the PPA between 3 commercially available serology assays as well as a neutralization assay titer of 50. Samples testing positive on both the Diazyme and Roche assays or the Diazyme and Abbott assays had PPA values of 79.2% and 78.4%, respectively. Unfortunately, owing to the methodologic differences between the 2 articles, a direct comparison of data is not possible.

These early studies correlating automated serology assay signal with the neutralization titer are encouraging; however, additional studies using semiquantitative or quantitative assays are needed to determine if a universal threshold indicating immunity is possible.

ANTIBODY RESPONSE

Early publications supported a classic viral response pattern after infection with SARS-CoV-2[21,22]. In this model, IgM antibodies are first detected within 1 week after infection, and IgG antibodies develop several days after that. Instead, IgG antibodies to SARS-CoV-2 appear before or at the same time as IgM antibodies[23,24]. In the classic viral response model, IgG antibodies were predicted to increase over time, peak around 1 month after an infection, and remain detectable for 1 to 6 years[22]. Although antibody longevity may not be confirmed for several years, many research groups have investigated the time to initial antibody detection and ongoing studies are monitoring antibody response over time.

Determining antibody seroconversion rates after a SARS-CoV-2 infection can be difficult because the exact day of infection is often unknown. The window period between infection and the presence of detectable antibodies ranged from less than 4 days to several weeks after a confirmed infection[16,23–27]. Seroconversion kinetics may also depend on disease severity. People with mild or asymptomatic infections generally had a weaker immune response than those with symptomatic or severe infection[23,26]. However, it has also been reported that asymptomatic patients seroconvert more quickly compared with those are who are symptomatic[27]. Interindividual variation combined with the novelty of the SARS-CoV-2 virus have contributed to an incomplete understanding of the humoral response.

As described elsewhere in this article, the antibody response pattern over time varies widely with the analytical platform being used[14–17]. However, differing antibody trends are at least partially attributed to whether antinucleocapsid or antispike antibodies are being monitored. Previous reports have demonstrated that, although nucleocapsid antibodies continue to increase over time, antibodies to the spike protein begin to decrease within 1 to 4 months after symptom onset[15,28,29]. This phenomenon has been observed on several different test platforms. Despite this finding, antibodies to both the spike and nucleocapsid antibodies remain detectable for several months after infection. Future studies should continue to monitor the longevity of antibodies to both the nucleocapsid and spike proteins after natural infection.

Neutralizing antibodies can block infection by the SARS-CoV-2 virus. Because the spike protein engages angiotensin-converting enzyme 2 receptors to initiate infection, antibodies to the spike protein have been theorized to correlate with antibody neutralization[5,19,20]. After a natural infection, spike antibodies were moderately associated ($R^2 = 0.46$) with neutralizing antibody titers but suffered from a poor negative percent agreement[19]. Interestingly, the correlation between antinucleocapsid antibodies with neutralizing antibodies was assay dependent, but ranged from a coefficient of determination of 0.29 to 0.47. After vaccination, antibodies to the spike protein also exhibited a moderate association ($R^2 = 0.39$) with neutralizing titers[20]. Current vaccinations only elicit a humoral response against the spike protein of SARS-CoV-2 and, therefore, would not have any association with nucleocapsid antibody response.

As a result of the COVID-19 global pandemic, vaccine development through multinational collaborations has occurred at an unprecedented rate. Antibody response after vaccination will be an important consideration when establishing reimmunization intervals. At the time of this publication, all vaccines currently granted EUA by the World Health Organization target the spike protein and, therefore, only elicit antispike antibodies. In these cases, vaccination status should be monitored with an antispike assay. However, there are vaccines currently under development that contain live, attenuated, or inactivated virus that would induce both a nucleocapsid and spike antibody response, similar to a natural infection[30]. In these cases, vaccination antibody response could be monitored with either an antispike or antinucleocapsid assay and would remain indistinguishable from a natural infection. Currently available vaccines result in antibody titers that exceed those seen after a natural infection[31–33]. Although this robust response is promising, antibody longevity after vaccination remains unknown and may vary with vaccine technology. Understanding how each vaccine works will be an important consideration when monitoring antibody titers to determine reimmunization frequency.

COVID-19 VACCINES

After the COVID-19 outbreak in December 2019, the entire genomic sequence of SARS-CoV-2 was published in January 2020. By March 2020, vaccines were developed, shipped to appropriate testing sites, and early phase clinical and preclinical trials were underway. As of June 2021, nearly 300 vaccine candidates were under clinical or preclinical development[30]. These vaccines use a variety of technologies, including adenovirus vectors, viral-like particles, inactivated or attenuated virus, and synthetic DNA or RNA. Dosing schemes range from 1 to 3 doses given over zero to 56 days. Although more than a dozen vaccines have already been cleared for emergency use by the World Health Organization, only 3 vaccines were granted FDA EUA status for use in the United States. These vaccines are manufactured by Pfizer-BioNTech, Moderna, and Janssen Biotech, Inc.

Pfizer-BioNTech Vaccine

Pfizer-BioNTech produced 2 RNA-based vaccines formulated in lipid nanoparticles. The first, BNT162b1, encoded a trimerized SARS-CoV-2 receptor-binding domain of the spike glycoprotein whereas the second, BNT162b2, encoded a membrane-anchored full-length spike glycoprotein stabilized in the prefusion conformation[31,34,35]. During phase I clinical trials, immunogenicity and safety were monitored for various dosing paradigms of BNT162b1 and BNT162b2. Although both vaccines were found to be effective and exhibited tolerability profiles similar to other messenger RNA (mRNA)-based vaccines[36], BNT162b2 had a milder systemic reactogenicity profile while exhibiting a similar antibody response to BNT162b1. Both vaccines exhibited a strong dose-dependent response, and the 2-dose series of 30 μg BNT162b2 vaccine was selected as the candidate to advance to phase II and III clinical trials[31].

The Pfizer-BioNTech BNT162b2 vaccine was submitted for EUA to the FDA on November 20, 2020[37]. The vaccine series consisted of 2 doses given 21 days apart. The submission included data from ongoing clinical trials consisting of 44,000 participants and the vaccine was found to be 95% effective at preventing SARS-CoV-2 infection with no major safety concerns identified. On December 11, 2020, this became the first COVID-19 vaccine to receive EUA clearance from the FDA in the United States. In May 2021, the FDA expanded the EUA to allow for vaccination in children as young as 12 years of age.

Moderna Vaccine

Similar to Pfizer-BioNTech BNT162b2, the Moderna mRNA-1273 vaccine is also a lipid nanoparticle–encapsulated mRNA-based vaccine encoding a stabilized prefusion trimer of the spike glycoprotein. In early clinical trials, participants received 2 injections of either a 25, 100, or 250 μg dose 28 days apart[32,38]. Two doses were deemed necessary to elicit sufficient pseudovirus neutralizing activity. The median antibody response was similar between the 100 μg and 250 μg dose groups but the 100 μg dose group had a more favorable reactogenicity profile. Therefore, the 100 μg dose was chosen to advance into additional clinical trials.

Moderna submitted the mRNA-1273 COVID-19 vaccine (2 doses of 100 μg, administered 1 month apart) to the FDA for EUA on November 30, 2020, for adults 18 years of age or older[39]. The phase III clinical trials consisted of 30,400 participants and demonstrated a greater than 94% efficacy at preventing COVID-19[40]. Adverse reactions were reported frequently, but were considered mild, with injection site arm pain, fatigue, and headache being the most common. One week after Pfizer-BioNTech, the Moderna mRNA-1272 vaccine was issued EUA from the FDA for use in adults on December 18, 2020.

Janssen Biotech, Inc, Vaccine

The Janssen Biotech, Inc (Johnson & Johnson) Ad26.COV2.S vaccine is an adenovirus vector encoding a variant of the SARS-CoV-2 spike protein. Beginning in July 2020, Janssen conducted multicenter phase I clinical trials with doses of 5×10^{10} or 1×10^{10} viral particles per milliliter given as a single dose or on a 2-dose schedule[33,41]. All dosing schemes had an acceptable safety and reactogenicity profile and more than 90% of participants demonstrated the presence of both S-binding and neutralizing antibodies after a single dose of either potency vaccine. Interestingly, adverse events were more common after the first dose, a finding that contrasted both the Pfizer-BioNTech and Moderna mRNA-based vaccines[33]. Although a second vaccine dose exhibited slightly increased immunogenicity, Janssen recognized the logistical advantages of a single-dose vaccine and decided to proceed with a single dose of the 1×10^{10} viral particles per milliliter vaccine in phase III clinical trials. This decision was further supported by nonhuman primate studies that demonstrated complete or near-complete protection against SARS-COV-2[42]. More recently, it was discovered that the Ad26.COV2.S vaccine may offer some protection against other SARS-CoV-2 variants of concern[43].

Janssen Biotech, Inc, submitted the Ad26.COV2.S single dose vaccine consisting of 5×10^{10} viral particles for EUA by the FDA on February 4, 2021[44]. Phase III clinical trials of more than 40,000 participants demonstrated that this vaccine was both safe and at least 66% effective in preventing the development of COVID-19 in adults 18 years of age or older. On February 27, 2021, the FDA issued an EUA for the Janssen the Ad26.COV2.S single dose vaccine, making it the third approved for use in the United States. However, on April 23, 2021, the FDA amended the EUA to include information about the rare occurrence of cerebral venous sinus thrombosis in women after vaccination.

As more vaccines are developed, it will become increasingly important to monitor reactogenicity and immunogenicity in addition to efficacy. Differences in immune response and frequency of adverse events may help to personalize vaccine selection, with potent vaccines preferred in individuals who may produce a suboptimal immune response, and single-dose vaccines preferred for those who are prone to adverse reactions after vaccination.

SARS-CoV-2 ANTIGEN TESTING

Nucleic acid amplification tests detecting the presence of SARS-CoV-2 RNA are considered the gold standard for the diagnosis of symptomatic patients by the Centers for Disease Control and Prevention[45]. Although these assays offer optimal sensitivity and specificity, their implementation can be hindered by the limited availability of reagents or other consumables, they require capital investment in the necessary instrumentation, and they must be performed by specialized and highly trained laboratory personnel. Owing to the centralized nature of this testing model, results are often returned several hours or days after specimen collection, complicating efforts to limit further viral spread.

To overcome these limitations, several manufacturers have developed rapid, lateral flow devices that detect SARS-CoV-2 antigen (typically the nucleocapsid protein) in nasal or nasopharyngeal swabs with results available in 15 to 30 minutes. Briefly, viral proteins present on the test swab are suspended by mixing in a buffer solution, which is transferred to the test cartridge. Labeled antibodies bind to the viral protein of interest and the buffer-suspended antibody–antigen complex migrates through an internal membrane toward the test and control lines. The test line consists of a capture antibody attached to the solid phase that recognizes a different epitope on the viral protein, immobilizing the antigen detector–antibody complex and forming a visible line. Any unbound detector antibody flows past the test line and accumulates at the control line, indicating a valid test. Result interpretation varies by device, but typically follows 1 of 2 models. In the first, after the introduction of patient sample, each device is placed into a reader that evaluates the signal intensity at the test and control lines and produces a digital "detected" or "not detected" result. In the second, test and control line signal intensity is evaluated visually after a manufacturer-defined incubation period. Result interpretation outside of this window can lead to erroneous results.

Although these rapid antigen devices are not considered the gold standard for SARS-CoV-2 diagnosis, they may offer several advantages, including limited expense, capacity for rapid implementation without extensive infrastructure, short turnaround time, and high specificity in populations with a high prevalence of disease. At the time of release for clinical use, the performance of these devices was largely unknown beyond the manufacturers' validation studies described in the package inserts. However, after implementation in a variety of clinical settings, several recent publications have described the performance characteristics of rapid antigen tests relative to concurrently performed nucleic acid testing as the reference method.

BinaxNOW

The Abbott BinaxNOW COVID-19 antigen card is a lateral flow device granted EUA by the FDA in August 2020. Results are interpreted visually between 15 and 30 minutes after the introduction of the resuspended patient sample to the test card. Analytical sensitivity has been estimated to fall between 4 and 8×10^4 copies per swab, roughly approximating a generic reverse transcriptase (RT)-PCR cycle threshold value of 29 to 30[46].

One study compared the performance of the BinaxNOW lateral flow antigen test to the Thermo Fisher TaqPath COVID-19 Combo kit in 2645 asymptomatic students at the University of Utah using 2 concurrent nasal swabs self-collected by study participants under the supervision of trained, nonmedical personnel[47]. Antigen testing was performed at the collection site by trained nonmedical personnel while RT-PCR testing was performed at a reference laboratory. SARS-CoV-2 RNA was detected by RT-PCR in 1.7% of the study participants. Relative to RT-PCR, the BinaxNOW antigen test demonstrated a sensitivity of 53.3% and a specificity of 100%.

A second study summarized the performance of the BinaxNOW antigen device relative to the Clinical Research Sequencing Platform (CRSP) SARS-CoV-2 RT-PCR assay in specimens collected at a drive-through community testing site in Massachusetts[7]. Two nasal swabs were collected from each participant by trained medical personnel, with 1 swab used to perform BinaxNOW testing on-site in a dedicated testing tent while the other swab was sent to an off-site reference laboratory for RT-PCR testing. In this study population, 974 of 1380 adults (71%) and 829 of 928 children (89%) were asymptomatic. Among symptomatic participants, the BinaxNOW device demonstrated a sensitivity of 96.5% in adults and 84.6% in children (ages 7–17 years) and a specificity of 100% in both age groups. Among asymptomatic participants, the sensitivity was 70.2% in adults and 65.5% in children and the specificity was 99.6% in adults and 99.0% in children.

A third study compared the BinaxNOW antigen device to either the CDC or Fosun SARS-CoV-2 RT-PCR assay using concurrently collected nasal (antigen) and nasopharyngeal (RT-PCR) samples from participants in 2 community testing centers in Pima County, Arizona[48]. Antigen testing was performed on site according to the manufacturer's instructions and RT-PCR testing was performed within 24 to 48 hours at an off-site laboratory. Of the 3419 participants, 827 (24.2%) reported at least 1 symptom consistent with SARS-CoV-2 infection. SARS-CoV-2 RNA was detected in 161 participants (4.7%): 113 of 827 were symptomatic (13.7%) and 48 of 2592 were asymptomatic (1.9%). In symptomatic participants presenting within 7 days of symptom onset, the sensitivity and specificity of the BinaxNOW device were 71.1% and 100%, respectively. In asymptomatic participants, the sensitivity and specificity were 35.8% and 99.8%, respectively.

Sofia

The Quidel Sofia SARS-CoV-2 lateral flow antigen assay was granted EUA in May 2020 and is intended for use within 5 days of symptom onset. Results are introduced into a device reader that reports digital results as positive or negative between 15 and 30 minutes.

One study performed on 2 college campuses in Wisconsin compared the performance of the Sofia antigen device to either the Centers for Disease Control and Prevention or Thermo Fisher TaqPath COVID-19 Combo RT-PCR assays[49]. At University A, all persons tested for screening or diagnostic purposes were eligible to participate in the study. At University B, participation was limited to only those quarantined after a known COVID-19 exposure. Two concurrent nasal swabs were collected from participants in both groups (medical personnel collect at University A, self-collect at University B). Limited information was provided regarding the logistics of antigen test performance, with the authors indicating only that testing was performed according to the manufacturer's instructions. Of the 1098 participants, 227 (20.7%) reported at least 1 symptom; 871 (79.3%) were asymptomatic. Overall RT-PCR positivity was 5.2% (40 symptomatic and 17 asymptomatic participants). The sensitivity, specificity, positive predictive value, and negative predictive value were 80.0%, 98.9%, 94.1%, and 95.9%, respectively, in the symptomatic group and 41.2%, 98.4%, 33.3%, and 98.8%, respectively, in the asymptomatic group.

A second study evaluated the performance of the Sofia antigen device in the emergency department of a tertiary medical center in Los Angeles, California[50]. Paired nasal (antigen) and nasopharyngeal (RT-PCR) specimens were collected by medical personnel for all patients admitted to the hospital through the emergency department. RT-PCR testing was performed using the Fulgent COVID-19 assay and antigen testing was performed on-site in the emergency department. Of the 2039 participants, 307 (15.1%) reported at least 1 symptom. SARS-CoV-2 RNA was detected in 68 of 307 symptomatic participants (22.1%) and 81 of 1732 asymptomatic participants (4.7%). Relative to RT-PCR, the sensitivity and specificity of the Sofia antigen test were 72.1% and 98.7%, respectively, in the symptomatic group and 60.5% and 99.5%, respectively, in the asymptomatic group.

A third study evaluated the performance of the Sofia antigen device relative to the Hologic Aptima SARS-CoV-2 TMA assay in symptomatic individuals presenting to an urgent care center in West Bend, Wisconsin[51]. Concurrently collected nasal (antigen) and nasopharyngeal samples (TMA) were collected by medical staff in the urgent care center, with both specimens sent to a clinical laboratory for testing. SARS-CoV-2 RNA was detected in 18% of symptomatic patients seen in the clinic in the month before the implementation of antigen testing and this positivity rate remained constant throughout the study period. Of the 298 patients tested within 5 days of symptom onset, the sensitivity, specificity, positive predictive value, and negative predictive value were 82.0%, 100%, 100%, and 96.5%, respectively. Of the 48 patients tested more than 5 days after symptom onset, antigen test performance decreased, with a sensitivity, specificity, positive predictive value, and negative predictive value of 54.5%, 97.3%, 85.7%, and 87.8%, respectively.

Becton Dickinson Veritor

The Becton Dickinson (BD) Veritor lateral flow antigen device was granted EUA in July 2020 and is intended for use with nasal swabs collected from patients suspected of SARS-CoV-2 infection within 5 days of symptom onset. Results are generated by a cartridge reader at least 15 minutes after introduction of the sample to the test device and are reported qualitatively as positive or presumptive negative.

One study evaluated the performance of the BD Veritor device relative to the Simplexa COVID-19 Direct EUA RT-PCR assay in paired nasal (antigen) and nasopharyngeal (RT-PCR) samples from 1384 patients with known SARS-CoV-2 exposure within 5 days of symptom onset presenting to a hospital system in Winston-Salem, North Carolina[52]. Antigen testing was performed at the site of collection according to the manufacturer's instructions, whereas RT-PCR testing was performed in a central laboratory. SARS-CoV-2 RNA was detected in 116 of 1384 specimens (8.4%). Relative to RT-PCR, the BD Veritor demonstrated a sensitivity, specificity, positive predictive value, and negative predictive value of 66.4%, 98.8%, 83.7%, and 97.0%, respectively.

A second study with 2 parts evaluated the BD Veritor relative to the Lyra RT-PCR assay in concurrently collected nasal (antigen) and nasopharyngeal or oropharyngeal swabs (RT-PCR) in 251 symptomatic individuals within 7 days of symptom onset presenting to 21 geographically diverse study locations (part 1)[53]. RT-PCR testing was performed at a commercial reference laboratory and antigen testing was performed at a laboratory operated by the device manufacturer. SARS-CoV-2 RNA was detected in 38 of 251 part 1 study participants (15.1%). In participants with 2 or more symptoms, the sensitivity, specificity, positive predictive value, and negative predictive value were 88%, 100%, 100%, and 97.3%, respectively. In participants with 1 symptom, values were 67%, 100%, 100%, and 97.7%, respectively. In part 2, concurrently collected nasal swabs from 377 symptomatic participants at 5 study sites were tested at an off-site commercial reference laboratory on the BD Veritor and Sofia devices according to the manufacturer's instructions. Using the Sofia device as the reference method, the BD Veritor demonstrated a sensitivity and specificity of 97.4% and 98.1%, respectively.

Effectiveness of Antigen Testing in Controlling Viral Spread

Many have advocated for the implementation of serial SARS-CoV-2 antigen testing to facilitate rapid identification of infected individuals and permit timely self-quarantine to prevent further viral spread. Although antigen testing is consistently less sensitive than molecular diagnostic techniques, the short turnaround time and capacity for repeated testing may support efforts at viral containment more effectively than single sample nucleic acid testing with a long turnaround time. To date, relatively few studies have tested this hypothesis.

One publication describing the implementation of the Sofia antigen device in routine monitoring of intercollegiate athletes documented 2 separate SARS-CoV-2 outbreaks attributed to false-negative antigen test results[54]. In outbreak A, 32 confirmed cases were traced to contact during a team meeting with a single infectious individual whose antigen test result was negative on the morning of the meeting. Viral RNA sequences were closely related, supporting transmission from a single individual to the other team members. The authors note that viral transmission was not interrupted until the implementation of RT-PCR testing, which led to the identification of an additional 21 confirmed SARS-CoV-2 infections, 18 of which were not detected by concurrent antigen testing. In outbreak B, 12 confirmed cases were documented in 2 teams competing against each other, all of whose participants received negative antigen test results on the day of competition. Viral RNA sequences were closely related and distinctly different from strains circulating in one of the teams' communities, supporting transmission from one team to the other.

Antigen Conclusions

To decrease the rates of viral transmission, SARS-CoV-2 diagnostic test methods must be analytically accurate, accessible, and reported in a timely and effective manner. Antigen methods generate rapid results and their high specificity and positive predictive value allows SARS-CoV-2–positive individuals to quickly self-isolate, minimizing the risk of further viral spread. However, the lower sensitivity of antigen testing relative to nucleic acid methods increases the likelihood of further transmission in high interaction environments by individuals with false-negative antigen results. With this limitation in mind, confirmation of negative antigen results by nucleic acid testing is recommended, particularly in patient populations with a high disease prevalence.

In addition to the test method used, the environment in which testing is performed is a primary determinant of the effectiveness of SARS-CoV-2 testing efforts. The majority of studies evaluating antigen test performance described dedicated testing spaces staffed by trained operators with no other competing responsibilities. Little is known about how antigen devices perform when implemented in patient care settings with testing performed by clinical personnel who are also actively caring for patients. The limited available data using the BD Veritor device suggest improved performance in a controlled laboratory setting relative to an active patient care environment[52,53]. However, this observation is complicated by differences in reference method and disease prevalence in the study populations.

SUMMARY

Laboratory medicine professionals play an integral role in the global response to SARS-CoV-2 through the development and implementation of test methods to identify infected individuals and monitor the immune response to vaccination and natural infection. SARS-CoV-2 antibody test methods can be used to confirm past infection and, pending further correlation with neutralizing antibody assays, may help to guide personalized vaccine selection or the establishment of revaccination intervals. Antigen test methods offer rapid turnaround time and improved access to testing as well as high specificity, but their limited sensitivity requires confirmation of negative results by nucleic acid testing, particularly in populations with high disease prevalence.

CLINICS CARE POINTS

- Antigen tests exhibit lower sensitivity relative to nucleic acid testing and increase the risk of further transmission by patients with false-negative antigen results.
- SARS-CoV-2 antibody test methods lack harmonization and correlation with neutralizing antibodies, limiting their clinical usefulness.

- Current vaccines result in higher antibody titers than natural infection, and antibodies made after vaccination should be monitored with antispike antibody assays.

DISCLOSURE

The authors have nothing to disclose.

REFERENCES

1. Park SE. Epidemiology, virology, and clinical features of severe acute respiratory syndrome -coronavirus-2 (SARS-CoV-2; Coronavirus Disease-19). Clin Exp Pediatr 2020;63(4):119–24.
2. Dutta NK, Mazumdar K, Gordy JT. The nucleocapsid protein of SARS–CoV-2: a target for vaccine development. J Virol 2020;94(13). https://doi.org/10.1128/JVI. 00647-20.
3. Cong Y, Ulasli M, Schepers H, et al. Nucleocapsid protein recruitment to replication-transcription complexes plays a crucial role in coronaviral life cycle. J Virol 2020;94(4). https://doi.org/10.1128/JVI.01925-19.
4. Burbelo PD, Riedo FX, Morishima C, et al. Detection of nucleocapsid antibody to SARS-CoV-2 is more sensitive than antibody to spike protein in COVID-19 patients. J Infect Dis 2020. https://doi.org/10.1093/infdis/jiaa273.
5. Garcia-Beltran WF, Lam EC, Astudillo MG, et al. COVID-19-neutralizing antibodies predict disease severity and survival. Cell 2021;184(2):476–88.e11.
6. Esbin MN, Whitney ON, Chong S, et al. Overcoming the bottleneck to widespread testing: a rapid review of nucleic acid testing approaches for COVID-19 detection. RNA 2020. https://doi.org/10.1261/rna.076232.120. rna.076232.120.
7. Pollock NR, Jacobs JR, Tran K, et al. Performance and implementation evaluation of the Abbott BinaxNOW Rapid antigen test in a high-throughput drive-through community testing site in Massachusetts. J Clin Microbiol 2021;59(5). https:// doi.org/10.1128/JCM.00083-21.
8. Health C for D and R. EUA Authorized Serology Test Performance. FDA. 2021. Available at: https://www.fda.gov/medical-devices/coronavirus-disease-2019-covid-19-emergency-use-authorizations-medical-devices/eua-authorized-serology-test-performance. Accessed June 16, 2021.
9. Hicks J, Klumpp-Thomas C, Kalish H, et al. Serologic cross-reactivity of SARS-CoV-2 with endemic and seasonal betacoronaviruses. J Clin Immunol 2021. https://doi.org/10.1007/s10875-021-00997-6.
10. Jaimes JA, André NM, Chappie JS, et al. Phylogenetic analysis and structural modeling of SARS-CoV-2 spike protein reveals an evolutionary distinct and proteolytically sensitive activation loop. J Mol Biol 2020;432(10):3309–25.
11. Burbelo PD, Riedo FX, Morishima C, et al. Sensitivity in detection of antibodies to nucleocapsid and spike proteins of severe acute respiratory syndrome coronavirus 2 in patients with coronavirus disease 2019. J Infect Dis 2020;222(2): 206–13.
12. Gussow AB, Auslander N, Faure G, et al. Genomic determinants of pathogenicity in SARS-CoV-2 and other human coronaviruses. Proc Natl Acad Sci U S A 2020; 117(26):15193–9.
13. Kang S, Yang M, Hong Z, et al. Crystal structure of SARS-CoV-2 nucleocapsid protein RNA binding domain reveals potential unique drug targeting sites. Acta Pharm Sin B 2020;10(7):1228–38.

14. Hubbard JA, Geno KA, Khan J, et al. Comparison of two automated immunoassays for the detection of SARS-CoV-2 nucleocapsid antibodies. J Appl Lab Med 2021;6(2):429–40.

15. Poore B, Nerenz RD, Brodis D, et al. A comparison of SARS-CoV-2 nucleocapsid and spike antibody detection using three commercially available automated immunoassays. Clin Biochem 2021. https://doi.org/10.1016/j.clinbiochem.2021.05.011.

16. Suhandynata RT, Hoffman MA, Kelner MJ, et al. Multi-platform comparison of SARS-CoV-2 serology assays for the detection of COVID-19. J Appl Lab Med 2020;5(6):1324–36.

17. Tang MS, Hock KG, Logsdon NM, et al. Clinical performance of two SARS-CoV-2 serologic assays. Clin Chem 2020;66(8):1055–62.

18. Suhandynata RT, Hoffman MA, Huang D, et al. Commercial serology assays predict neutralization activity against SARS-CoV-2. Clin Chem 2021;67(2):404–14.

19. Tang MS, Case JB, Franks CE, et al. Association between SARS-CoV-2 neutralizing antibodies and commercial serological assays. Clin Chem 2020. https://doi.org/10.1093/clinchem/hvaa211.

20. Suhandynata RT, Bevins NJ, Tran JT, et al. SARS-CoV-2 serology status detected by commercialized platforms distinguishes previous infection and vaccination adaptive immune responses. medRxiv 2021. https://doi.org/10.1101/2021.03.10.21253299.

21. Guo L, Ren L, Yang S, et al. Profiling early humoral response to diagnose novel coronavirus disease (COVID-19). Clin Infect Dis 2020;71(15):778–85.

22. Galipeau Y, Greig M, Liu G, et al. Humoral responses and serological assays in SARS-CoV-2 infections. Front Immunol 2020;11. https://doi.org/10.3389/fimmu.2020.610688.

23. Long Q-X, Liu B-Z, Deng H-J, et al. Antibody responses to SARS-CoV-2 in patients with COVID-19. Nat Med 2020;1–4. https://doi.org/10.1038/s41591-020-0897-1.

24. Suhandynata RT, Hoffman MA, Kelner MJ, et al. Longitudinal monitoring of SARS-CoV-2 IgM and IgG seropositivity to detect COVID-19. J Appl Lab Med 2020;jfaa079. https://doi.org/10.1093/jalm/jfaa079.

25. Long Q-X, Tang X-J, Shi Q-L, et al. Clinical and immunological assessment of asymptomatic SARS-CoV-2 infections. Nat Med 2020;26(8):1200–4.

26. Jiang C, Wang Y, Hu M, et al. Antibody seroconversion in asymptomatic and symptomatic patients infected with severe acute respiratory syndrome coronavirus 2 (SARS-CoV-2). Clin Transl Immunology 2020;9(9):e1182.

27. Zhao J, Yuan Q, Wang H, et al. Antibody responses to SARS-CoV-2 in patients of novel coronavirus disease 2019. medRxiv 2020. https://doi.org/10.1101/2020.03.02.20030189. 2020.03.02.20030189.

28. Ibarrondo FJ, Fulcher JA, Goodman-Meza D, et al. Rapid decay of anti–SARS-CoV-2 antibodies in persons with mild Covid-19. N Engl J Med 2020. https://doi.org/10.1056/NEJMc2025179.

29. Perreault J, Tremblay T, Fournier M-J, et al. Waning of SARS-CoV-2 RBD antibodies in longitudinal convalescent plasma samples within 4 months after symptom onset. Blood 2020;136(22):2588–91.

30. COVID-19 vaccine tracker and landscape. Available at: https://www.who.int/publications/m/item/draft-landscape-of-covid-19-candidate-vaccines. Accessed June 14, 2021.

31. Walsh EE, Frenck RW, Falsey AR, et al. Safety and immunogenicity of two RNA-based covid-19 vaccine candidates. N Engl J Med 2020;383(25):2439–50.

32. Anderson EJ, Rouphael NG, Widge AT, et al. Safety and immunogenicity of SARS-CoV-2 mRNA-1273 vaccine in older adults. N Engl J Med 2020;383(25):2427–38.

33. Sadoff J, Le Gars M, Shukarev G, et al. Interim results of a phase 1–2a trial of Ad26.COV2.S Covid-19 vaccine. N Engl J Med 2021. https://doi.org/10.1056/NEJMoa2034201.

34. Sahin U, Muik A, Derhovanessian E, et al. COVID-19 vaccine BNT162b1 elicits human antibody and T H 1 T cell responses. Nature 2020;586(7830):594–9.

35. Mulligan MJ, Lyke KE, Kitchin N, et al. Phase I/II study of COVID-19 RNA vaccine BNT162b1 in adults. Nature 2020;586(7830):589–93.

36. Feldman RA, Fuhr R, Smolenov I, et al. mRNA vaccines against H10N8 and H7N9 influenza viruses of pandemic potential are immunogenic and well tolerated in healthy adults in phase 1 randomized clinical trials. Vaccine 2019;37(25):3326–34.

37. Covid P-B. Vaccines and Related Biological Products Advisory Committee Meeting December 10, 2020. 53.

38. Jackson LA, Anderson EJ, Rouphael NG, et al. An mRNA Vaccine against SARS-CoV-2 — Preliminary report. N Engl J Med 2020. https://doi.org/10.1056/NEJMoa2022483.

39. Vaccines and Related Biological Products Advisory Committee December 17, 2020 Meeting Announcement - 12/17/2020 - 12/17/2020. FDA. 2021. Available at: https://www.fda.gov/advisory-committees/advisory-committee-calendar/vaccines-and-related-biological-products-advisory-committee-december-17-2020-meeting-announcement. Accessed June 15, 2021.

40. Baden LR, El Sahly HM, Essink B, et al. Efficacy and safety of the mRNA-1273 SARS-CoV-2 vaccine. N Engl J Med 2021;384(5):403–16.

41. Stephenson KE, Le Gars M, Sadoff J, et al. Immunogenicity of the Ad26.COV2.S vaccine for COVID-19. JAMA 2021;325(15):1535–44.

42. Mercado NB, Zahn R, Wegmann F, et al. Single-shot Ad26 vaccine protects against SARS-CoV-2 in rhesus macaques. Nature 2020;586(7830):583–8. https://doi.org/10.1038/s41586-020-2607-z.

43. Alter G, Yu J, Liu J, et al. Immunogenicity of Ad26.COV2.S vaccine against SARS-CoV-2 variants in humans. Nature 2021. https://doi.org/10.1038/s41586-021-03681-2.

44. Covid J. Vaccines and Related Biological Products Advisory Committee Meeting February 26, 202. 62.

45. CDC. Labs. Centers for Disease Control and Prevention. 2020. Available at: https://www.cdc.gov/coronavirus/2019-ncov/lab/resources/antigen-tests-guidelines.html. Accessed June 16, 2021.

46. Perchetti GA, Huang M-L, Mills MG, et al. Analytical sensitivity of the Abbott BinaxNOW COVID-19 Ag card. J Clin Microbiol 2021;59(3). https://doi.org/10.1128/JCM.02880-20.

47. Okoye NC, Barker AP, Curtis K, et al. Performance characteristics of BinaxNOW COVID-19 antigen card for screening asymptomatic individuals in a university setting. J Clin Microbiol 2021;59(4). https://doi.org/10.1128/JCM.03282-20.

48. Prince-Guerra JL, Almendares O, Nolen LD, et al. Evaluation of Abbott BinaxNOW rapid antigen test for SARS-CoV-2 Infection at two community-based testing sites - Pima County, Arizona, November 3-17, 2020. MMWR Morb Mortal Wkly Rep 2021;70(3):100–5.

49. Pray IW, Ford L, Cole D, et al. Performance of an antigen-based test for asymptomatic and symptomatic SARS-CoV-2 testing at two university campuses - Wisconsin, September-October 2020. MMWR Morb Mortal Wkly Rep 2021;69(5152):1642–7.

50. Brihn A, Chang J, OYong K, et al. Diagnostic performance of an antigen test with RT-PCR for the detection of SARS-CoV-2 in a hospital setting - Los Angeles County, California, June-August 2020. MMWR Morb Mortal Wkly Rep 2021; 70(19):702–6.
51. Beck ET, Paar W, Fojut L, et al. Comparison of the Quidel Sofia SARS FIA test to the hologic aptima SARS-CoV-2 TMA test for diagnosis of COVID-19 in symptomatic outpatients. J Clin Microbiol 2021;59(2). https://doi.org/10.1128/JCM.02727-20.
52. Kilic A, Hiestand B, Palavecino E. Evaluation of performance of the BD Veritor SARS-CoV-2 chromatographic immunoassay test in patients with symptoms of COVID-19. J Clin Microbiol 2021;59(5). https://doi.org/10.1128/JCM.00260-21.
53. Young S, Taylor SN, Cammarata CL, et al. Clinical evaluation of BD veritor SARS-CoV-2 point-of-care test performance compared to PCR-based testing and versus the Sofia 2 SARS antigen point-of-care test. J Clin Microbiol 2020;59(1). https://doi.org/10.1128/JCM.02338-20.
54. Moreno GK, Braun KM, Pray IW, et al. SARS-CoV-2 transmission in intercollegiate athletics not fully mitigated with daily antigen testing. Clin Infect Dis 2021. https://doi.org/10.1093/cid/ciab343.

UNITED STATES POSTAL SERVICE®

Statement of Ownership, Management, and Circulation (All Periodicals Publications Except Requester Publications)

1. Publication Title	2. Publication Number	3. Filing Date
CLINICS IN LABORATORY MEDICINE	000 – 713	9/18/2022

4. Issue Frequency	5. Number of Issues Published Annually	6. Annual Subscription Price
MAR, JUN, SEP, DEC	4	$283.00

7. Complete Mailing Address of Known Office of Publication (Not printer) (Street, city, county, state, and ZIP+4®)

ELSEVIER INC.
230 Park Avenue, Suite 800
New York, NY 10169

Contact Person
Malathi Samayan

Telephone (include area code)
91-44-4299-4507

8. Complete Mailing Address of Headquarters or General Business Office of Publisher (Not printer)

ELSEVIER INC.
230 Park Avenue, Suite 800
New York, NY 10169

9. Full Names and Complete Mailing Addresses of Publisher, Editor, and Managing Editor (Do not leave blank)

Publisher (Name and complete mailing address)

DOLORES MELONI, ELSEVIER INC.
1600 JOHN F KENNEDY BLVD, SUITE 1800
PHILADELPHIA, PA 19103-2899

Editor (Name and complete mailing address)

STACY EASTMAN, ELSEVIER INC.
1600 JOHN F KENNEDY BLVD, SUITE 1800
PHILADELPHIA, PA 19103-2899

Managing Editor (Name and complete mailing address)

PATRICK MANLEY ELSEVIER INC.
1600 JOHN F KENNEDY BLVD, SUITE 1800
PHILADELPHIA, PA 19103-2899

10. Owner (Do not leave blank. If the publication is owned by a corporation, give the name and address of the corporation immediately followed by the names and addresses of all stockholders owning or holding 1 percent or more of the total amount of stock. If not owned by a corporation, give the names and addresses of the individual owners. If owned by a partnership or other unincorporated firm, give its name and address as well as those of each individual owner. If the publication is published by a nonprofit organization, give its name and address.)

Full Name	Complete Mailing Address
WHOLLY OWNED SUBSIDIARY OF REED/ELSEVIER, US HOLDINGS	1600 JOHN F KENNEDY BLVD, SUITE 1800 PHILADELPHIA, PA 19103-2899

11. Known Bondholders, Mortgagees, and Other Security Holders Owning or Holding 1 Percent or More of Total Amount of Bonds, Mortgages, or Other Securities. If none, check box ▶ ☐ None

Full Name	Complete Mailing Address
N/A	

12. Tax Status (For completion by nonprofit organizations authorized to mail at nonprofit rates) (Check one)
The purpose, function, and nonprofit status of this organization and the exempt status for federal income tax purposes:
☒ Has Not Changed During Preceding 12 Months
☐ Has Changed During Preceding 12 Months (Publisher must submit explanation of change with this statement)

PS Form 3526, July 2014 [Page 1 of 4 (see instructions page 4)] PSN: 7530-01-000-9931   PRIVACY NOTICE: See our privacy policy on www.usps.com.

---

13. Publication Title	14. Issue Date for Circulation Data Below
CLINICS IN LABORATORY MEDICINE	JUNE 2022

15. Extent and Nature of Circulation			Average No. Copies Each Issue During Preceding 12 Months	No. Copies of Single Issue Published Nearest to Filing Date
a. Total Number of Copies (Net press run)			85	68
b. Paid Circulation (By Mail and Outside the Mail)	(1)	Mailed Outside-County Paid Subscriptions Stated on PS Form 3541 (Include paid distribution above nominal rate, advertiser's proof copies, and exchange copies)	33	26
	(2)	Mailed In-County Paid Subscriptions Stated on PS Form 3541 (Include paid distribution above nominal rate, advertiser's proof copies, and exchange copies)	0	0
	(3)	Paid Distribution Outside the Mails Including Sales Through Dealers and Carriers, Street Vendors, Counter Sales, and Other Paid Distribution Outside USPS®	17	15
	(4)	Paid Distribution by Other Classes of Mail Through the USPS (e.g. First-Class Mail®)	0	0
c. Total Paid Distribution (Sum of 15b (1), (2), (3), and (4))		▶	50	41
d. Free or Nominal Rate Distribution (By Mail and Outside the Mail)	(1)	Free or Nominal Rate Outside-County Copies Included on PS Form 3541	21	12
	(2)	Free or Nominal Rate In-County Copies Included on PS Form 3541	0	0
	(3)	Free or Nominal Rate Copies Mailed at Other Classes Through the USPS (e.g. First-Class Mail)	0	0
	(4)	Free or Nominal Rate Distribution Outside the Mail (Carriers or other means)	0	0
e. Total Free or Nominal Rate Distribution (Sum of 15d (1), (2), (3) and (4))		▶	21	12
f. Total Distribution (Sum of 15c and 15e)		▶	71	53
g. Copies not Distributed (See Instructions to Publishers #4 (page 6#3))		▶	14	15
h. Total (Sum of 15f and g)		▶	85	68
i. Percent Paid (15c divided by 15f times 100)		▶	70.42%	77.35%

* If you are claiming electronic copies, go to line 16 on page 3. If you are not claiming electronic copies, skip to line 17 on page 3.

PS Form 3526, July 2014 (Page 2 of 4)

16. Electronic Copy Circulation	Average No. Copies Each Issue During Preceding 12 Months	No. Copies of Single Issue Published Nearest to Filing Date
a. Paid Electronic Copies ▶		
b. Total Paid Print Copies (Line 15c) + Paid Electronic Copies (Line 16a) ▶		
c. Total Print Distribution (Line 15f) + Paid Electronic Copies (Line 16a) ▶		
d. Percent Paid (Both Print & Electronic Copies) (16b divided by 16c × 100) ▶		

☒ I certify that 50% of all my distributed copies (electronic and print) are paid above a nominal price.

17. Publication of Statement of Ownership

☒ If the publication is a general publication, publication of this statement is required. Will be printed
in the DECEMBER 2022 issue of this publication.   ☐ Publication not required.

18. Signature and Title of Editor, Publisher, Business Manager, or Owner	Date
Malathi Samayan *Malathi Samayan* - Distribution Controller	9/18/2022

I certify that all information furnished on this form is true and complete. I understand that anyone who furnishes false or misleading information on this form or who omits material or information requested on the form may be subject to criminal sanctions (including fines and imprisonment) and/or civil sanctions (including civil penalties).

PS Form 3526, July 2014 (Page 3 of 4)   PRIVACY NOTICE: See our privacy policy on www.usps.com

Printed and bound by CPI Group (UK) Ltd, Croydon, CR0 4YY

03/10/2024

01040477-0002